Hearing in Children

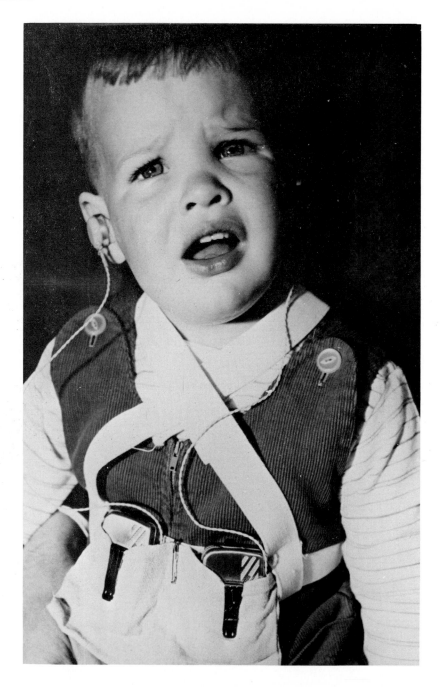

We have measured, described, researched, catalogued, analyzed, and synthesized the entity of hearing loss. Now we must busy ourselves with the prevention of its devastating effects on children (JLN and MPD).

Hearing in Children

by

Jerry L. Northern, Ph.D.

Associate Professor
Department of Otolaryngology
University of Colorado
Medical Center
Denver, Colorado

and

Marion P. Downs, M.A.

Assistant Professor
Department of Otolaryngology
University of Colorado
Medical Center
Denver, Colorado

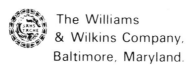 The Williams & Wilkins Company, Baltimore, Maryland.

Made in the United States of America

Reprinted 1975

Library of Congress Cataloging in Publication Data

NORTHERN, JERRY L
HEARING IN CHILDREN.

    1. Hearing disorders in children. I. Downs, Marion P., joint author. II.
Title. [DNLM: 1. Hearing disorders—In infancy and childhood. 2. Hearing tests—In infancy and childhood. WV270 N874h 1974] RF122.5.C4N67
617.8   74-615
ISBN 0-683-06569-6

Composed and printed at the
Waverly Press, Inc.
Mt. Royal and Guilford Aves.
Baltimore, Md. 21202, U.S.A.

PREFACE

Why a book about the hearing of children?

Long ago the function of hearing became the building stone upon which our intricate human communication system was built. If pre-dawn man had not inherited an ear, he might have resorted instead to signing with his fingers or scratching marks upon the sand, to share his thoughts with others. The result would have been an awkward method of communication that could have slowed, for millennia, our so-called progress. For good or bad, we have developed the ear and the vocal mechanism as the media through which language is communicated.

The structure of language is unique to *Homo sapiens*. Recent experiments have demonstrated that signed symbols and other visual language forms could be taught to chimpanzees, but in essence it has been on a conditioned basis (Gardner and Gardner, 1969; Premack and Premack, 1972). This kind of signalization is far removed from the higher conceptualization and syntax of human language. Between the laboriously learned signal response of the chimpanzee and the first voluntary sentence of the 18-month-old baby lies, as Langer stated (1957), a whole day of creation.

The auditory-linked acquisition of language is further unique to human beings because it is a time-locked function, related to early maturational periods in the infant's life. The longer auditory language stimulation is delayed, the less efficient will be the language facility. Critical periods exist for the development of biological functions, and these are responsible for the dependency of language acquisition on time. A baby who is deprived of appropriate language stimulation during his first 3 years of life can never fully attain his best potential language function, whether the deprivation is from lack of hearing or from lack of high quality language experience. There is a lesson to be learned from these facts when we consider the ills of society today.

No complete textbook has been written on the audiologic problems of children. Chapters on this topic have appeared in other books, but, in our opinion, nowhere has the entire subject been covered in a comprehensive way. The reason is that until recent years there has been an aura of magic around the audiologic evaluation of very young children. Few people were willing to work with this population because of the myth that the very young could not be tested subjectively—nor, indeed, it was felt, could anything beneficial be done for the infant who was found to have a hearing loss. All this has been changed, and we now find that many disciplines are interested in understanding childhood deafness, its causes, and its audiologic diagnosis.

Pediatricians are concerned with how they can identify early deafness in babies and what can be done for such children; otolaryngologists want to learn the techniques of testing such a population and what the audiologic manifestations are; audiologists are interested in the *how* of testing young children and the relationship of the auditory findings to pathology; rehabilitation people want to know how to relate audiologic data with their expectations of the hearing-impaired children they work with.

We hope this book will provide new information for the practicing physician, audiologist, and educator. It will hopefully be valuable in the university training centers for resident programs in otolaryngology and pediatrics, audiologic training programs, and curricula in deaf education on both the graduate and undergraduate levels as a basic textbook or reference source.

Our book's purpose is to give a comprehensive description of the current state of knowledge of the audiologic problems of children; to present a medically oriented point of view in the testing and management of deaf children; and to provide a practical reference source on testing procedures for children and on the interpretation of test data.

But the chief goal of this book is to demonstrate how we can help children with hearing losses gain their fundamental right to attain the best potential language skills possible for them. If language could be acquired easily for the first time at 10 years of age, or at 6 years, or even at 3 years, it would make our task a good deal lighter. Indeed, one of the erroneous assumptions made in the past is that at any age we can start to teach language to the deaf child who has not had language exposure, and expect successful results. A multitude of failures remains to admonish us that we must find a better way.

The better way is to be forever vigilant: identify hearing loss at every age; apply appropriate tests for the child's age; and secure for each child the habilitation program that will most effectively permit his optimal language development. The aim of this book is to help the pediatrician, otolaryngologist, deaf educator, audiologist, and speech pathologist understand what hearing problems in children are all about, and what can be done about them. Our book presupposes some knowledge about the audiometer, audiologic testing, and general orientation to the anatomy and physiology of the ear. Our main intent is to convey an audiologic philosophy in regard to hearing impairment in children. We invite all interested specialists to enter our world of children's hearing.

JLN and MPD

ACKNOWLEDGMENT

A book of this magnitude cannot be assembled and written without the help of many other people. We would like to pay special tribute and thanks to five of our colleagues and good friends who gave graciously of their valuable time and personal material for our benefit—LaVonne Bergstrom, M.D.; Isamu Sando, M.D.; Janet M. Stewart, M.D.; Marlin Weaver, M.D.; and Winfield McChord, Jr., M.S.

Many others responded to our needs, willingly and unselfishly, to provide requested information at a moment's notice: Carol Amon, M.A.; Owen Black, M.D.; Carol Cox, M.A.; Kathleen O. Foust, M.A.; William K. Frankenberg, M.D.; W. G. Hemenway, M.D.; Brian Hersch, M.D.; Aram Glorig, M.D.; Mrs. Page T. Jenkins; Darrel Teter, Ph.D.; Pat Tesauro, M.A.; and Harold Weber, M.A. Connie H. Knight, M.A., Audiologist at the Georgia Retardation Center, Atlanta, was our Research Associate and gathered much of the material presented in the "Index of Selected Birth Defect Syndromes," Sharon Mraz was our Editorial Assistant. Patricia Jenkins Thompson, M.A., diligently proofread and critiqued our efforts.

Y. Oishi, M.D., served as our primary photographer; Miriam Eliachar illustrated the chapter pictures and embryology figures; and Anita McGuire typed the entire manuscript. We would also like to acknowledge the cooperation of the publishing staff at The Williams & Wilkins Company, especially William R. Hensyl who encouraged us to write this textbook.

And finally, we would like to extend our appreciation and thanks to our spouses, families, children, and friends, who will long remember (as will we!) this period of time during which we were too busy, too preoccupied, or too tired—our Year of the Book, 1973.

JLN and MPD

CONTENTS

Hearing in Children

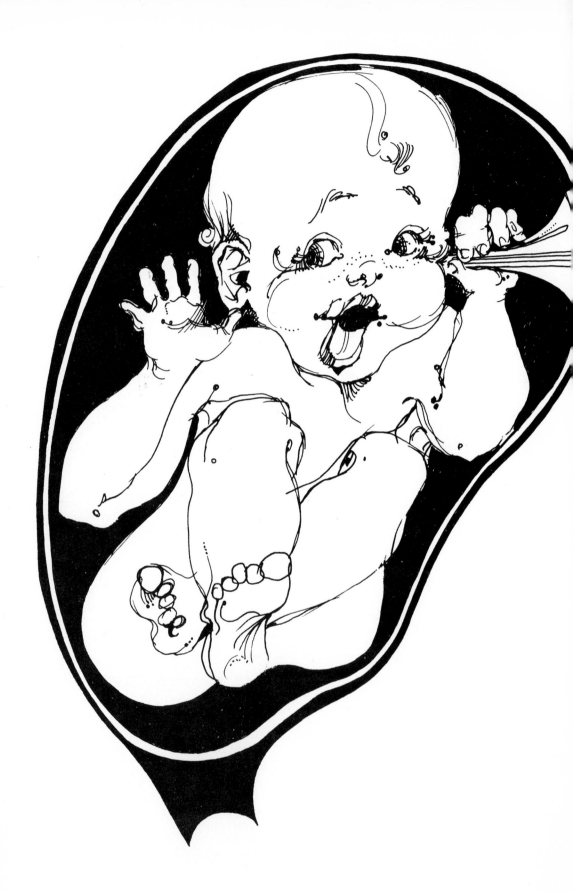

1 DEVELOPMENT OF THE AUDITORY MECHANISM

The embryologic development of the ear is of more than academic interest to the clinician. An understanding of embryologic relationships helps the physician in his diagnosis and the audiologist in his plan for early identification and management of hearing loss. If one is aware of the timetable of prenatal development and the association of the various structures with each other, the suspicion of deafness and its subsequent diagnosis and treatment become easier. Although the major changes in the development of the ear take place in the mother's womb, first as an embryo and later as a fetus, the baby becomes a more progressively complex structure with time. Several mechanical processes occur concurrently to produce the final structure including enlargements, constrictions, and foldings which are further modified by evaginations and invaginations. However, development of the auditory structure does not cease, nor is it totally complete, at the time of birth.

Knowledge of the origins of auditory structures can be diagnostically significant to the clinician. For example, when an infant presents with a congenital skin disorder, one considers the fact that the skin and the otocyst both originate from ectoderm. It may then be logical to suspect that anomalies of the cochlear structures could have occurred contiguously with the skin disorder and that a search for severe sensorineural deafness is in order.

Similarly, the timing of development of the various organ systems guides us to suspect that a hearing loss may have occurred at the same time that other systems were affected. A noxious influence on the fetus at 2 months gestation may result in a malformation of the pinna which is developing at that time. The pinna malformation, however, does not necessarily imply malformation of the ossicles of the middle ear. Although the ossicles of the middle ear share partially the same time clock as the pinna in embryologic development, the origins of the structures are different. On the other

hand, an insult to one may well result in a related insult to the other.

Principles such as these allow us to look for the occult symptom of hearing loss whenever an overt embryologically-related symptom becomes evident. The prognosis for auditory function can then be estimated from what is known of the origin and the expected pathology. A simple review of the embryologic development of the ear and its related structures will clarify some of these principles.

Phylogeny

Unfortunately, "ears" and "hearing" are often synonyms to the naive student who may be unaware that the ability to hear is actually a secondary acquired characteristic of the ear. The major responsibility of the auditory organ is maintaining equilibrium. The study of comparative anatomy confirms that hearing is only important to higher forms of vertebrates, but the basic function of equilibrium remains essentially unchanged in the phylogenetic evolution between fish and man (Van Bergeijk et al., 1960; Romer, 1962).

In many fish, amphibians, and reptiles the paired internal ears are devoted primarily to functions related to equilibrium. In these creatures the membranous labyrinth of the inner ear is filled with endolymph, and two distinct sac-like structures are generally present, the utricle and saccule. An endolymphatic duct extends upward from these two sacs and terminates within the brain case as the endolymphatic sac. A structure known as the lagena, which is actually the forerunner of the cochlea, is formed as a depression pocket in the floor of the saccule. Even in these lower vertebrates, branches of the auditory nerve are associated in the sensory sacs with end organs known as macula.

The macula-type of sensory cell is found in all vestibular systems and is the basic means of transforming equilibrium information into

3

neural codes. These sensory end organs, much like the human cochlear hair cells, have hair-like projections embedded in an overlying gelatinous material, the cupula. In the utricular and saccular maculae, and often in the primitive lagena, this gelatinous material becomes a thickened structure in which are deposited crystals of calcium carbonate, to form an "earstone" or otolith (Romer, 1962).

An interesting equilibrium system utilized by the crayfish is described by Storer and Usinger (1957). The crayfish has a small sac known as the statocyst located at the base of each antennae. The statocyst contains a ridge of sensory hairs to which sand grains are attached by mucus to form structures called statoliths. The action of gravity on the statoliths causes the sensory hairs to bend, informing the crayfish of his present orientation. Each time the crayfish molts, it loses the statolith lining and must acquire new grains of sand to deposit in the statocyst. The crayfish shows disorientation in an aquarium with no foreign debris particles following molting. When iron filings are placed in the aquarium, the crayfish will pick some up for use in his statocyst and then his equilibrium may be controlled with a magnet held in various positions along the sides of the aquarium.

All vertebrates are, of course, dependent on information concerning turning movements provided by the semicircular canals. In every jawed vertebrate, three such canals arise from each utricle. The three canals are at right angles to each other and represent the three planes of space. Each canal has an enlargement at one end known as an ampulla. Within the ampulla is a sensory end organ, the crista. Displacement of the endolymph in the semicircular canal causes displacement of the cupula which is attached to the cristae, bending the sensory hairs and initiating neural impulses.

Some fish and amphibians have a peculiar sensory system termed the lateral line system. The receptor organ of the lateral line is the neuromast, a generalized name applied to nerve receptors that demonstrate a hair-like projection enclosed in a flexible mass of gelatinous material—the cupula. Neuromasts are generally located on the surface skin of the water-dwelling organism, and the question exists whether this system is really sensitive to "sound." Romer (1962) suggests that evidence of embryonic development of the sensory endings in the human cochlea—which closely resembles the externally placed neuromast organs—may indicate that the internal ear originated phylogenetically as a specialized, deeply sunk portion of the lateral line system.

As animals evolved to become land-dwelling creatures, adaptations in the hearing sense organ were necessitated to process airborne sound waves. Changes were in order to transmit sounds and amplify them to the inner ear which was usually set deeply in the skull. The middle ear of amphibians, reptiles, and birds is quite similar, in the sense that the hyomandibular bone seen in the fish has changed its function to become a rod-like stapes or columella. The columella crosses the middle ear between the tympanic membrane and the oval window of the inner ear. This columellar-type middle ear ossicle is of particular interest since human middle ear malformations may show this type of deformity. It makes one wonder if this is a throwback to our primitive evolutionary forebears (Fig. 1.1). An abnormal structure reminiscent of normal structures in "lower" animals, such as a cervical fistula or a columella ossicle, is known as a reversion structure or atavism (Moody, 1953).

In the mammals the external ear becomes a prominent structure known as the pinna. A more fundamental change occurs in the middle ear where, instead of a single bone, an articulated series of three ossicles between the eardrum and oval window exist. According to Romer (1962) the origin of this series of ossicles has been long debated. The question existed as to whether the three ossicles were really due to subdivisions of the columella. Careful study, however, of paleontology, and comparative anatomy led to the conclusion that only the mammalian stapes is related to the lower vertebrate columella. Mammals have developed a new specialized jaw system and the "older" jaw elements have been developed into the other two middle ear ossicles. The reptile eardrum lies close to a jaw joint known as the articular which becomes the malleus in mammals. A second jaw bone, the quadrate, is attached to the articular in the reptile, and to

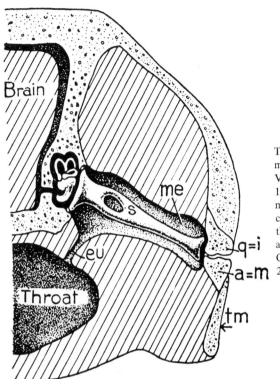

Fig. 1.1. Example of an otic reversion structure. Top, ventricle cross-section of the normal reptile middle ear. (With permission from A. S. Romer: The Vertebrate Body, Philadelphia, W. B. Saunders Co., 1962.) Bottom, horizontal cross-section of a human middle ear from a Treacher Collins patient, showing congenital columella-type of stapes with absence of the malleus and incus. (With permission from I. Sando and R. P. Wood: Congenital middle ear anomalies. Otolaryngol. Clin. North Am. (Symposium) 4: 29–318, 1971.)

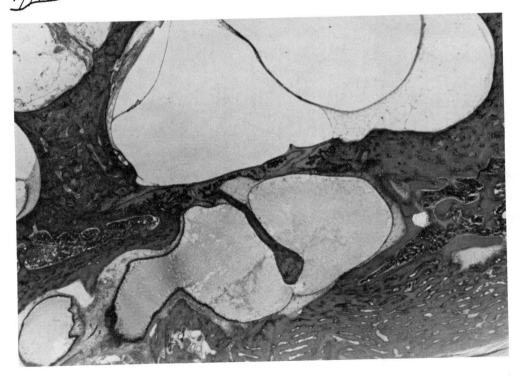

the hyomandibular bone (forerunner of the stapes in the fish). The quadrate retains these primitive connections and becomes the incus in mammals. Thus, these bones which were originally part of the gill structure in fish develop into the jaw structure of reptiles and finally into ear structures in mammals. In Romer's words, the breathing aids of the fish developed into feeding aids in reptiles and finally into "hearing aids" in mammals!

The inner ear in birds and mammals functions from nearly identical physiologic mechanisms—auditory sensory structures vibrated by movements of a membrane located beneath them. Birds and mammals refined their hearing abilities with the advanced development of a cochlea. The number of coils present in the cochlea may vary among mammalian species. As indicated earlier in this phylogenetic discussion, the portions of the inner ear devoted to balance show little change in evolutionary development. Additional information regarding the evolutionary development of the ear may be found in the book *Sound and Hearing* in the Life Science Library. (Stevens and Warshofsky, 1965).

Basic Embryology

Most audiologists have not had training or coursework in the field of embryology so some basic background information is essential to fully appreciate the development of the ear. The reader is also referred to Zemlin (1968) for a very good discussion of the embryonic development of the facial, head, and neck regions.

All growth is the result of cell division of pre-existing cells. Through a process known as mitosis, changes take place in the nucleus of a cell which produce a specific number of double structures. The cell and nucleus then subdivide into two identical "daughter" cells. At the same time "organizers" exist in the embryo which stimulate development of associated areas, and create specific differentiation of cells in the developmental process.

One of the earliest organizational developments in the embryo is the differentiation of cells into three superimposed, cellular plates

called germ layers. These germ layers are known as ectoderm, mesoderm, and endoderm. Ectoderm is generally responsible for development of the outer skin layers, but also gives rise to the nervous system and the sense organs. Mesoderm is associated with skeletal, circulation structures, kidneys, and reproductive organs. Endoderm creates the digestive canal and respiratory organs. These germ layers are actually not quite so specific in their functions as outlined above; but, as you will see, the outer and inner portions of the ear do indeed develop from ectodermal tissue, while the middle ear ossicles and the bone surrounding the inner ear originate from mesodermal tissue.

It is often difficult for the embryologist to determine the exact age of a human embryo, and likewise it may be a problem to establish the exact time of development for specific structures. In circumstances of exogenous injury to the fetal ear, however, it may be possible to determine at what point in the gestation period the injury occurred (Sando and Wood, 1971). The embryonic period actually begins at the end of the second week when a cellular disc exists composed of the three germ layers. By the end of the first month of life, the embryo is only about a fourth of an inch long. The embryonic period terminates around the eighth week when the structure assumes a "human" appearance, and is known as a fetus for the remainder of the gestation period (Moody, 1953).

The ear begins its development during the early life of the embryo, so some discussion of the detailed growth of the embryo itself is worthwhile. The embryonic disc is split by a primitive streak at about 25 hours, which leads the way for development of the ectodermal-lined primitive groove and primitive fold (Fig. 1.2). The primitive groove deepens into a primitive pit, which in turn becomes the neural groove and neural fold (Fig. 1.3). An enlargement exists (the primitive knot) at the cephalic end of the primitive streak which is destined to become the head of the organism. The ectodermal-lined neural folds come together to close off the neural groove, which is now known as the neural tube. It is during the stage of the neural tube that the earliest beginnings of the ear are seen.

Development of the Ear

Inner Ear

Only the basic gross essentials in the development of the ear are presented here. Readers interested in an excellent, in-depth presentation on embryology of the ear are referred to Anson (1973).

The earliest demarcations of the ear in the human embryo are seen early in the third week as thickenings in the superficial ectoderm on either side of the open neural plate. These thickenings are the auditory or otic placodes and are obvious by the middle of the third week (Fig. 1.4a). About the 23rd day, the auditory placodes begin to invaginate into the surface ectoderm and are known as the auditory or otic pits. When the mouth of each auditory pit closes on or about the 30th day, it becomes the auditory vesicle or otocyst and appears as an ectodermal cavity lined with epithelium lateral to the now closed neural tube as shown in Figure 1.4c.

The auditory vesicle proceeds to differentiate through a series of folds, evaginations, and elongations and takes on an elongated shape divided into a utricular-saccule area and a tubular extension known as the endolymphatic duct. By 4½ weeks the portion of the auditory vesicle connected to the endolymphatic duct can be recognized as the future vestibular

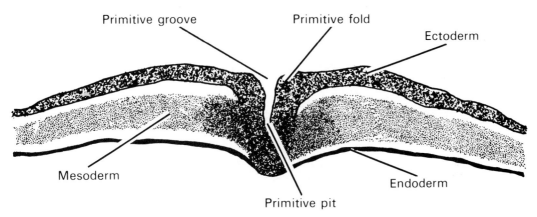

Fig. 1.2. Early life of the embryo. The embryonic disc is split at about 25 hours. This drawing is made from a transverse cut through a seven-segment chick embryo. (Modified with permission from L. B. Arey: Developmental Anatomy. Philadelphia, W. B. Saunders Co., 1940.)

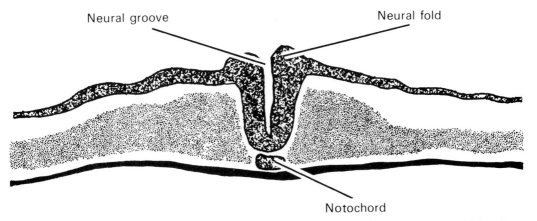

Fig. 1.3. A cephalic transverse section through the fifth pair of somites in a seven-segment chick embryo. (Modified with permission from L. B. Arey: Developmental Anatomy. Philadelphia, W. B. Saunders Co., 1940.)

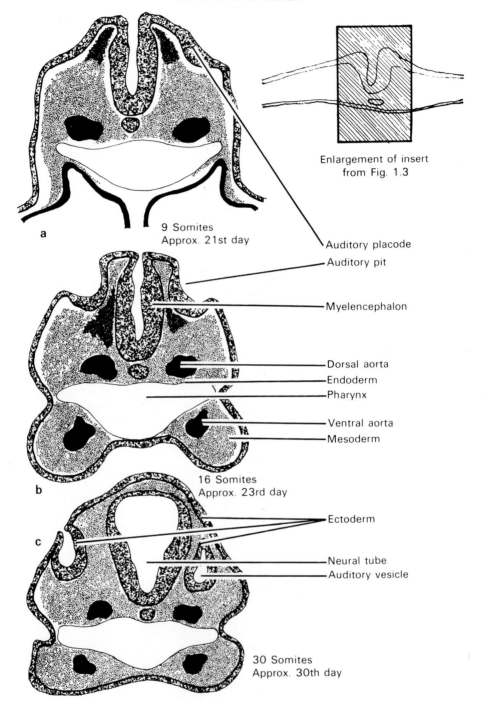

Enlargement of insert
from Fig. 1.3

9 Somites
Approx. 21st day

Auditory placode

Auditory pit

Myelencephalon

Dorsal aorta
Endoderm
Pharynx

Ventral aorta
Mesoderm

16 Somites
Approx. 23rd day

Ectoderm

Neural tube
Auditory vesicle

30 Somites
Approx. 30th day

Fig. 1.4. Early development of inner ear in human embryo. (Modified with permission from L. B. Arey: Developmental Anatomy. Philadelphia, W. B. Saunders Co., 1940.)

portion of the labyrinth, while the more slender portion of the vesicle begins to elongate from the saccular area as the future cochlea (Fig. 1.5a). At the end of the sixth week, three arch-like outpockets are visible and destined to become the semicircular canals. At this same time the utricle and sacculus become two definitive areas through a deepening constric- tion of the vestibular portion of the auditory vesicle (Fig. 1.5b).

By the end of the seventh week, the elon- gated outpocketing of the saccular por- tion of the auditory vesicle has completed one coil of the future cochlea. During the 8th through 11th week, the two and a half coils of the cochlea are completed. The cochlear duct

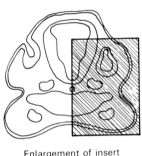

Enlargement of insert from Fig. 1.4

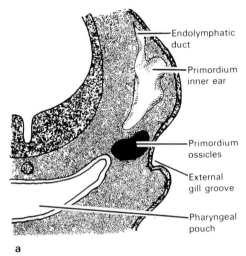

Endolymphatic duct

Primordium inner ear

Primordium ossicles

External gill groove

Pharyngeal pouch

a

Approx. 4½ weeks

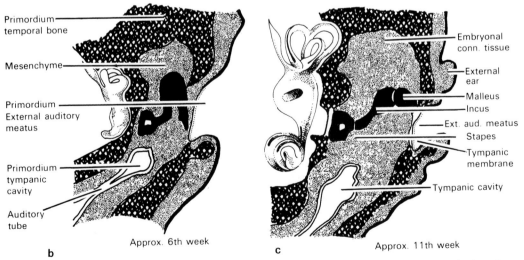

Primordium temporal bone

Mesenchyme

Primordium External auditory meatus

Primordium tympanic cavity

Auditory tube

b

Approx. 6th week

Embryonal conn. tissue

External ear

Malleus

Incus

Ext. aud. meatus

Stapes

Tympanic membrane

Tympanic cavity

c

Approx. 11th week

Fig. 1.5. Schematic development of inner and middle portions of the auditory mechanism from approximately 4½ to 11 weeks. (Modified with permission from B. M. Patten: Human Embryology, 3rd ed. New York, McGraw-Hill Book Co., 1968.)

continues to be attached to the vestibular area by means of a narrow tube known as the ductus reuniens. The cochlear division of the eighth nerve follows the elongation and coiling of the cochlear duct, and fans its fibers out to be distributed along the duct's entire length.

During the seventh week, the complicated convolutions of the otic labyrinth continue to develop, and sensory end organs first appear as localized thickenings of epithelium in the utricle and saccule. Similar localized epithelial thickenings are found in the ampullated ends of the semicircular canals during the eighth week and in the floor of the cochlear duct at 12 weeks. These epithelial thickenings show differentiation into two types of cells including sensory cells with bristle-like hairs and supporting cells at one end. Complete maturation of the sensory and supporting cells in the cochlea does not occur until the fifth month when the entire cochlear duct has shown considerable growth and expansion.

The membranous labyrinth of the inner ear reaches its full adult configuration by the early part of the third month. At this time the otic capsule, which has been encased in cartilage, begins to ossify through a complex system of 14 different endochondral ossification centers in the petrous portion of the temporal bone. The inner ear is the only sense organ to reach full adult size and differentation by fetal midterm. However, it should be noted that the cochlear portion of the inner ear is the last inner ear end organ to differentiate and mature. Thus, the cochlea may be subject to more possible developmental deviations, malformations, and acquired disease than the vestibular end organs.

Middle Ear

During the period of time that the sensory portion of the auditory system—the inner ear—is developing, the transmission portion of the auditory mechanism is developing as the middle ear. Unlike the inner ear which originates from ectodermal tissue, the middle ear is an endodermal structure. The middle ear cavity begins its development during the third week while the auditory pit is sinking into the neural plate to become the auditory vesicle. The tympanic cavity and the auditory tube (later known as the eustachian tube) come from an elongation of the lateral-superior edge of the endodermal-lined first pharyngeal pouch. This elongation is called the tubotympanic recess (Fig. 1.5b).

By the time the human embryo is in its fourth week, a series of five branchial grooves or "gill slits" has appeared. These grooves are in the lower head and neck region on the outside of the embryo. On the inside of the embryo a corresponding series of pharyngeal pouches develops and the collective structures are identified as "arches." In the fish these grooves from the outside ultimately meet the corresponding pouches on the inside to form "gills" as part of their respiratory mechanism. In humans, most of the branchial grooves do not form slits with the pharyngeal pouches; however, the embryo's passing through this developmental stage is an example of our inheritance of embryonic structure from aquatic ancestors. It is of interest that in the human embryo one of the gill pouches does actually become perforated, forming a passageway from the pharynx to the outside of the head. This passageway becomes the external ear canal and eustachian tube. The eardrum forms a barrier between these two portions of a passageway, which otherwise would directly connect the pharynx and the exterior as does the gill slit of a fish (Moody, 1953). Occasionally an additional opening will occur, forming a cervical fistula or branchial cyst which is an opening on the throat between the pharynx and the surface of the neck. The exact position of the fistula depends on which of the pouches is involved.

During the second month the tubotympanic recess approaches the embryo surface between the first and second branchial arches, known as Meckel's (or hyoid) and Reichert's (or mandibular) cartilages, respectively. By the eighth week, the tympanic cavity is present in the lower half of the future middle ear, while the upper half is filled with cellular mesenchyme (Fig. 1.5b). The classical theory of ossicle origin holds that the malleus and incus arise from Meckel's cartilage and the stapes comes from Reichert's cartilage. More recent observations, however, suggest a more complex and dual origin for the ossicles (Pearson et al., 1970). Currently the first branchial arch is credited for most of the body structure in the malleus and incus, while the second branchial arch gives rise to the lenticular process of the incus, the handle of the malleus, and the stapes. The middle ear cavity itself also has a dual origin with the anterior area coming from the first arch and the posterior area coming from the second arch. It is of interest to note that the mandible also arises from the first arch.

By 8½ weeks, the incus and the malleus have attained complete cartilaginous form similar to an adult (Fig. 1.5c). The stapes grows as a cartilaginous structure until the 15th week. By the 15th through the 16th week, ossification begins to occur in the cartilaginous surface of the malleus and incus, which have nearly reached completion by the 32nd week. The stapes does not begin to ossify until the 18th week and continues to develop even after ossification is complete. The stapes develops further during life. Surgeons recognize the stapes in a child to be more bulky and less delicate than the normal stapes seen in the adult.

As the ossicles begin to ossify, the surrounding mesenchymal tissue becomes loose, less cellular, and is absorbed into the mucoperiosteal membrane of the middle ear cavity. When the ossicles are free from mesenchyme, mucous membrane connecting each ossicle to the walls of the middle ear cavity remains to eventually become the ossicular supporting ligaments.

By the 30th week, development of the tympanum proper is almost complete. The middle ear cavity antrum is pneumatized by the 34th through 35th week, and the epitympanum is pneumatized during the last fetal month (36th to 38th week). The air cells of the temporal bone develop as outpouchings from the middle ear cavity during the 34th week. Air does not actually enter the middle ear cavity until the onset of respiration immediately after birth.

External Ear and Eardrum

The auricle develops during the third or fourth week from the first and second branchial arches (Fig. 1.6a). Actually, the auricle is derived primarily from the second branchial arch, and only the tragus seems to originate from the first branchial arch. This is about the same time that the auditory vesicle is formed in the development of the inner ear.

During the sixth week, six hillocks or tissue thickenings form on both sides of the first branchial groove (Fig. 1.6b), arranged as three hillocks on each facing border. The ultimate shape and configuration of the adult auricle depends on the development of these six growth centers; thus many divergent forms of the auricle are within the extremely wide range of normal (Fig. 1.6c). Darwin's tubercle forms in some people as an irregularity in the posterior margin of the helix or outer edge of the auricle as shown in Figure 1.6d. At this time the mesenchymal folds of the auricle are beginning to become cartilage. From the 7th to the 20th week, the auricle continues to develop, moving from its original ventromedial position to be slowly displaced laterally by the growth of the mandible and face. At the 20th week the auricle is in the adult shape (Fig. 1.6d), but continues to grow in size until the individual is 9 years of age.

The external auditory meatus is derived from the first branchial groove during the fourth to fifth week. At this time, the ectodermal lining of the first branchial groove is in brief contact with the endodermal lining of the first pharyngeal pouch. Mesodermal tissue, however, soon grows between the two layers and separates the pharyngeal pouch from the branchial groove. In the eighth week, the primary auditory meatus sinks toward the middle ear cavity and becomes the outer one-third of the auditory canal surrounded ultimately by cartilage.

The ectodermal groove continues to deepen toward the tympanic cavity from the external surface until it meets a thickening of epithelial cells known as the meatal plug which has arisen from surface ectoderm. Mesenchyme grows between the meatal plug and the epithelial cells of the tympanic cavity. These three layers of tissue, then, become the tympanic membrane composed of inner circular fibers, the fibrous middle layer of tissue, and the outer radial fiber layer, before the ninth week. The solid meatal plug, however, keeps the external auditory canal closed until the 21st week. By this time the inner and middle ear structures are well formed and ossified. The meatal plug disinte-

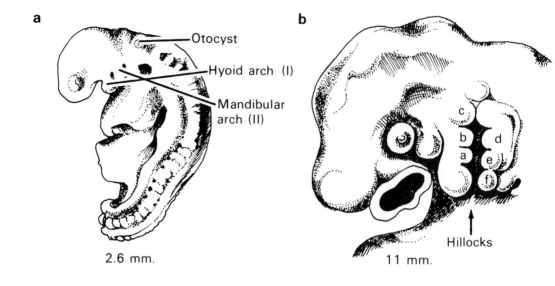

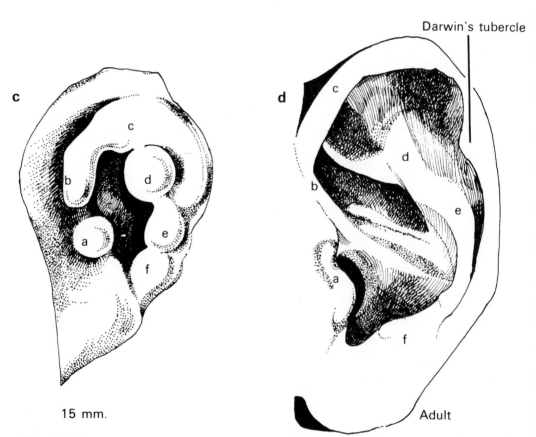

Fig. 1.6. Schematic development of auricle from third or fourth week to adult stage. (Modified with permission from L. B. Arey: Developmental Anatomy. Philadelphia, W. B. Saunders Co., 1940; and B. J. Anson: An Atlas of Human Anatomy, 2nd Ed. Philadelphia, W. B. Saunders Co., 1963.)

grates and forms a canal, with the innermost layer of meatal plug epithelium becoming the squamous epithelial layer of the tympanic membrane. The external auditory canal continues to develop until the ninth year. At birth the floor of the external auditory canal has no bony portion. In the infant, the external auditory canal is short and straight, while in the adult the canal is longer and curves. This suggests that the infant tympanic membrane might be easier to observe than the eardrum of the adult. That is not the case, however, because the infant tympanic membrane is in an oblique or almost a horizontal position and difficult to visualize. The bony portion of the external canal is not complete until about the seventh year. A summary of major embryologic features and their time sequence is presented in Table 1.1.

A young patient with evidence of multiple congenital anomalies related to first and second branchial arch origins is shown in Figure 1.7. This patient has been diagnosed to have Möbius syndrome, sometimes termed aplasia of the sixth and seventh cranial nerve (Ford, 1966). Her cranial deformities include obvious malformations of the external ear, bilateral facial weakness producing a consistent mask-like appearance, submucous cleft palate with a bifed uvula, and macrostomia or a greatly exaggerated width of the mouth resulting from failure of proper union of the maxillary and mandibular processes. She has no measurable hearing and is a student in a residential school for the deaf. Radiographic tomographic studies reveal symmetric middle ear anomalies including malleus and incus deformities, the absence of the oval window bilaterally, and mastoid dysplasia. The cochlea and semicircular canal system appear normal on the x-ray study, but the internal auditory canals are hypoplastic measuring only 1.5 mm in diameter instead of the normal diameter of approximately 8.0 mm.

Anatomy of the Ear Through Temporal Bone Study

Knowledge concerning the anatomy of the temporal bone is becoming increasingly more important to the clinician who deals with hearing loss patients. More and more journal articles and oral presentations at meetings include histologic temporal bone sections to demonstrate some aspect of deafness. Many of the significant advances in our knowledge about the etiology of deafness have come from careful study of temporal bone histological sections. This new information has influenced many areas of clinical services including hearing aid fittings, educational recommendations and referrals, genetic counseling, and patient progress estimation.

Most speech and hearing training programs have infrequent access to normal or pathologic temporal bone sections. In fact, only a handful of nonmedical clinicians are experienced enough with this technical discipline to teach through the use of histologic sections. Yet this method of instruction enables the student to achieve an understanding of the anatomy of the structures of the ear and vestibular system, as well as an appreciation for the complexity of the hearing mechanism. An understanding of the anatomy of the normal temporal bone will provide the clinician with new insight into the etiology and pathology of deafness.

The paucity of temporal bone anatomic sections available for the benefit of hearing and speech students has prompted us to include this section of histologic samples from a normal temporal bone prepared in our laboratory at the University of Colorado Medical School. Our own understanding of deafness has been enhanced greatly by careful study of temporal bone anatomy and pathology, and we feel that it is important for students to examine fully the normal temporal bone sections presented in this chapter. These normal histologic samples may be used as a comparative reference for pathologic temporal bone sections shown in other chapters of this book. The clinician can extrapolate from what is known about the pathology of a given ear disease or genetic entity to other similar cases or patients. As example, knowledge of the temporal bone pathology of meningitis deafness can suggest that when little or no hearing can be detected in a child who has had meningitis, the probability of destruction of cochlear structures is quite high. Temporal bone studies of rubella deafness often demonstrate sections of nearly normal tissues that suggest the possibility of real residual hearing in a youngster with this disorder, despite clinical failures in obtaining measurable audiometric responses.

Temporal Bone

The temporal bone forms part of the lateral wall and base of the skull, as shown in Figure 1.8. It articulates with other bones of the skull including the sphenoid, parietal, and occipital bones. The petrous part of the temporal bone is the most dense bone of the body, and contains among other things, most of the structures of

Table 1.1. Embryology summary of the ear

Fetal Week	Inner Ear	Middle Ear	External Ear
3rd	Auditory placode; auditory pit	Tubo-tympanic recess begins to develop	
4th	Auditory vesicle (otocyst); vestibular-cochlear division		Tissue thickenings begin to form
5th			Primary auditory meatus begins
6th	Utricle and saccule present; semicircular canals begin		6 hillocks evident; cartilage begins to form
7th	One cochlear coil present; sensory cells in utricle and saccule		Auricles move dorso-laterally
8th	Ductus reuniens present: sensory cells in semi-circular canals	Incus and malleus present in cartilage; lower half of tympanic cavity formed	Outer cartilagenous third of external canal formed
9th		3 tissue layers at tympanic membrane are present	
11th	2½ cochlear coils present; VIII nerve attaches to cochlear duct		
12th	Sensory cells in cochlea; membranous labyrinth complete; otic capsule begins to ossify		
15th		Cartilagenous stapes formed	
16th		Ossification of malleus and incus begins	
18th		Stapes begins to ossify	
20th	Maturation of inner ear; inner ear adult size		Auricle is adult shape, but continues to grow until age 9
21st		Meatal plug disintegrates exposing tympanic membrane	
30th		Pneumatization of tympanum	External auditory canal continues to mature until age 7
32nd		Malleus and incus complete ossification	
34th		Mastoid air cells develop	
35th		Antrum is pneumatized	
37th		Epitympanum is pneumatized	
		Stapes continues to develop until adulthood; tympanic membrane changes relative position during first 2 years of life	

the ear. The temporal bone is generally divided into four sections—the squamous, mastoid, petrous, and tympanic areas (Anson and Donaldson, 1967). In general terms, the squamous portion of the temporal bone is superior to the external auditory meatus; the mastoid area is posterior; while the tympanic portion forms the anterior, inferior, and part of the posterior walls of the external auditory meatus.

The petrous portion of the temporal bone extends medially from the external auditory canal, and its middle third contains the structures of the middle and inner ear. In the petrous bone it is important to note that the cochlear portion of the inner ear is situated anteriorly and medially to the internal auditory meatus and the vestibular portion of the inner ear. The internal auditory meatus houses the facial nerve (seventh) which lies superior to the auditory portion of the acoustic nerve (eighth) and anterior to the superior vestibular branch of the eighth cranial nerve. The petrous bone is shown in Figure 1.9 as part of the base of the skull as seen from above.

Preparation of Temporal Bone Histologic Sections. The density of the temporal bone and intricacy of the inner ear structures make preparation of suitable histologic slides from the gross bone specimen very difficult. Some 35 laboratories in the United States are capable of processing temporal bone specimens into adequate slides for examination.

The processing of a temporal bone into slides is a difficult, demanding, precise, time-consuming, and expensive procedure as shown in Figure 1.10. Initially, the temporal bone must

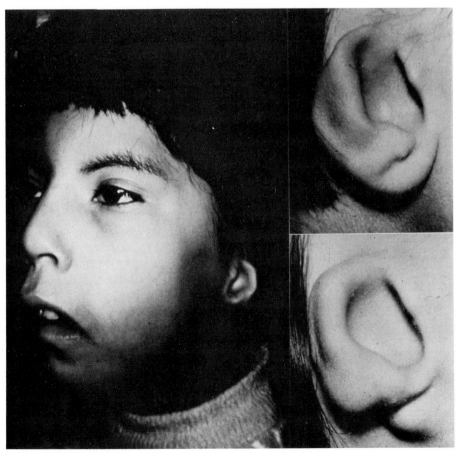

Fig. 1.7. A patient with Möbius syndrome, with first and second branchial arch anomalies as described in the text.

be removed from the skull of the donor within 24 hours of death or the inner ear structures undergo necrosis. The bone is immediately submerged in formalin for 2 or 3 weeks for fixation of structures. An extensive decalcification process follows for some 5 weeks in an adult bone to remove the dense calcium from the temporal bone. Infant temporal bones that are hours or days old may not show the presence of calcium after the first or second week in the decalcification solutions. Excess bone is then pared from the gross structure, and the decalcification chemicals are neutralized and the bone carefully washed.

The temporal bone is then dehydrated with ethyl alcohol solutions, infiltrated, and embedded into varying solutions of celloidin for nearly 3 months. The celloidin provides support for the bone tissues to permit sectioning with a microtome.

The temporal bone is sliced into sections of $20\text{-}\mu$ thickness, forming some 400 sections from each temporal bone. Only every 10th section is initially stained with dyes, generally hematoxylin and eosin to give the various tissues color for ease in identification. The dyed sections are mounted on microscope slides, ready for reading.

Examination of the stained sections of the temporal bone under high-powered magnification takes expert skills and knowledge gained only through experience and thorough study. The entire procedure involved in preparation of a single temporal bone may involve some five

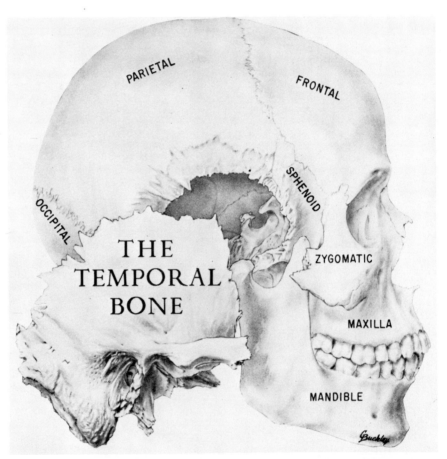

Fig. 1.8. The temporal bone section of the human skull. (With permission from B. J. Anson and J. A. Donaldson: The Surgical Anatomy of the Temporal Bone and Ear. Philadelphia, W. B. Saunders Co., 1967.)

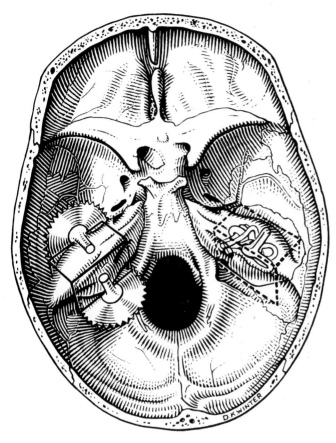

Fig. 1.9. Petrous portion of temporal bone shown as part of the skull viewed from above. (With permission from J. C. Gallagher: Histology of the human temporal bone. American Registry of Pathology. Washington, D.C., Armed Forces Institute of Pathology, 1967.)

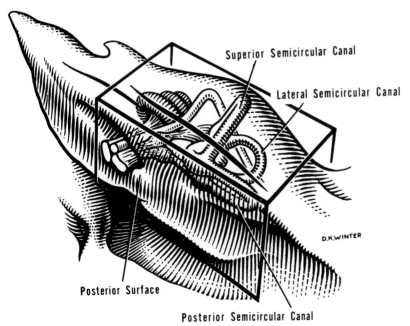

Superior Semicircular Canal

Lateral Semicircular Canal

Posterior Surface

Posterior Semicircular Canal

individuals, 9 months of time, and is estimated to cost several hundred dollars.

The method of horizontal section study of temporal bone anatomy is by no means the only, or necessarily the best means of preparing inner ear tissue. Johnsson and Hawkins (1967) use a surface preparation initially described by Bredberg et al. (1965) in which the otic capsule is lifted from the temporal bone, infused with fixative solutions, and examined as a whole surface preparation structure which can be studied within a few hours (Fig. 1.11). Johnsson and Hawkins point out that their surface preparation technique avoids postmortem changes of tissue, shrinkage, and inordinate time delay problems associated with stained horizontal, temporal bone preparation.

Anatomy of a Normal Temporal Bone. An understanding of normal temporal bone structures is necessary before one can appreciate the

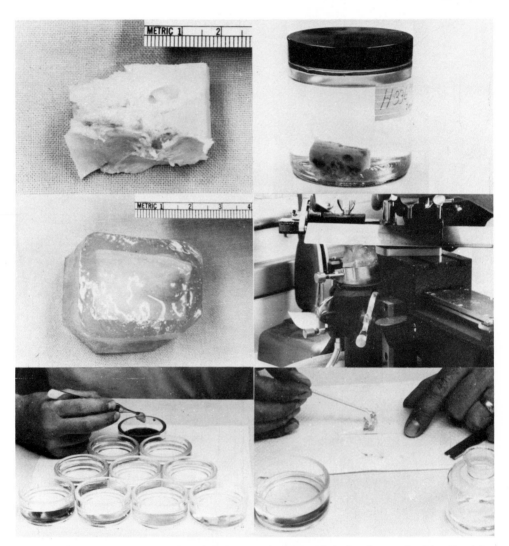

Fig. 1.10. The stages of processing a temporal bone into histopathologic microscopic slides. Top left, raw petrous portion of temporal bone as removed from cadaver; top right, lengthy decalcification process; middle left, petrous bone block in celloidin; middle right, microtome slicing bone into thin tissue sections; bottom left, staining of tissue sections; and bottom right, mounting stained tissue on microscope slides.

abnormalities found in temporal bones from patients with various kinds of deafness. Temporal bone study is usually reserved for residents in otolaryngology or physiologists interested in studying mechanisms of hearing, but there seems sufficient reason for all students of hearing disorders to have some familiarity with anatomy as demonstrated by horizontally cut, temporal bone histopathologic sections.

Typically, temporal bone sections are cut in the horizontal plane. Vertical sections may be prepared, but horizontal sections seem to be the general standard cuts utilized in journal articles. One must keep in mind the general level of the section under study as it was taken from the inner ear, or temporal bone block. Figure 1.12 shows the general gross structure of the inner ear. Imagine a horizontal line drawn through the most superior portion of the inner ear and you will see that the only structure represented might be the arch of the superior semicircular canal. As the microtome cuts off horizontal sections from a temporal bone block, the superior semicircular canal will be the initial structure to be sectioned. One must then imagine how a horizontal slice of temporal

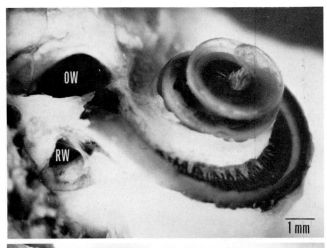

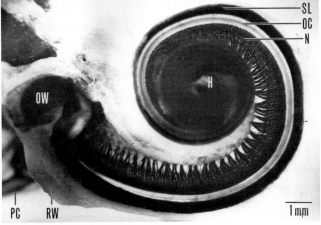

Fig. 1.11. Top, the human cochlea in "semiprofile" after removal of the otic capsule to expose the scala vestibuli in the surface preparation technique, oval window (OW), and round window (RW); bottom, final stage of surface cochlea dissection showing normal-appearing cochlea, oval window (OW), round window (RW), posterior canal (PC), spiral ligament (SL), organ of Corti (OC), network of nerve fibers (N), helicotrema (H).
(With permission from L. Johnsson and J. E. Hawkins, Jr: Sensory and neural degeneration with aging, as seen in micro-dissections of the human inner ear. Ann. Oto. Rhin. Laryng., 81: 179–193, 1972).

bone tissue will appear when placed on a microscope slide and viewed from above. The student of temporal bone anatomy must have a draftsman's ability to imagine three-dimensional structures from a two-dimensional picture.

Sample sections from a horizontally-sectioned petrous portion of a temporal bone are shown in the next few pages. The sections have been selected because they show specific portions of the inner ear that are of interest to audiologists. Photographs of the midmodiolar section of the cochlear and a single coil, or turn of the cochlea, have been included at higher magnification, so readers can appreciate these interesting structures. These temporal bone sections are presented through the courtesy of Isamu Sando, M.D., Director of the Temporal Bone Research Laboratory, University of Colorado Medical Center, Division of Otolaryngology.

Figure 1.13: Well pneumatized mastoid in the posterior (or left) area of this section. The ampulla of the superior semicircular canal is shown as a nearly round structure enclosing the membranous labyrinth. The crista is noticeable on the anterior edge of the superior semicircular canal ampulla. The facial nerve and its genu are very clearly shown in this slide, which has cut across the superior portion of the internal auditory canal. Immediately anterior to the genu of the facial nerve is the dense bone of the

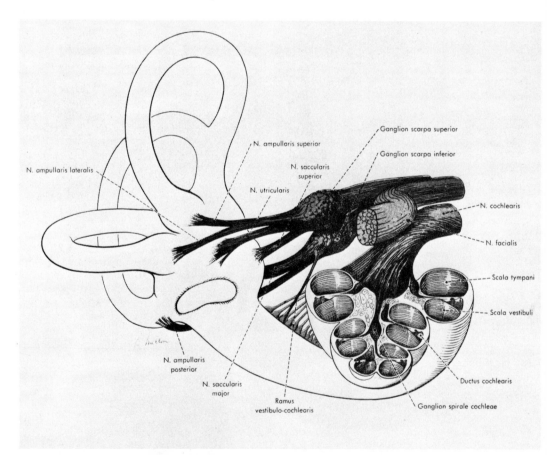

Fig. 1.12. The inner ear. Note the position of the facial nerve to the cochlear nerve and to the superior and inferior vestibular nerve. The cochlea is open to illustrate the midmodiolar view as observed in temporal bone sections. (With permission from B. J. Melloni: Some Pathological Conditions of the Eye, Ear, and Throat: An Atlas. Chicago, Abbott Laboratories, 1957.)

otic capsule which contains the cochlea. The lateral semicircular canal and its membranous labyrinth is also present at the peripheral edges of the structure.

Figure 1.14: This section is approximately 1 mm below the previous slide. The middle ear cavity is now obvious in this section and contains a cross-section view of the malleus and incus joined by the malleoincudal joint. The facial nerve is now encased in the facial canal. The upper portion of the basal turn of the cochlea is now present anteriorly and medially to the facial nerve. The superior branch of the vestibular nerve is visible in the internal auditory meatus, and is shown passing to the macula of the utricle. The endolymphatic duct is also present.

Figure 1.15: A section approximately 1 mm below the section shown in the previous figure. The middle ear cavity shows the malleus and incus with its short process pointing posteriorly toward the aditus and antrum into the mastoid air spaces. The anterior mallear ligament can

also be seen. The large space immediately medial to the facial nerve and canal contains the utricle. This section passes through the basal and middle turns of the cochlea which extend laterally. Reissner's membrane, the basilar membrane, and spiral ligament are obvious, even at this magnification. The modiolus is evident in the center of the basal turn of the cochlea. The inferior division of the vestibular nerve and the cochlear branch of the auditory nerve are shown in the internal auditory meatus. The endolymphatic sac is apparent in the posterior-medial portion of the photograph.

Figure 1.16: This section is about 1 mm lower than the section shown in Figure 1.15. This section passes through the bony modiolus of the basal and middle turns of the cochlea and now includes the final cochlear turn, the apical coil. In the middle ear, the malleus and incus are no longer touching. The large tensor tympani muscle in its canal is very obvious immediately adjacent to the cochlea and run-

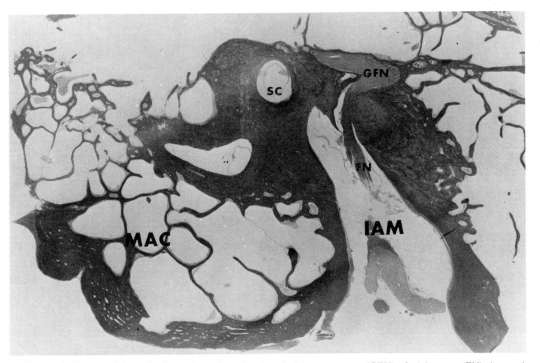

Fig. 1.13. Temporal bone horizontal section showing facial nerve genu (GFN), facial nerve (FN), internal auditory meatus (IAM), ampulla of superior semicircular canal (SC), and mastoid air cells (MAC). (Courtesy of I. Sando, University of Colorado Medical Center.)

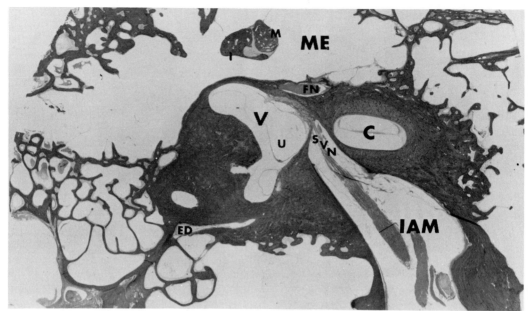

Fig. 1.14. Horizontal section of normal temporal bone showing malleus (M) and incus (I) in attic of middle ear (ME), utricle (U), basal turn of the cochlea (C), and superior vestibular nerve (SVN) feeding into vestibule (V) from the internal auditory meatus (IAM). The endolymphatic duct (ED) is seen at lower left corner. (Courtesy of I. Sando, University of Colorado Medical Center.)

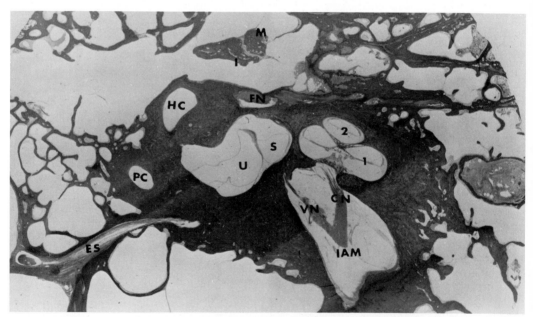

Fig. 1.15. Horizontal section from normal temporal bone showing two cochlear turns, basal (1) and middle (2); vestibular (VN) and cochlear (CN) portions of the eighth nerve in the internal auditory meatus (IAM), the endolymphatic sac (ES) is shown at lower left. The uricle (U) and the saccule (S) may be seen in the vestibule. The horizontal (HC) and posterior (PC) semicircular canals are also identified. (M) Malleus; (I) incus; (FN) facial nerve. (Courtesy of I. Sando, University of Colorado Medical Center.)

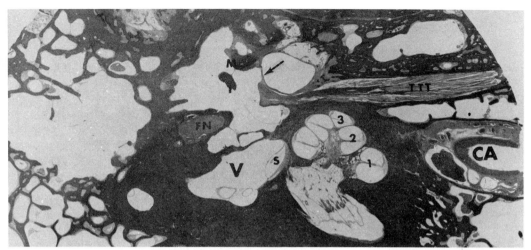

Fig. 1.16. Cochlear midmodiolar horizontal section of normal temporal bone. All three coils of cochlea (1, 2, and 3) are evident; the malleus (M) is attached to tympanic membrane; the tensor tympani muscle (TTT) extends through the processus cochlearformis with tensor tympani tendon (identified by arrow) attached to malleus. (FN) facial nerve; (V) vestibule; (CA) internal carotid artery; (I) incus; (S) saccule. (Courtesy of I. Sando, University of Colorado Medical Center.)

ning anterior-posterio. This section shows the processus cochleariformis extending posteriorly into the middle ear cavity from which the small tensor tympani tendon can be seen attaching to the anterior surface of the malleus. Part of the stapedial cura can be seen with the stapes footplate in the oval window niche. (An enlargement of the stapes in the oval window with the attachment of the stapedial tendon is shown in Figure 1.17.) The saccule and its innervation can be seen clearly in the vestibule along with the lateral semicircular canal and utricle. The large circular structure at the anterior edge of the section is the internal carotid artery. All three ossicles are difficult to demonstrate on one temporal bone section because they are not lined up equally on a single horizontal plane level.

Figure 1.18: An enlargement of the cochlea as viewed in Figure 1.16. It may be useful to the reader to review the gross view of the inner ear in Figure 1.12 to see how this exposure of the cochlea is obtained. This is a midmodiolar section of the cochlea showing the basal, middle, and apical turns. The nerve fibers are easily seen in the internal auditory meatus, and the ganglion cells of the spiral ganglion may be seen in Rosenthal's canal. The osseous spiral lamina extends radially from the modiolus in

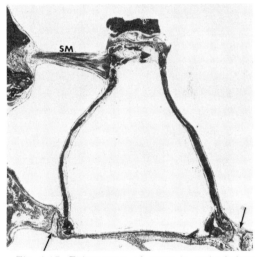

Fig. 1.17. Enlargement of stapes in oval window and stapedial tendon (SM). Note normal attachment of stapes footplate in oval window by annular ligament (arrows). (Courtesy of E. L. Grandon, M.D., Cedar Rapids, Iowa.)

each turn. The basilar membrane can be seen extending from the osseous spiral lamina to the spiral ligament and stria vascularis. Reissner's membrane is seen in each coil of the cochlea, separating the scala vestibuli from the scala media. The basilar membrane supports the organ of Corti which can just barely be seen at this magnification.

Figure 1.19: The classic view of a cochlear turn, emphasizing the structures of the scala media. These structures can be observed on any good temporal bone section by increasing the

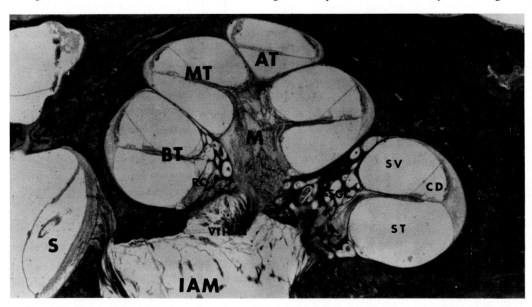

Fig. 1.18. Enlargement of cochlea from horizontal temporal bone section shown in Figure 1.16. Note auditory nerve (VIII N) in internal auditory meatus (IAM) with ganglion cells (SGC) in Rosenthal's canal (RC). The cochlear basal turn (BT), the middle turn (MT), and apical turn (AT) are clearly shown. Three ducts are seen in each turn, the scala vestibuli (SV), cochlear duct (CD), and scala tympani (ST); the saccule is also obvious in this view (S) with its innervation. (M) Modiolus. (Courtesy of I. Sando, University of Colorado Medical Center.)

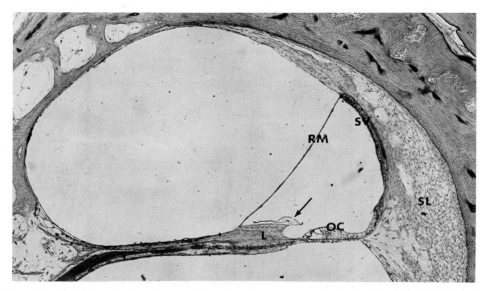

Fig. 1.19. Higher magnification of one cochlear duct showing organ of Corti (OC), spiral ligament (SL), stria vascularis (SV), Reissner's membrane (RM), tectorial membrane (arrow), and limbus (L). (Courtesy of I. Sando and L. Bergstrom, University of Colorado Medical Center.)

magnification on a single cochlear turn. The cochlear nerve fibers are shown under the spiral osseous lamina at the left of the photograph. The limbus supports one end of the tectorial membrane, which in its natural position should extend over the outer hair cells. The tectorial membrane, however, is very often seen in distorted position as an artifact of the temporal bone preparation procedure. Reissner's membrane extends from the limbus (crista spiralis) to the edge of the spiral ligament and stria vascularis. The curve between the limbus and the organ of Corti is the internal sulcus. The lower edge of the limbus, pointing and extending toward the organ of Corti, is known as the tympanic lip, which has numerous holes termed the habenula perforata. The habenula perforata permit cochlear nerve fibers to enter the organ of Corti from below the osseous spiral lamina.

The basilar membrane supports the organ of Corti (Fig. 1.20) which includes inner hair cells, outer hair cells, and the tunnel of Corti. The tunnel of Corti is formed by inner and outer pillar cells. Various supporting cells are seen next to the hair cells. Hensen's and Claudius' supporting cells are found between the outer hair cells and the external sulcus formed by the lower curve of the stria vascularis. Nuel's space may be seen between the outer pillar and the first row of outer hair cells. The outer hair cells are supported by outer phalangeal cells (Deiters' cells). Thus, the outer hair cell rests on a Deiters' cell and extends hairs from its upper surface toward the tectorial membrane. The lower portion of the stria vascularis contains a bulge known as the spiral prominence, which contains a blood vessel, the vas prominens.

Physiology of Hearing

In order to fully appreciate the intricacies of hearing impairment, one must understand the normal physiology of the hearing mechanism and the nature of hearing loss. These concepts are presented lightly here only as background material so that we may develop discussion regarding the pathologies of hearing impairment in the following chapter.

The phenomenon of hearing is the result of a complex series of events. Sound energy, originating as vibration and transmitted through an elastic medium such as air, impinges on the tympanic membrane causing it to vibrate. The vibrations are transmitted to the oval window of the otic capsule by the three middle ear ossicles. In addition to serving as a conductor to

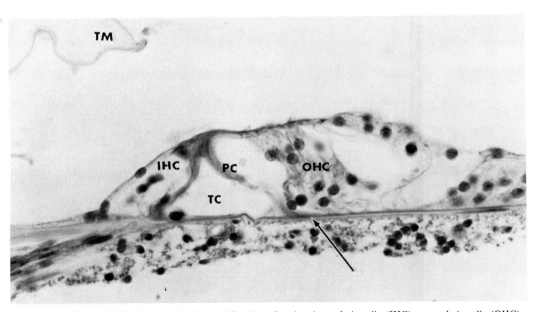

Fig. 1.20. Organ of Corti under high magnification showing inner hair cells (IHC), outer hair cells (OHC), tunnel of Corti (TC), pillar cells (PC), basilar membrane (arrow), and a displaced tectorial membrane (TM). (Courtesy of I. Sando, University of Colorado Medical Center.)

the sound energy, the tympanic membrane and ossicles amplify the sound by two simple mechanical principles consisting of a slight lever action of the ossicles and the areal surface relationship between the surface area of the tympanic membrane and the funneling of sound energy onto the smaller surface area of the stapes footplate. This middle ear amplification amounts to approximately 30 dB, and may be lost when defects or pathologies inhibit either or both of the amplifying mechanisms.

The vibration transmitted by the stapes to the oval window induces motion in the fluids of the cochlea. Perilymph fluid fills two ducts within the cochlea known as the scala vestibuli and the scala tympani. These parallel scalae communicate with each other at the helicotrema in the apical tip of the cochlear coils. When sound vibration displaces the stapes inward into the scala vestibuli, a simultaneous outward motion occurs in the scala tympani at the round window membrane which is termed the round window reflex.

The vibratory fluid motion ultimately causes a nerve impulse, with the cochlear neural epithelium acting as a mechanical transducer. This cochlear epithelium is composed of some 25,000 hair cells arranged neatly into one row of inner hair cells and three or four rows of outer hair cells. The hair cells rest on supporting cells which in turn rest on the basilar membrane, and extend into a third cochlear duct, filled with endolymph fluid known as the scala media or cochlear duct. This third duct is interposed between the scala vestibuli and scala tympani throughout the entire two and a half turns of the cochlea. Hair cells have a very orderly arrangement related to sound frequency. Hair cells that respond to high frequency above 2000 Hz are located in the basal turn of the cochlea, while hair cells that are tuned to stimulating frequencies below 2000 Hz are found in the middle and apical cochlear coils.

The peripheral neurons of the cochlear nerve are distributed to hair cells from beneath the basilar membrane and its supporting shelf, the osseous spiral lamina. The fluid motion of the scala tympani displaces the basilar membrane in a traveling wave pattern, producing torsion on the hair-like processes of the cell and creating some type of mechanical-chemical change re-sulting in peripheral nerve-ending stimulation. Thus, the vibratory energy transmitted by the tympanic membrane is transformed into neural impulse code.

Auditory Nerve

The nerve fibers that innervate the hair cells have their cell bodies in the bipolar spiral ganglion which is located in Rosenthal's canal. Axons from the spiral ganglion cells join in the modiolus and collect as the auditory, or cochlear, branch of the eighth nerve. Just outside the cochlea the vestibular portion of the eighth nerve coming from the semicircular canals, utricle, and saccule, joins the cochlear portion. The two portions of the eighth nerve come together like a rope and pass through the internal auditory meatus toward the medulla. The structure of the auditory nerve is very orderly, with fibers from the apical quarter of the cochlea forming the core of the nerve, and around them the fibers from the apex of the cochlea twisting one way, while the fibers from the middle turn of the cochlea twist the other way. Fifty per cent of the fibers from the cochlea come from the basal coil, and represent sensory elements that respond to frequencies above 2000 Hz.

Recent work by Spoendlin (1967, 1969) has shown that most of the afferent neurons come from the inner hair cells, whereas only some 10% of the fibers come from the outer hair cells. Each outer hair cell is, however, innervated by several different neurons, while one neuron innervates a large number of outer hair cells. The inner hair cells are innervated by a large number of different neurons, but each neuron innervates only one inner hair cell.

The eighth nerve divides again, however, before it reaches the medulla. The auditory portion divides into dorsal and ventral branches which go to corresponding nuclei in the brain stem wherein the second-order afferent auditory neuron cell bodies are located.

Experimenters have found that fibers in the eighth nerve are "tuned" to certain frequencies. That is, certain fibers are most responsive to certain stimulating frequencies. This fact is determined by inserting microelectrodes into single nerve fibers and determining the threshold for the action potential "spike" of that nerve fiber for a variety of frequencies, then plotting what is known as the response area for that particular fiber. The threshold sensitivity of a fiber increases gradually and is most sensitive at its "tuned" frequency—which can then be used to name the fiber, such as a "7000 Hz fiber." Most of the auditory fibers are high frequency units, usually above 1000 Hz. Some individual units fire spontaneously, without a specific stimulus controlled by the experimenter (Tasaki, 1954). It is remarkable that only a few fibers of the eighth nerve are required to preserve good hearing. The auditory nerve must be sectioned more than half-way to have a measurable effect on hearing, and then, if indeed hearing is left, it is predominantly low frequency hearing (Neff, 1947; Wever and Neff, 1947). To click stimuli, the individual nerve responses, tuned to different frequencies, fire in close synchrony, so that the amplitude of the action potential is representative of the number of fibers that respond (Davis, 1961).

Brain Stem Pathways

Much of the brain stem auditory pathway can be seen in Figure 1.21. The higher auditory pathways are rather complex and often escape significance with students who tend only to memorize the names of the relay stations and major neuronal paths. It is important to realize that although first-order neurons from the cochlea reach the brain stem in the cochlear nuclei, most of the activity that ultimately reaches the cortex is by the way of fourth-order neurons. This seemingly too complex system seldom breaks down because of alternate paths to the cerebral cortex.

Two pairs of cochlear nuclei exist, a dorsal

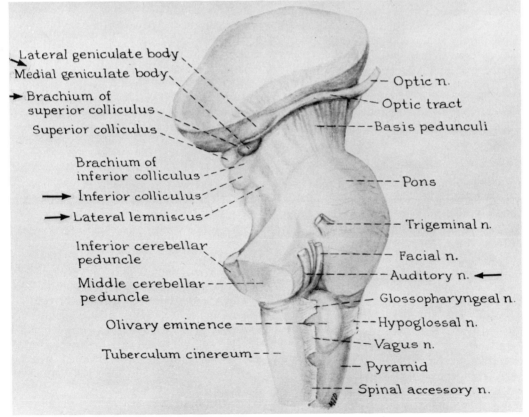

Fig. 1.21. This view of the dorsal-lateral portion of the medulla oblongata, or brain stem, shows much of the auditory pathway including the auditory nerve, lateral lemniscus, the inferior colliculus and its branchium, and the medial geniculate body. (With permission from N. B. Everett: Functional Neuroanatomy. Philadelphia, Lea and Febiger, 1965.)

and a ventral cochlear nucleus on each side of the medulla, but are referred to collectively as the cochlear nuclei of the medulla. Although some of the neurons of the cochlear nuclei ascend to higher nuclei on the same side of the system, most cross over to the opposite side in the trapezoid body. Auditory units in the cochlear nuclei are also sensitive to specific frequencies as we noted previously with auditory nerve fibers. Inhibitory units have also been reported in the cochlear nuclei, which under certain circumstances actually inhibit response rather than excite the unit under examination (Galambos and Davis, 1943, 1948). Thus a particular frequency stimulus may excite certain neurons of the auditory system, while inhibiting other units from firing. What starts out in the cochlea as the excitation of the relatively large group of hair cells is narrowed down to a smaller group of neurons through the process of inhibition. In addition, the cochlear nuclei, like the cochlea, exhibit tonotopic organization, or an orderly arrangement of responsiveness to different frequencies. In fact, Rose et al. (1959) report one unrolling of the cochlear frequency distribution in the dorsal cochlear nucleus and two separate complete frequency patterns in the ventral nuclei. The number of discharges from a single cochlear nucleus unit is apparently related to the intensity of the acoustic stimulus (Galambos and Davis, 1943).

The principal terminations of second-order afferent auditory neurons are in the nuclei of the trapezoid body and superior olivary body. The superior olive is the first structure in the medulla which receives fibers from both ears, and may play a role in the localization of sound. From here, neurons originate that course upward in the loosely compacted neurons of the lateral lemniscus to another principal relay station, the inferior colliculus. Collaterals of second- and third-order neurons are given off to the reticular formation which provides an indirect, diffuse, sensory pathway to the cerebral cortex. The reticular formation is closely related to arousal and attention during sleep, and may be responsible for the fact that a crying baby may wake only mother, but no one else in family. Or one may sleep soundly through a barrage of noise but wake suddenly upon hearing a soft familiar voice.

Most of the fibers in the lateral lemniscus pathway terminate in the inferior colliculus, but some may bypass and end in the next relay station, the medial geniculate body. So far as is known, all direct projections to the auditory cortex are relayed in the medial geniculate body (Morgan, 1965). The auditory cortex is, of course, responsible for the fine discrimination that is necessary in the understanding of speech. The "tuning" function of the higher auditory centers, including the inferior colliculus, the medial geniculate body, and the auditory cortex, has been summarized by Ades (1959): some units at higher levels in the auditory system are frequency specific and some are not; many units respond only to clicks with a complex spectrum and are unresponsive to pure tone signals; many units show spontaneous firing which can sometimes be inhibited by acoustic stimuli; and of the units that are frequency-specific, the response areas of the units higher up in the auditory system tend to be narrower than those units found in lower auditory centers.

Attempts to map the cortical responses to auditory stimuli have identified the temporal lobe as the responsive area, sometimes further localized as Brodmann's areas 41 and 42. The cortex has at least two tonotopic frequency projections which are the reverse of each other. Kryter and Ades (1943) established a very important fact with significant clinical implication. They showed that under appropriate conditions, cortical lesions have no appreciable effect on the absolute thresholds of pure tone stimuli. This is true even when extensive bilateral cortical lesions are made. Thus, the ability to respond to tones is not dependent upon cerebral cortex. These same investigators reported that removal of the inferior colliculi created an approximate 15-dB loss in pure tone sensitivity; destruction of the entire auditory system from the midbrain to the cortex created a pure tone loss of about 40 dB. It may be concluded that the most important aspect of auditory sensitivity to pure tones is due to intact neurons below the inferior colliculi, and a nearly normal audiogram may be obtained with a loss of 75% of the neurons of the auditory nerve.

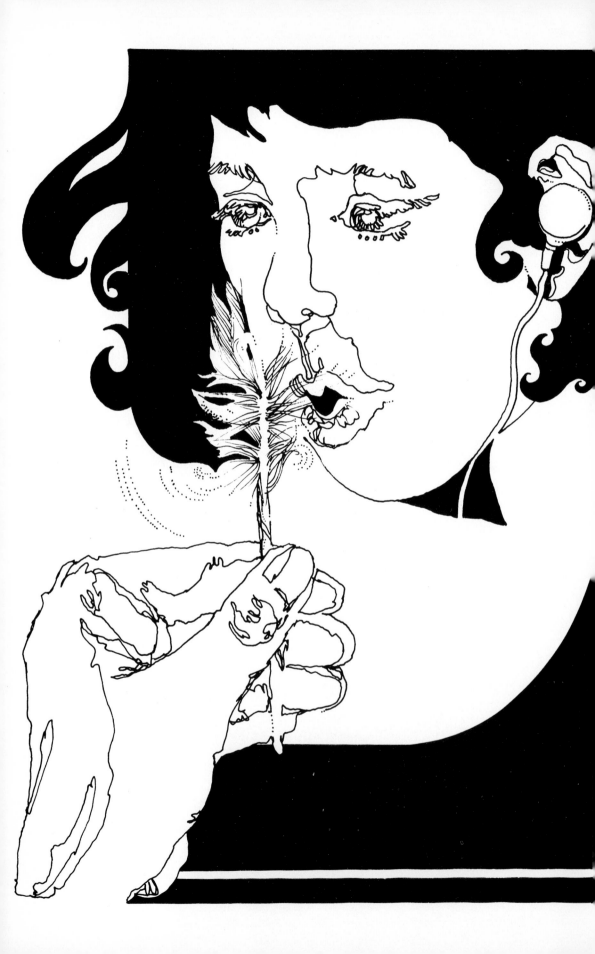

2 HEARING LOSS IN CHILDREN

The Nature of Hearing Loss

Hearing losses are generally identified as conductive or sensorineural. When a combination of both types of hearing loss occurs, we speak of a mixed type hearing loss. When auditory dysfunction can be shown to exist, yet peripheral hearing mechanisms are within normal limits, the loss is categorized as a central auditory defect.

Conductive Hearing Loss

Interference of any sort in the transmission of sound from the external auditory canal to the inner ear causes conductive hearing loss. The inner ear, in such cases, is capable of normal function, but the sound vibration is not able to stimulate the cochlea via the normal air conduction pathway.

The conductive-type loss is characterized by a hearing loss for air-conducted sounds, while sounds conducted to the inner ear directly by bone conduction of the skull and temporal bone are heard normally. When the air conductive pathway is totally blocked as in atresia, stenosis, complete stapes fixation, or ossicular discontinuity, a maximal 60-dB air conduction hearing loss will exist. Although conductive hearing losses may resolve spontaneously, frequently some residual of the pathologic condition may remain for long periods of time. Most conductive hearing losses can be corrected through medical treatment or surgery.

Sensorineural Hearing Loss.

Hearing impairment occurs when damage has been sustained by the sensory end organ or cochlear hair cells, or the dysfunction may be the fault of the auditory nerve. Traditionally, damage to the sensory end organ is not easily differentiated from neuronal damage, so the resultant hearing loss is lumped under the category "sensorineural." New testing techniques such as electrocochleography offer promise as an objective means of differentiating between sensory and neural hearing impairment.

In sensorineural hearing losses the air and bone conduction thresholds are nearly the same. Sensorineural hearing losses may easily be overlooked during physical examination since the external auditory canal and tympanic membrane will appear normal. This type of hearing loss is nearly always irreversible.

Mixed Hearing Loss

When both a sensorineural loss and a conductive hearing loss are present, the result is a mixed hearing loss. The audiogram shows less-than-normal bone conduction thresholds which are closer to normal levels than the air conduction thresholds. A significant air conduction/bone conduction gap between threshold levels may exist, which should disappear when the conductive portion of the hearing loss is ameliorated. The mixed hearing loss, however, improves only as much as the degree of air/bone gap, and hearing levels are not likely to return to normal limits (Jordan and Eagles, 1961).

Central Auditory Dysfunction

This type of impairment is not necessarily accompanied by a decrease in auditory sensitivity but tends to manifest itself in varying degrees as a decrease in auditory comprehension. For example, the child may have a rather normal audiogram, but be unable to recognize or interpret speech. Central auditory dysfunction is a complex topic and is discussed more fully in Chapter 3.

Degree and Severity of Hearing Loss

An important consideration of any hearing loss is its degree of impairment. Common descriptive terms used to identify degree of hearing loss include mild hearing loss (15 to 30 dB), moderate hearing loss (31 to 50 dB), severe hearing loss (51 to 80 dB), profound hearing loss (81 to 100 dB), and anacusis or total hearing loss. Sometimes borderline categories of hearing impairment are described with a combination of terms such as "moderately severe" hearing loss.

Additional consideration regarding the severity of the hearing loss must be given to its unilateral or bilateral presence. The child with a totally dead ear on one side but with a normal ear on the other side may function quite well in most situations. He will fail the school screening test, however, and offers special problems to the audiologist who tests his hearing. This youngster's auditory abilities will be lacking in circumstances where sound localization is needed or in instances when noise exists to compete with the signal of interest.

A complete description of a youngster's hearing loss should include its presence as unilateral or bilateral, in addition to a term which identifies its degree of auditory impairment, as well as a statement regarding the type of loss as conductive, sensorineural, or mixed. From the physician's diagnosis a description of the cause of the hearing loss can be made. Samples of hearing loss descriptions might include unilateral, severe sensorineural hearing loss due to mumps, or a bilateral, moderate conductive hearing loss due to otitis media.

Disorders Associated with Hearing Loss

Detailed descriptions of disorders associated with hearing loss are presented in most elementary textbooks in otolaryngology. Audiology textbooks may offer material on hearing pathology, but usually in a nonmedical manner so that insufficient information is available to audiologists who work with medical personnel. The material presented below is not as complete as that found in otolaryngology textbooks, but hopefully is more pertinent to childhood disorders than that commonly found in basic audiology books. For information regarding treatment and diagnosis of these disorders of hearing, the reader is referred to a most informative chapter on ear, nose, and throat problems written by Weaver and Downs (1972) in *Current Pediatric Diagnosis and Treatment.*

Stenosis and Atresia of the External Auditory Canal

Stenosis, or narrowing, of the external auditory canal may occur as a result of trauma, surgery, congenital anomaly, or chronic infection. If it is due to congenital anomaly, the pinna may be normal or abnormal. A canal that is very narrow is easily clogged with cerumen or ectodermal debris. Atresia, or closure of the external auditory meatus, may be due to congenital malformation or result from surgical misadventure. Children with these defects usually suffer conductive-type hearing losses and may do well with bone conduction hearing aids if medical or surgical treatment is not in order.

Collapse of the ear canal during audiometric testing can produce a hearing loss from pressure of the earphones against the pinna, tragus, and opening to the external auditory meatus. This problem is very common in children with stenotic ear canals that close down when an earphone is pressed over the pinna (Hildyard and Valentine, 1962; Bess, 1971). Audiometric testing will show an erroneous air-bone gap, or conductive hearing loss, that is not confirmed by impedance audiometry or physical examination of the ear. Such children can be shown to have normal hearing when retested with hollow auditory canal plugs used under the earphone or when tested under sound field conditions (Ventry et al., 1961).

Otitis Externa

Patients often present with a complaint of drainage from the ear. Although the audiologist may quickly assume that such drainage suggests an infected middle ear with perforation of the eardrum, the exudate is often from otitis externa. This condition is due to dermatitis of the external ear canal from bacterial infection. The presence of water in the ear canal against the tympanic membrane provides ideal circumstances for the development of bacterial growth. The patient may complain of tenderness when the earphone is placed over the pinna, or acute inflammation may be easily noted in the concha or opening of the external auditory canal.

Cerumen and Foreign Bodies

Cerumen, or ear wax, is a combined product of the apocrine and sebaceous glands and is supposed to protect the ear canal by its adhesive properties. Hearing loss may result from massive accumulation of wax that completely occludes the ear canal or when the wax is pressed against the tympanic membrane by an aggressive parent armed with a Q-tip.

Children are the leading candidates to appear with a foreign object in their ear canal—objects which may include broken crayons, food, small toys, or pieces of jewelry. Hearing loss is not a major concern in such cases unless the foreign object has ruptured the tympanic membrane. Referral to a medical specialist for removal of the object is, of course, mandatory.

Bullous Myringitis

Blisters occasionally form on the tympanic membrane in association with a coincident upper respiratory infection. The blisters, or bullae, represent an accumulation of fluid between the layers of the tympanic membrane and may appear to the untrained observer as acute otitis media. This disorder is extremely painful and accompanied by a feeling of pressure in the ear. Hearing levels may be within normal limits.

Perforations of the Tympanic Membrane

Perforations may occur from some sort of trauma such as a blow to the side of the head, a water-skiing fall, diving, or sudden changes in air pressure, or from middle ear problems such as acute otitis media. The tympanic membrane is about 8 mm in diameter and perforations from acute otitis media are usually much smaller, 1 to 2 mm in diameter. Often these perforations will heal spontaneously.

Conductive hearing loss occurs as a consequence of poor vibration of the tympanic membrane. The degree of loss, however, is variable and dependent upon the size of the perforation and its location on the tympanic membrane. Small perforations may be obvious with hearing levels within normal limits. Impedance audiometry may be used very effectively as described in Chapter 6 to identify children with perforated tympanic membranes. Complications from perforations may be very serious and all such children should be immediately referred to a medical specialist. Parents should be advised to practice aural hygiene by keeping water out of the child's ear when swimming or bathing until proper medical care of the ear has been taken.

Otitis Media

Otitis media is properly differentiated into serous, acute, and chronic otitis media. The terms refer to various conditions of fluid in the middle ear space which when inflamed may be coincident with mastoiditis (inflammation of the mastoid air cells) since the mastoid air cell system openly communicates with the middle ear.

Serous otitis media occurs when the eustachian tube becomes closed or blocked thus creating a closed middle ear space. Under these circumstances, the air of the middle ear is absorbed creating negative middle ear pressure and transudation of fluid into the cavity. Hearing impairment may be present due to the retracted tympanic membrane and negative middle ear pressure, or due to the presence of fluid. Hearing levels may be relatively normal and impedance audiometry utilized to identify this condition. Tympanograms will be of the Jerger Type B or C variety, and acoustic reflexes will probably be absent from the probe tip ear (see Chap. 6 for full explanation). Serous otitis media is very common in children aged 3 to 8 years and may be rather recalcitrant to medical treatment. If pain is present in this disease, it is usually intermittent and rather mild.

Acute otitis media generally presents suddenly with ear pain, which may as suddenly subside when the tympanic membrane ruptures. The middle ear secretion in this disorder is purulent. The pain which accompanies this ear condition often makes audiometry and impedance testing difficult, if not impossible. Parents often describe young children as "pulling at their ears," but this does not seem to be a very reliable or consistent diagnostic clue in our experience.

Chronic otitis media includes purulent discharge from an ear with a perforation of the tympanic membrane. Chronic otitis media is a recurrent disease. The tissues of the middle ear intermittently undergo destruction, healing, and scarring during the recurrent infections. The pathology of chronic otitis media is characterized by a lack of uniformity among diseased ears. The disease may also be the result of cholesteatoma.

The size of the perforation may vary considerably from a very small to a large area. Occasionally, the entire tympanic membrane and portions of the annulus may be absent. Spontaneous healing may result with a growth of squamous epithelium over the perforation. Should the epithelium invade the middle ear, a cholesteatoma may ensue. Also, during healing the middle ear and tympanic membrane may develop tympanosclerosis, which is hyalinized and calcified scar tissue. Tympanosclerosis deposits may cause stiffening of the tympanic membrane or fusion and fixation of the

ossicular chain. Middle ear granulation tissue, polyps, and monomeric membranes are also associated with various forms of chronic otitis media as shown in Figure 2.1.

Chronic otitis media most often has its onset in early childhood, between the ages of 5 and 10 years. Recurrent otitis media may halt or reverse the process of mastoid pneumatization, or cause mastoid sclerosis. Severe forms of otitis media may, or may not, damage the middle ear ossicles, depending on the severity and duration of the disease. Severe otitis media may produce areas of osteitis in the mastoid septae, resulting in a continuous foul discharge.

Paparella and Brady (1970) reviewed 232 patients with chronic suppurative otitis media and mastoiditis. They found a definite increase in the incidence of sensorineural hearing loss which they suggested was due to a cochlear biochemical change created by toxic materials passed into the inner ear through the round window resulting in gradual destruction of the organ of Corti. English et al. (1973) evaluated 404 patients with various forms of otitis media and reached conclusions in accord with the Paparella and Brady study. English et al. found

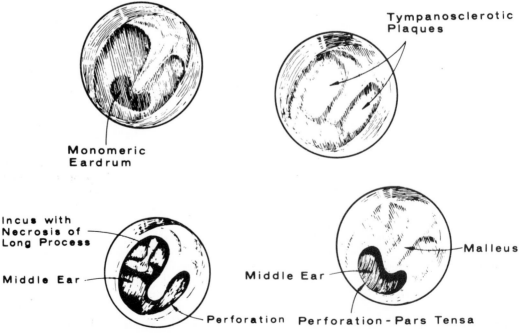

Fig. 2.1. Otoscopic views of the tympanic membrane showing some sequelae of chronic otitis media. (Courtesy of Gerald M. English, M.D., Denver, CO.)

that bone conduction thresholds worsened with the severity and duration of disease. Post-treatment bone conduction thresholds were unchanged from pretreatment tests, leading these authors to conclude that sensorineural hearing loss can be a natural sequela of chronic otitis media.

Cholesteatoma

The continuing maturation and persistent growth of squamous epithelium (skin) often can create problems in the ear. When the growing skin from the ear canal finds its way into the middle ear cavity or mastoid through a tympanic membrane perforation, the material accumulates and forms a cholesteatoma. A cross-section diagram in Figure 2.2 shows an attic and a middle ear cholesteatoma. Moisture and bacteria may gain access to the cholesteatoma (which is really a deposit of desquamated keratin) and foul-smelling ear drainage may ensue. The disease process may cause erosion of surrounding bone or create meningeal complications or fistulae of the otic capsule.

Cleft Palate

Deformities of the lip and palate are among the most common major congenital malformations, occurring once in 900 newborns. A substantial number of articles have been published concerning the otologic and audiologic

problems of children with overt cleft palate. The incidence of recurrent otitis media in such children is quite high and has been reported from 50% to 90% by various investigators (Holborow, 1962; Graham, 1963; Stool and Randall, 1967; Paradise and Bluestone, 1969). Complications such as cholesteatoma and adhesive otitis may accompany middle ear effusions in cleft palate children. Hearing loss as a secondary problem to the middle ear disorder related to cleft palate is also very common, and may exist in 90% of such patients (Pannbacker, 1969; Yules, 1970). Goetzinger et al. (1960) and Graham (1963) indicate that the incidence and severity of middle ear problems related to the cleft palate decrease as the patient grows older.

Otologic and hearing problems associated with submucous cleft palate have been reviewed by Bergstrom and Hemenway (1971). The submucous cleft palate is described as an imperfect union of muscle across the soft palate that tends to "tent" when the patient phonates. The area may appear bluish since it is covered by only nasal and oral mucosa. The dehiscence of muscle and bone may be obvious with palpation and is often accompanied by a bifid uvula. From a study of 58 patients with submucous cleft palate, Bergstrom and Hemenway reported an incidence of 39% with recurrent or chronic disease of the middle ear ranging in severity between serous otitis media

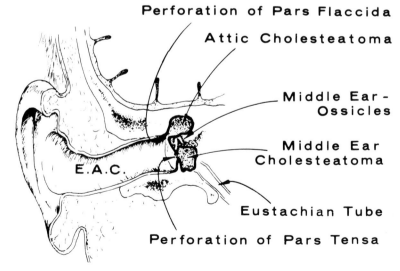

Perforation of Pars Flaccida

Attic Cholesteatoma

Middle Ear - Ossicles

Middle Ear Cholesteatoma

E.A.C.

Eustachian Tube

Perforation of Pars Tensa

Fig. 2.2. Cross-section of the external and middle ear showing an attic cholesteatoma through a perforation of the pars flaccida portion of the tympanic membrane; a perforation of the pars tensa portion of the tympanic membrane may lead to development of a middle ear choleasteatoma. (With permission from G. M. English, J. L. Northern, and T. J. Fria: Chronic otitis media as a cause of sensorineural hearing loss. Arch. Otolaryngol. 98: 17-22, 1973.)

to cholesteatoma. Conductive hearing loss was demonstrated by 34% of the group, while an additional 25% had either pure sensorineural or mixed type hearing loss. They suggest that the presence of submucous cleft palate indicates the possibility of accompanying middle ear disease, and likewise the presence of persistent or recurring middle ear disease makes the patient suspect for undiscovered submucous cleft palate.

Although numerous ideas have been offered to explain the high incidence of hearing problems associated with overt and submucous cleft palate children, most clinicians agree that the deficiency of palate musculature is the probable cause of poor eustachian tube function. This results in inadequate middle ear ventilation, effusion of fluid, tympanic membrane retraction, and hearing loss. Such disease of the middle ear is most common in children between 3 and 8 years of age which also corresponds to the increased exposure and susceptability to upper respiratory infections found in this age group (Halfond and Ballenger, 1956; Bennett et al., 1968).

Clinicians should be sensitive to this increased incidence of hearing difficulty and recurrent middle ear disease in children with cleft palate. The hearing of such patients should be monitored on a regular basis with close medical follow-up. Our experiences with cleft palate children have exposed numerous youngsters with recurrent episodes of otitis media accompanied by significant hearing loss who undoubtedly miss much auditory information at school and home. Immediate medical treatment is often necessary for these children who may qualify for repeated myringotomy and ventilation tubes. Mild to moderate power hearing aids may be in order for children who do not respond well to medical treatment, especially during the important school years.

Impedance audiometry is an especially valuable clinical procedure in children with cleft palate. The overt cleft palate is diagnosed within the first few days of life, although the submucous cleft palate may not be diagnosed until years later. Impedance audiometry may identify conductive impairments in even very young infants, not readily amenable to bone conduction testing, and who have sufficient hearing sensitivity to respond well to air conduction hearing tests.

Ototoxic Hearing Loss

Certain medications may permanently injure or destroy the hair cells of the cochlear creating sensorineural hearing impairment. Kanamycin and neomycin are the worst ototoxic drugs. However, other pharmaceutical members of the antibiotics, diuretics, and antimalarials, especially other members of the streptomyces family such as gentamycin, vancomycin, etc., are also known to be ototoxic. Streptomycin is most often destructive to the vestibular system, but may also cause cochlear insult (Hawkins, 1967a). There is considerable individual susceptibility to these ototoxic drugs, which is usually, but not always, bilaterally symmetrical and of varying degree and severity. Impaired renal function permits abnormally high blood levels of these drugs, tending to increase the chance of ototoxic hearing loss. Aspirin, quinine, and diuretics are the only drugs which produce temporary hearing loss which often recovers when the patients are taken off these medications. Hawkins (1967b) has published an excellent treatise on ototoxic deafness in children.

Ingestion of ototoxic drugs by pregnant women can result in a multitude of congenital abnormalities and deformities in their child (Moya and Thorndyke, 1963). Skeletal malformations, cleft palate, dental anomalies, ocular malformations of cardiovascular system, urinary tract anomalies, genital tract anomalies, intestinal tract malformations, and abnormalities of the ear have all been reported as a result of ingestion of drugs during pregnancy. Of the drugs known to cause hearing impairment, the most common associated with prenatal deafness are cholorquine (Matz and Naunton, 1968), thalidomide (d'Avignon and Barr, 1964; Jorgensen and Kristensen, 1964), quinine, salicylates, as well as a number of antibiotics, particularly those of the "mycin" group, including streptomycin (Robinson and Cambon, 1964). Severity and type of resulting malformations and anomalies can be traced to time of intake of the ototoxic drugs.

Ingestion of such drugs during first trimester,

especially the sixth and seventh weeks of pregnancy, is most devastating to the developing embryo. Damage to the auditory system resulting from maternal ingestion of drugs includes outer and inner hair cell damage, middle ear anomalies, absence of seventh and eighth nerves, dysplasia of organ of Corti, and decreased number of ganglion cells. Aplasia of inner ear has been reported. The audiogram may typically show flat, high tone, or saucer-shaped configuration with mild to profound sensorineural loss. Conductive loss has also been observed due to ossicular malformation of the middle ear.

Cochlear Trauma

Skull fracture involving the occipital or squamous portion of the temporal bone may extend into the petrous portion of the temporal bone and involve the otic capsule. Should the fracture line cross the external auditory canal, laceration of the skin and bleeding of the external canal may occur with little permanent loss of hearing. More medial fractures may produce bleeding in the middle ear or disruption of the ossicular chain which would create a maximal 60-dB conductive-type hearing loss.

Should a fracture line occur through the cochlea, total deafness may result in the involved ear. Trauma to the side of the head creates a sensorineural hearing loss on the opposite side, which often takes the form of a 4000-Hz dip in the audiogram. Hearing loss due to concussion may recover totally or partially, while hearing loss due to fracture of the cochlea is irreversible.

Noise-Induced or Noise Trauma Hearing Loss

Loud sound produces destruction of the hair cells in the organ of Corti. The most common exposure in childhood is related to single, identifiable, noise experiences such as an explosion of a firecracker, etc. Usually such hearing loss consists of a sensorineural loss in the audiogram at 4000 Hz, regardless of the type of noise exposure. Tremendous individual susceptibility to hearing loss from noise exposure exists. Some children, who hunt or operate noisy farm machinery will show evidence of noise-induced hearing loss. These youngsters should be fitted with adequate ear protection and protected against additional unnecessary noise exposure. Hearing loss due to noise may be reversible in the early stages or may proceed to permanent hearing damage. Weber et al. (1967) evaluated 1000 children from Colorado with hearing loss and found 249 males and 51 females with the noise exposure characteristic audiogram.

Viral Diseases

Viral diseases have long been recognized as a cause of deafness. Both prenatal and postnatal infections have been identified as a cause of hearing loss. Maternal rubella has been the cause of large numbers of deaf children, with some 10,000 to 20,000 children affected by the epidemics of the early and mid-1960's. The sequelae of maternal rubella are discussed further in the "Index of Audiologic Disorders" in Chapter 9. Congenital deafness has also been attributed to meningoencephalitis, chicken pox, and other viruses.

Postnatal viruses as a cause of early acquired deafness commonly result in profound bilateral deafness. Infectious meningitis which causes deafness as the result of bilateral labyrinthitis due to extension of infection from the meninges was early recognized as a leading cause of profound bilateral deafness (Vernon, 1967a, b). The infecting agent has been found to pass from the meninges to the inner ear through the cochlear aqueduct and along vessels and nerves from the internal auditory meatus (Paparella and Suguira, 1967). Bacterial postnatal infections known to result in deafness due to meningogenic spread include streptococcus, pneumococcus, and staphylococcus.

Common viruses of later postnatal period known to or suspected to cause deafness and/or vestibular symptoms include mumps, measles, chicken pox, influenza, and viruses of the common cold. Here again deafness results from damage to the inner ear due to direct infiltration via the internal meatus. Disease may be limited to the endolymphatic system with the inflammatory process beginning in the vascular beds (Lindsay, 1967a).

The viral diseases usually cause mild to profound sensorineural hearing loss. Histopathologic effects of viral infections reported have included extensive destruction of organ of Corti, degeneration of saccule, damage or complete destruction of stria vascularis and tectorial membrane, damage or obliteration of vestibular system, and atrophy or destruction of neural pathways (Lindsay, 1967b).

Maternal infections have been demonstrated as the cause of a host of other congenital malformations and abnormalities. However, congenital infections often cause fetal death and miscarriage. Damage to the fetus attributed to congenital viral infections has included congenital malformations such as club foot; intrauterine growth; retardation; damage to nervous system including anencephaly, encephalocele, and spina bifida; congenital heart disease; and disease of other organs such as the liver, pancreas, and adrenals.

Residuals of postnatal viral infections include nerve atrophy, notably the optic nerve, cerebral palsy, mental retardation, disturbances of respiration, muscular atrophy or paralysis, convulsions, disturbances of autonomic system, and disturbances of metabolism.

Congenital Syphilis

Early manifestations include nasal discharge (snuffles), rash, anemia, jaundice, and osteochondritis. Later manifestations include saddle nose, saber skin, Hutchinson teeth, mulberry molars, and other dental anomalies. Congenital syphilis may demonstrate a multitude of central nervous system abnormalities including vestibular dysfunction, sensorineural hearing loss, and occasionally aortic valvulitis. Possible accompanying mental retardation depends on severity of neurologic damage.

Auditory impairment may not be present at birth. Onset of hearing loss is generally in early childhood, usually sudden bilaterally symmetrical causing severe to profound impairment. The hearing loss is usually not accompanied by marked vestibular manifestations. Poor hearing function and limited use of hearing aid can be expected due to neural atrophy. The general treatment of congenital syphilis consists of prompt treatment of infant with penicillin. Treatment may be done in utero prior to delivery when an infected mother is identified (Karmody and Schuknecht, 1966).

Cytomegalic Inclusion Disease

This viral infection is disseminated widely in certain geographic areas. It shows little pathogenicity in adults but when transmitted in utero the conceptus may be associated with a spectrum of infections possibly including severe systemic disease of the brain, lungs, liver, spleen, and bone marrow. Manifestations include intrauterine growth retardation, jaundice, erythroblastemia, microephaly, pneumonia, cerebral calcifications, mental retardation, and seizures. Infection beyond the neonatal stage may result in failure to thrive, an infectious mononucleosis-like syndrome, or severe pulmonary infection (Meyers and Stool, 1968; Ward et al., 1965).

Rh Incompatibility

The condition is believed to involve the destruction of Rh positive blood cells of the fetus by maternal antibodies. Complications of Rh incompatibility account for about 3% of profound hearing loss among school age deaf children. Resulting pathology is known as erythroblastosis fetalis, or if the brain is affected, kernicterus. The causes of erythroblastosis fetalis and kernicterus are debatable (Matkin and Carhart, 1966, 1968). The disorder is commonly associated with Rh and other blood incompatibility, or may include drugs, neonatal sepsis, and enzyme abnormalities of either red blood cells or the liver.

Clinical symptoms develop during the immediate neonatal period, and include elevated bilirubin, jaundice, and brain damage. Most infants having kernicterus die during the first week with 80% of those surviving having complete or partial deafness. Other common residuals reported include cerebral palsy, mental retardation, epilepsy, aphasia, and behavioral disorders.

The cause of the associated hearing loss is still open to question. Reports are contradictory, indicating pathology in cochlear nuclei, cochlea, and/or central nervous system involvement. Audiometric findings typically show mild to profound sensorineural hearing loss characterized by a "cookie-bite" or "saucer-shaped" curve. Hearing loss is usually sensorineural and bilaterally symmetrical (Goodhill, 1967).

Acoustic Nerve Tumors

Tumors arising from the eighth nerve and extending into the cerebellar-pontine angle have been reported in children. Tumors in this area are usually neuromas originating from the vestibular portion of the eighth nerve. The hearing loss is usually unilateral, progressive sensorineural type and may be difficult to identify, especially in children. The ultimate diagnosis is made from the middle cranial fossa myelograms which outline the tumor with dye. Audiometric tests and vestibular procedures may contribute information to the ultimate diagnosis. Cases of acoustic tumors in children, although rather rare, have been presented by Craig et al. (1954), Bjorkesten (1957), Krause and McCabe (1971), and Anderson and Bentinck (1972). The total number of published cases of children with acoustic nerve tumors is approximately 10.

An interesting personal communication from Weaver (1972) relates the history of an acoustic tumor in a 9-year-old girl. This youngster was seen in a private otolaryngology office with a history of total hearing loss in the right ear for 3 months previously. Her hearing in the left ear was within normal limits and she reported having mumps 5 years previously. In addition, she had spasm of the facial muscles on the right side beginning some 8 months prior to the initial office visit.

Audiometry confirmed normal hearing in the left ear and total hearing loss in the right ear. With a Mueller speaking tube in the right ear and Bárány noisemaker in the left, she was able to repeat spondee (bysyllabic) words. An ice water caloric produced symmetrical reactions within normal limits.

An electronystagmogram showed diminished response in the right ear. Petrous pyramid polytomography showed widening of the right internal auditory meatus. A posterior fossa myelogram demonstrated a small acoustic neuroma which was successfully excised (Fig. 2.3). This youngster had been examined by other clinicians who felt that the unilateral hearing loss was probably related to the episode of mumps.

Medical Referral or Treatment

It is the audiologist's responsibility to insist that regular medical examinations be obtained for the hearing-impaired child. Until the child is 8 or 10 years of age, an otolaryngologic examination should be insisted upon every 6 months.

An erroneous assumption is that after a child has sustained a hearing loss, nothing more can happen to his ears. Not only is this belief incorrect, but there is some evidence suggesting that even sensorineural hearing impairment may be accompanied by increased susceptibility to other ear disease, to noise-induced loss, or to ototoxity (Falck, 1972). In addition, the demonstrated relationship of progressive sensorineural loss with otitis media poses a threat to the child who cannot afford to lose more hearing (Paparella and Brady, 1970; English et al., 1973). Therefore it is imperative that the hearing-impaired child be monitored more regularly than the normal hearing child. The importance of every dB of residual hearing that the child possesses may be in exponential ratio to each dB of hearing loss.

At the same time an otologic examination is made, a recheck audiologic evaluation should be done. Monitoring the degree of loss pays dividends in information on changes in hearing that are pertinent for the habilitation program. A change in hearing aids, or a revision of the gain-output-frequency response of the aid may be indicated. A more extensive otologic and physical examination may be suggested when deterioration of the auditory threshold or the speech discrimination is found.

The kinds of changes that should be watched for include the following:

Progression of the Sensorineural Hearing Level

Genetic deafness is known to be subject to deterioration, either gradual or rapid. An example of the progression of a recessive hereditary hearing loss is shown in Figure 2.4. The hearing first deteriorated slowly for 4 years, then very rapidly in a period of 2 months.

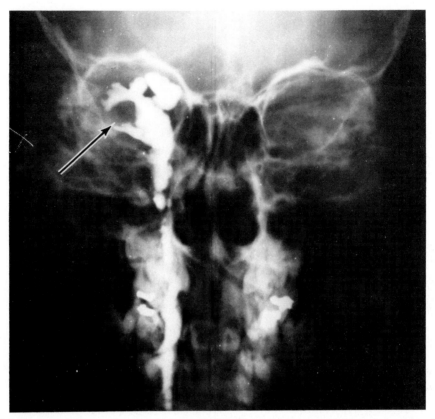

Fig. 2.3. Posterior fossa myelogram which clearly identifies a 7-mm acoustic tumor (arrow) in a 9-year-old patient. (Courtesy of Marlin Weaver, M.D., Denver, CO.)

Maternal rubella can also result in progressive hearing loss as seen by us in a child whose mother had had rubella. The child had normal hearing at birth and was tested at regular intervals until the age of 18 months, at which time she presented with a severe sensorineural loss. In two other children in our clinic this same early progression has been suspected, occurring in the first 8 months of life. Progression has also been seen by us to occur in an older rubella child who had a mild to moderate hearing loss that developed into profound deafness. Whether a persistence of the rubella virus in the cochlea is responsible for such progression, or whether it is due to another unknown factor is not presently understood.

Progression of the Air Conduction Hearing Level

It should not be necessary to point out that whenever a conductive loss appears, superimposed upon a sensorineural loss, immediate referral should be made to a physician. A problem arises in the case of profoundly deaf children whose bone conduction levels cannot be reached by the audiometer. The air conduction level may not change notably—the fragmentary responses could be tactile—and a conductive element may go unnoticed. For this reason it is always imperative that a tympanogram be obtained at every check-up of the child's hearing. Serious middle ear problems may be prevented by prompt referral of such patients to a physician's care.

Reports of Tinnitus, Dizziness, and Changes in the Quality of Sound

It has been confirmed in the older child, and suspected in the younger child, that symptoms resembling those of hydrops can occur with sudden onset. The child may complain of a ringing sound in one ear, which may or may not be accompanied by dizziness. It is often associated with reports of changes in the quality of the sound perceived in that ear. In one young adult case of rubella deafness, the ear in which the symptoms had appeared was no longer able to be used for amplification. The distortion of sound and the low tolerance level that developed prohibited the further use of that ear. This same youth several years later developed the same symptoms in the opposite ear. He was then immediately treated by an otolaryngologist on the basis of a hydrops diagnosis. The ear recovered and continues to receive good performance from amplification. Whether the treatment was responsible for the remission of symptoms, the case points up the urgency of making a medical referral immediately upon the report of such symptoms.

A 4-year-old child with a mild 30-dB sensorineural loss developed similar symptoms. He would stagger and would scream occasionally at the "loud sound in my ear." When brought to the clinic, his hearing loss had progressed to a 90- to 100-dB level. Medical treatment was immediately instituted, in the form of a stellate ganglion block. After a few weeks the symptoms had disappeared, but the hearing loss had only improved to a 70-dB level, where it remained permanently. The discrimination for speech continued to be remarkably good, considering the degree of loss. Again, it is a moot question whether the treatment was responsible for the remission and the small improvement of the hearing loss. Nonetheless, the physician is the person who must make the decision to treat or not to treat; the audiologist must get the patient to the physician for the diagnosis.

A case in which improvement occurred without treatment, but under an otolarynologist's care, demonstrated another bizarre symptom: a 14-year-old girl with only fragmentary hearing since birth appeared in the clinic suddenly unable to wear the hearing aid she had used successfully since 2 years of age. When the hearing aid was on, any sudden sound over 65 dB caused a Tullio phenomenon, a condition in which loud sounds cause giddiness, and possible nystagmus. This effect is presumably caused by a fistula leading into the inner ear, in the oval or round window. The physician's recommendation was to remove the hearing aid for a month, and to institute no treatment. After a month, the symptom subsided and the young girl was again able to

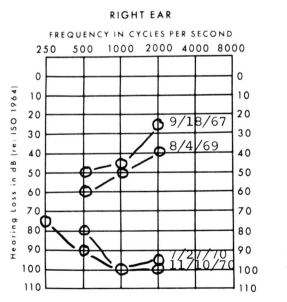
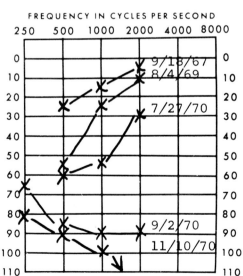

Fig. 2.4. Audiogram of a patient with documented progressive bilateral sensorineural hearing loss. This child had normal hearing by observation of responses from birth to age 2½ years.

tolerate the aid.

Whether the physician elects to give treatment, a child presenting with any unusual symptoms should be referred to a physician without delay. Serious ear disease such as cholesteatoma or eighth nerve tumor must always be ruled out through the physician's diagnosis. The audiologist is responsible for the child's receiving the proper kind of health care for his ears.

Genetics

Humans take great pride in identifying distinguishing traits from one generation to the next. We enjoy speculating on the resemblance of children to their parents, and question which child has its father's eyebrows or its mother's chin. With such observations begins the study of genetics and the submicroscopic structures known as genes.

Genes are found in the nuclei of the many cells which compose our body. Genes are concerned with the determination of what an individual's characteristics shall be, and they form the hereditary link between one generation and the next. The characteristics of an offspring are, to a large degree, determined by the genes he receives from his parents—from his mother through the ovum, or egg, and from his father through the sperm cell that fertilized that ovum at the time of conception. Genetic factors present at conception are largely unaltered throughout life. The genes are contained in chromosomes which occur in pairs. One member of each chromosome pair is inherited from the father, the other chromosome member is inherited from the mother.

The clinician concerned with hearing disorders should have some basic knowledge of genetics in hereditary inheritance. There is probably some genetic component in almost all disease processes, but the extent of this component varies. Some diseases are almost entirely determined by an individual's genetic constitution such as Down's syndrome, achondroplasia, and other individually rare conditions (Carter, 1969). The incidence of congenital abnormalities, serious disorders, or gross malformations has been estimated from 1% to 3% or as high as 5% of all births. This incidence

figure grows higher if the affected individual is followed into adult life.

The following presentation will include basic information concerning chromosomes and chromosome defects, patterns of inheritance, the genetics of deafness, and genetic counseling. Our goal is to acquaint the clinician who has had little or no formal course work in genetics with the fundamentals of this important aspect of life which contributes to many of the cases of deafness we see commonly in the patient population. We are greatly indebted to Janet Stewart, M.D. (1973), of the University of Colorado Birth Defects Clinic and Pediatric Department, for permission to use her previously published materials on genetic counseling as the basis of the following discussion.

Chromosomes and Chromosomal Defects

All hereditary material, in the form of deoxyribonucleic acid (DNA) is carried as genes on the chromosomes. All human body cells contain 23 pairs of chromosomes or 46 total chromosomes. Twenty-two of these pairs are known as autosomes; the remaining two chromosomes are called the sex chromosomes, two X chromosomes constituting a female (written as 46,XX in genetic nomenclature) and one X and one Y constituting a male (46,XY). The reproduction process of the body (or somite) cells is known as mitosis, while the reproduction of the germ (or sex) cells is called meiosis.

During the process of mitosis, each chromosome becomes shortened and thickened, and splits longitudinally into two chromatids joined at the point called the centromere. This is the form in which most chromosomes are pictured. They are then aligned and split longitudinally through the centromere, separating the two chromatids which then migrate to opposite ends of the cell. Cleavage then occurs in the cell to produce two genetically similar cells. Mitosis is an elegant, yet simple, mechanism for the replication of body cells (Fig. 2.5).

Man, like all forms of life, must reproduce if his species is to continue. An essential factor in the reproductive process is the formation of additional sperm and eggs by a special type of cell division (meiosis) which involves only the germ cells as shown in Figure 2.6.

In this process the chromosomes again shorten and thicken and split into two chromatids joined at the centromere as described in mitosis. Matching pairs are arranged together and at this time material may be exchanged between paired chromosomes. The paired chromosomes then separate (known as dysjunction) and move to opposite poles of the cell, forming two cells now with 23 chromosomes each (known as the haploid number). Each cell contains either an X or a Y. The next step in the process is simple mitotic division in which there is a longitudinal split at the centromere and migration of the chromatids to opposite poles. In this manner new ova and new sperm are formed, each with 23 chromosomes. At some future time of fertilization, one ovum and one sperm will unite to form a cell, known as the zygote, with a full 46 chromosome constitution.

Abnormalities may occur during meiotic or mitotic division, producing an individual with a chromosomal defect. These abnormalities may involve one of the autosomes or one of the sex chromosomes and consists of either too much or too little total chromosome material. In

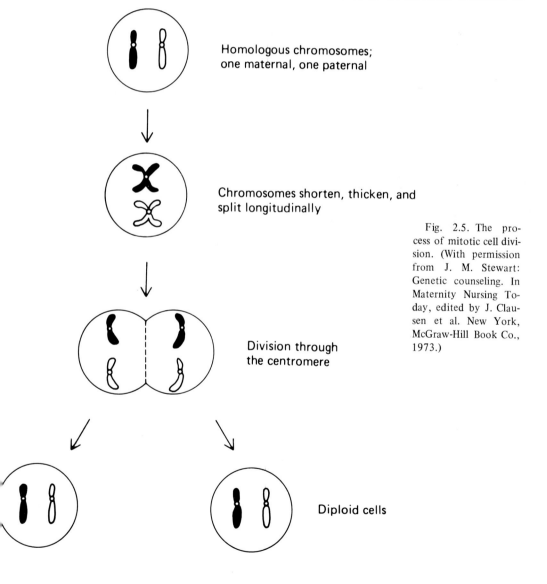

Homologous chromosomes; one maternal, one paternal

Chromosomes shorten, thicken, and split longitudinally

Division through the centromere

Diploid cells

Fig. 2.5. The process of mitotic cell division. (With permission from J. M. Stewart: Genetic counseling. In Maternity Nursing Today, edited by J. Clausen et al. New York, McGraw-Hill Book Co., 1973.)

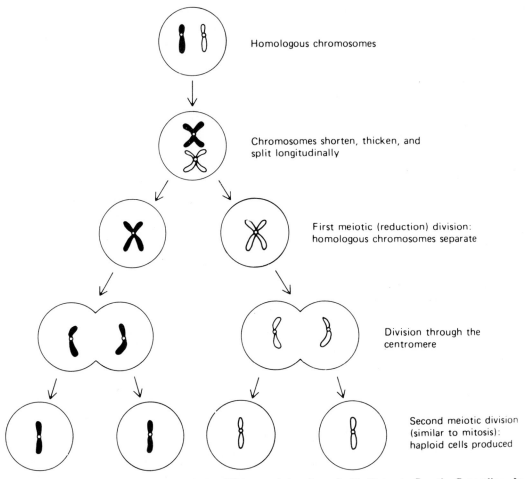

Homologous chromosomes

Chromosomes shorten, thicken, and split longitudinally

First meiotic (reduction) division: homologous chromosomes separate

Division through the centromere

Second meiotic division (similar to mitosis): haploid cells produced

Fig. 2.6. Germ cell division, or meiosis. (With permission from J. M. Stewart: Genetic Counseling. In Maternity Nursing Today, edited by J. Clausen et al. New York, McGraw-Hill Book Co., 1973.)

certain types of tissue, and under certain conditions, chromosomes are readily visible under high magnification. A photographic record of chromosomal constitution of a cell is called a karyotype (Figs. 2.7 and 2.8). The human karyotype is often described in terms of "Denver system," so-called because it was formulated at a meeting of cytologists in Denver, Colorado (Crispens, 1971). In the human karyotype the pairs of somatic chromosomes (autosomes) are identified by number (1 to 22) as nearly as possible in descending order of their length, and also divided into seven groups (usually designated as group A through group G). Each group is composed of chromosome pairs with similar morphologic features.

The sex chromosomes are identified by the symbols X and Y.

The most common autosomal defect is known as Down's syndrome, or mongolism. The affected individual has an extra number 21 chromosome (trisomy 21) for a total of 47 chromosomes. The clinical features of Down's syndrome are described in our "Index of Audiologic Disorders," Chapter 9. Down's syndrome can also occur in another form. An occasional child with Down's syndrome will have only 46 chromosomes, including one large abnormal chromosome which consists of the translocation of the extra 21 to another chromosome. Clinically, the child with the translocation type of Down's syndrome is indistinguishable from the child with the more common form, trisomy 21.

Hearing loss may also occur with trisomy 13 and trisomy 18, as described more fully in the "Index of Audiologic Disorders." These children usually have many severe abnormalities and rarely live beyond a few months of age. The total absence of an autosome is felt to be incompatible with life, although a few exceptions have been reported. For example, a deletion of the short arm of chromosome 5 results in severe mental retardation and a cat-like cry in infancy, comprising the cri du chat syndrome.

Unlike the loss of autosomal material, an individual may lose one of the sex chromosomes with surprisingly little defect. Sex chromosome defects do cause disorders usually less severe than autosomal defects, such as Turner's syndrome and Klinefelter's syndrome. About 1% of inmates of institutions for the retarded have sex chromosome anomalies (Robinson, 1972).

Patterns of Inheritance

The chromosomal defects that have been described above are all grossly obvious in a standard karyotype. Defects involving single genes, however, are much more discreet and invisible by any currently used technique. The determination of the hereditary nature of an abnormality is done primarily by the careful study of an individual's family.

Genes occur in pairs and are located on homologous chromosomes. One gene is maternal in origin and the other paternal. If the two genes have the same effect, the individual is said to be "homozygous" for the gene. If the effect is different, he is said to be "heterozygous" for the gene. The expression of each gene factor depends on its interaction with other genes and the environment. Genetic defects can be inherited in three well known ways and in a fourth less well understood, but commonly occurring, manner.

Autosomal Dominant

A condition or trait is said to be dominantly inherited if it is manifest in the heterozygous state. This is a type of inheritance with an affected individual having a 50% chance of passing the gene on to each of his offspring.

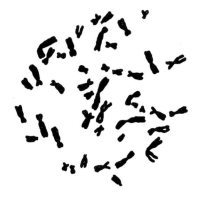

Fig. 2.7. Human male karyotype with normal chromosomes. (Courtesy of A. Robinson, M.D., Cytogenetics Laboratory, University of Colorado Medical Center.)

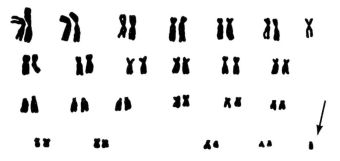

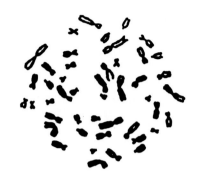

Fig. 2.8. Human female karyotype with normal chromosomes. (Courtesy of A. Robinson, M.D., Cytogenetics Laboratory, University of Colorado Medical Center.)

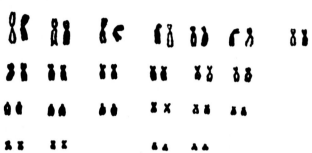

Every afflicted individual will have a similarly afflicted parent. An unaffected individual in most cases does not carry the abnormal gene, and all of his offspring will be normal. Dominantly inherited traits have several distinguishing characteristics. They are usually milder, since the gene is passed on by the affected individual who is capable of reproduction. There is much variation in the clinical manifestations of a dominant gene, which is known as "variation in expressivity." In other words, a few individuals are so very severely affected, while those at the other end of the spectrum may be so mildly affected that they have no obvious clinical manifestation of the gene problem. If this occurs, a gene is said to have "decreased penetrance." On occasion, a dominant trait will seem to appear as a spontaneous gene mutation. The parents of such a child are not at an increased risk for future pregnancies, although the affected individual himself would have a 50% chance of passing the trait on to his offspring.

Autosomal Recessive

A condition is said to be recessively inherited if it is manifest only when the individual is homozygous for the defective gene. This is a type of inheritance in which the carrier parents may often be asymptomatic with a 25% chance of producing an affected child. One half of their children will be carriers, like themselves, and 25% will be genetically normal. In many cases, recessive conditions are more severe than dominant conditions, as the abnormality is passed on by the asymptomatic carrier and the affected person need not reproduce. If a particularly recessive condition is rare, there is an increased incidence of consanguinity in the parents. Consanguinity, which refers to a marriage of parents with recent common ancestors, such as cousins, uncle-niece marriages, etc., has genetic significance in that there is a greatly increased chance that two parents who have a recent common ancestor may each have the same recessive gene inherited from that common ancestor. Each partner, then, could give a child this gene, so that it would possess two such genes and be homozygous for the abnormal gene (Brown, 1967). The pattern of this type of inheritance shows a cluster of affected individuals among brothers and sisters, with normal parents. It is not possible to identify such families in the general population until they have produced affected children. An example of an autosomal recessive disorder is Pendred's syndrome, a condition characterized by hearing loss and a goiter which appears in adolescence. Both parents in some circumstances might have normal hearing with no other family history of deafness.

Sex-linked

If the gene for a particular trait or abnormality is located on the X chromosome, the condition is said to be inherited in an X-linked or sex-linked manner. The condition then is X-linked recessive if it is manifest only in the male who is homozygous—that is, the abnormal gene on the single X chromosome is genetically unopposed. The female who has a normal gene on one X chromosome and an abnormal gene on the other is a carrier and usually asymptomatic. The carrier female passes the gene on to 50% of her sons who then manifest the abnormality, and 50% of her daughters who are also carriers but who will not manifest the abnormality. The cardinal feature of an X-linked trait is the lack of male-to-male transmission, since the male may only pass on his Y chromosome to his sons. The pattern of father-daughter alternation is characteristic because affected fathers have only one X chromosome, so they must pass the gene to their daughters, and none of their sons, who get the father's Y chromosome and the mother's X chromosome. Sex-linked inheritance patterns have been familiar since Biblical times when it was noted that hemophilia as well as color blindness seemed to be passed from unaffected females to males (Brown, 1967).

Polygenic

Many of the more common congenital abnormalities, such as cleft lip, cleft palate, and spina bifida are not inherited in one of the manners described above, and yet it is well known that these defects cluster in families. It has been postulated that multiple genes contribute to these defects and that each individual has a threshold above which the abnormality will be manifest. This condition is known as polygenic inheritance. The more severe the defect, the more the predisposing genes must present. Unlike single gene defects, the recurrence risk varies with the number of affected persons in the family.

Genetic Counseling

Genetic counseling is often given to parents who have had one abnormal child and who are interested in knowing the potential for having additional children with the same defect. Genetic counseling may also be offered to siblings of an abnormal individual and to the affected person himself as he approaches marriage age and possible parenthood. Genetic evaluation and counseling may be done effectively in many places by a variety of persons and is based on the absolutely imperative indication that the diagnosis of the individual is correct. Therefore, a referral to a genetic center is often advisable where various medical specialties are available to insure accurate diagnoses.

The steps of the genetic counseling vary with the complexity of the problem, but include a careful family, pregnancy, birth, and infancy history to find factors which might explain the abnormality, careful physical examination of the affected individual and other family members, and necessary laboratory work as required (Stewart, 1973). When the evaluation has been completed and the diagnosis reached, the parents return for the actual counseling sessions. Both parents are generally required to attend and the counseling is done in an unhurried and relaxed atmosphere. They are given the final diagnosis and the risk figures for future pregnancies. When possible an attempt is made by the genetic counselors to minimize guilt; however, in situations in which one parent is obviously the carrier of the gene causing the defect, it may be better to acknowledge the guilt and help the parent deal with it. In many instances more than one counseling session is necessary. There is good evidence that parents who seek genetic advice will usually make appropriate and expected decisions about future children.

The field of genetics is old yet it is filled with new discoveries. Only in 1956 were man's chromosomes accurately counted, and in 1959 the first chromosomal abnormality—the trisomy 21 associated with Down's syndrome—was accurately described. Progress has been rapid, however, in the last 15 years, and many of the new techniques are of practical significance in terms of genetic counseling. Since 1963, it has been possible to aspirate amniotic fluid from the uterus late in pregnancy to predict the involvement of an infant with an Rh incompatibility. More recently, amniotic fluid has been aspirated from the uterus earlier in pregnancy to diagnose a variety of chromosomal and metabolic disorders. This process is known as amniocentesis and is accomplished routinely under specific circumstances in large medical centers. Amniocentesis can identify several abnormalities in utero, including Hurler's and Hunter's syndromes (Stewart, 1973).

The diagrammatic construction of a family pedigree, which is a representation of the family medical history used to determine if the etiology of a disease is indeed familial, is helpful to indicate modes of inheritance. The pedigree may provide evidence to establish whether a trait carried by a single gene is dominant, recessive, or sex-linked. Simple pedigrees showing classic types of single gene inheritance are presented in Figure 2.9.

Hereditary Deafness

According to Proctor and Proctor (1967) hereditary deafness is a fairly common disease entity, occurring somewhere between 1 in 2000 and 1 in 6000 live births. We use the term "hereditary deafness" rather than "congenital deafness" in this section because we are referring to children with profound, irreversible, bilateral sensorineural hearing loss of early onset. Congenital deafness would include those children with conductive hearing loss due to osseous malformation in the middle ear. Such a condition usually creates a moderate hearing loss, often amenable to surgical intervention, and thus quite a different group of children from those we describe with hereditary childhood deafness (Fraser, 1971). Hereditary deafness is usually a bilateral disease entity (Kinney,

1950). Everberg (1960), researched nearly 200,000 school children in Copenhagen to conclude that hereditary factors were of importance in only 10%, or 12 cases of 122 patients with unilateral deafness. In studying a child with apparent congenital severe deafness, the clinician must be aware of possible exogenous, or outside, factors that can cause childhood deafness as summarized in Table 2.1.

A high percentage of congenital deafness is hereditary, according to Fraser et al. (1964) and Konigsmark (1972). About 40% of profound childhood deafness is autosomal recessive in origin; 10%, dominant transmission; and some 3%, due to a sex-linked gene. Since deaf persons tend to marry other deaf persons (Schein, 1965; Northern et al., 1971), statistics regarding their potential for producing deaf offspring are of interest. According to Bergstrom et al. (1971), the marriage of two deaf persons gives only a slightly increased risk of deafness in their children because there is small chance that two such persons would be affected by the same exact genetic deafness. Should the same recessive gene be carried by two normal hearing parents, theoretically one-fourth of their offspring would be affected and one-half of their children would be carriers. However, if both parents are overtly affected by the same recessive type of hereditary deafness, they are homozygous for the trait and therefore *all* their children will not only be affected but also capable of passing the trait on to some of their offspring in turn.

Several modern population studies of deafness have been conducted with rather large samples, and the results have been concisely summarized by Brown (1967) and are presented in Table 2.2. These studies represent data from Northern Ireland (Stevenson and Cheesman, 1956), Japan (Furusho, 1957), England (Fraser et al., 1964), Clarke School for the Deaf in the United States (Brown and Chung, 1964), and Germany (Kittel and Schmoll-Eskuche, 1963). Acquired deafness, for the purposes of Table 2.2, is defined as those individuals in whom a prenatal or postnatal environmental factor has been claimed as a cause of deafness. One must be impressed at the close relationship of population percentages, across these studies, of deaf

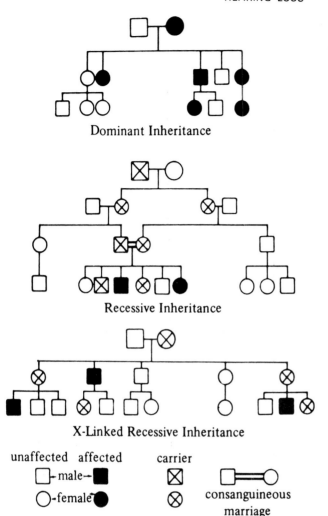

Dominant Inheritance

Recessive Inheritance

X-Linked Recessive Inheritance

unaffected affected   carrier

☐-male→■   ⊠

◯-female→●   ⊗   consanguineous
                          marriage

Fig. 2.9. Family pedigrees showing simple inheritance patterns of single gene factors. (With permission from A. Robinson: Genetic and chromosomal disorders. In Current Pediatric Diagnosis and Treatment, edited by C. H. Kempe et al. Los Altos, CA, Lange Medical Publications, 1972.)

individuals with hereditary and acquired deafness.

Another means of identifying the causes of deafness has been accomplished by interviewing large samples of adult deaf persons. The adult deaf, however, are unfortunately poorly informed regarding the cause of their hearing problems. Such analyses are usually obtained through a written questionnaire or personal interview, but in this type of population in which language and communication are problems, such information-gathering techniques suggest caution in data interpretation. We are reminded of the deaf father who told us that he lost his hearing between the ages of 1 and 2. His parents told him that he had cut his finger badly, and the doctor had stitched up the cut without use of anesthesia. The pain was apparently so severe, that his loud crying damaged his hearing. This story from a totally deaf man married to a deaf woman, the parents of three deaf children! A summary of results from two studies of deaf adults who were asked the cause of their hearing loss (Schein, 1965; Northern et al., 1971) is shown in Table 2.3.

Despite the large number of syndromes associated with dominant deafness, the great majority of human inherited deafness (about 90%) is of a recessive rather than dominant type (Proctor and Proctor, 1967). In the case of

Table 2.1. Summary of Known Exogenous Causes of Prelingual Deafness*

Preconception and prenatal causes
  Rubella
  Cytomegalovirus
  Ototoxic and other drugs, maternal alcoholism
  Hypoxia (and its possible causes: high altitude,
    general anesthetic, severe hemorrhage)
  Syphilis
  Toxemia, diabetes, other severe systemic
    maternal illness
  Parental irradiation
  Toxoplasmosis
Perinatal causes
  Hypoxia
  Traumatic delivery
  Maternal infection
  Ototoxic drugs
  Premature delivery
Neonatal and postnatal causes
  Hypoxia
  Infection
  Ototoxic drugs
  Erythroblastosis fetalis
  Infantile measles or mumps
  Otitis media (acute, chronic, serous)
  Noise-induced
  Meningitis
  Encephalitis

* With permission from L. Bergstrom, W. G. Hemenway, and M. P. Downs: A high risk registry to find congenital deafness. Otolaryngol. Clin. North Am. 4: 369-399, 1971.

Table 2.2. Ratio of Childhood Deafness from Several Population Studies*

	No. in Sample	Hereditary Deafness	Acquired Deafness
Northern Ireland	424	.513	
Japan	1561	.502	
England	2355	.517	.578
Clarke School, USA	1222	.512	.544
Germany	2788	.532	.606

* Modified with permission from K. S. Brown: The genetics of childhood deafness. In F. McConnell and P. H. Ward (Eds.), Deafness in Childhood, pp. 177-202. Nashville, Vanderbilt University Press, 1967.

recessively inherited deafness, both parents must be the carriers of the particular gene, in which event the chance of offspring being affected is only 25%. Most of these patients have no family history of deafness, thereby making the case for hereditary etiology difficult to prove.

Embryology of Hereditary Deafness

Proctor and Proctor (1967) present a very interesting discussion regarding the basic development of the sensory cells of the inner ear. Basic research in the early 1900's established the fact that the acoustic ganglion and sensory neuroepithelium were capable of complete differentiation even when the embryonic neural crest was removed. The acoustic ganglion was unique among all other cranial nerve ganglia, being the only nerve ganglion that did not develop directly from the central nervous system or neural crest.

Proctor and Lawrence (1959) established that the acoustic ganglion does indeed arise from the otic vesicle neuroepithelium. Soon after the ganglion cells have formed from the wall of the otic vesicle, innervation of the future sensory hair cells is established. After the connections are well accomplished between the auditory ganglia and sensory hair cells, the auditory ganglia migrate away from the otic vesicle.

With this sequence of embryonic events in mind, if genetic or toxic disturbances are exerted before the fifth week prior to the

Table 2.3. Etiology of Hearing Loss as Expressed by Manually Communicating Deaf Adults

	Percentage	
Etiology	Northern et al. (1971)	Schein (1965)
Unknown	35.8%	32.2%
Congenital	25.5%	10.5%
Meningitis	13.1%	12.7%
Scarlet fever	9.5%	4.6%
Result of a fall	8.1%	7.7%
Whooping cough	3.6%	2.3%
Measles	2.2%	3.4%
Pneumonia		2.3%
Mastoiditis		1.9%
Other	2.2%	16.7%
N =	137	1132

development of the auditory ganglion from the otic vesicle, one could expect damage to the entire vestibuloauditory complex, yet this clinical finding is rather rare. If the genetic or toxic effect were early and sufficiently severe to affect the self-differentiated cells of the auditory system, one would expect many developmental anomalies in other parts of the body.

In general, however, histologic examination of the temporal bone structures in cases of hereditary deafness, reveal that most such cases usually show affected hair cells, organ of Corti, and stria vascularis, with the auditory ganglion and auditory nerve affected to a much lesser degree. Phylogenetically, it may be recalled that the vestibular system was developed much earlier than the auditory system and is therefore more resistant to genetic defect. This view is supported by the fact that most patients with hereditary deafness have intact and functional vestibular systems.

According to the hypotheses of Proctor and Proctor, the lack of damage to the auditory nerve and ganglion cells demonstrates that the general causes of genetic deafness must occur after the ganglion and nerve have formed and migrated away from the otic vesicle. In view of this logic, the Proctors conclude that genetic defects probably occur from inherent biochemical influences in the labyrinthine fluids.

Obviously not all inherited deafness is due to biochemical defects. In Paget's disease, the internal auditory meatus is stenosed by the over-growth of bone; deafness in Von Recklinghausen's syndrome is due to neurofibromas on the auditory nerves; Pendred's deafness and goiter are due to endocrine abnormality related to the faulty metabolism of iodine. Yet, many other syndromes, often combined with mental retardation, are accompanied by metabolic dysfunction, including Hurler's, Herrmann's, and Refsum's syndromes.

With such basic knowledge and understanding of the possible causes of hereditary deafness, it seems likely that some forms of genetic deafness may some day be preventable. Such has been the case with other hereditary disease such as diabetes mellitus. The prevention of hereditary nerve deafness, however, will require more research into the genetic, physiologic, embryologic, and biochemical processes of the auditory mechanism.

Congenital Malformations

Congenital Malformations of the Inner Ear

Although wide variety exists in anatomic abnormalities of the inner ear, four classic types exist. These include (a) Michel, complete failure of development of the inner ear; (b) Mondini, incomplete development and malformation of the inner ear; (c) the Scheibe membranous cochleosaccular degeneration of the inner ear; and (d) the Alexander malformation of the cochlear membranous system. A Bing-Siebenmann classification has been suggested by Omerod (1960).

The Bing-Siebenmann anomaly is characterized by a normal bony capsule with malformed membranous components of the cochlea and vestibular mechanism. It has been reported in patients with mental retardation and retinitis pigmentosa. In terms of severity of aplasia, the Bing-Siebenmann deformity would be classified between the Mondini and Scheibe aplasias. These cases generally show profound hearing loss. These four inner ear anomalies have been described by many authors, including notable publications by Schuknecht (1967), Lindsay (1971a, b), and Hemenway and Bergstrom (1972). The question exists whether these malformations are due to embryonic developmental arrest, since in some instances the pathology does not represent any embryonic stage in development of the ear.

Aplasia of the inner ear implies failure of the ear to reach full development. Accordingly, inner ear aplasia is always a congenital malformation. The embryonic time of developmental failure, of course, determines the ultimate structure and appearance of the deformity. According to Schuknecht (1967), an individual may possess different degrees of aplasia in the two ears. Aplasia of the inner ear is a relatively uncommon aberration.

Michel-Type of Aplasia of the Inner Ear. The macroscopic description of this temporal bone anomaly was first described by Michel in 1863. This type of anomaly is represented by a complete absence of the inner ear and auditory nerve. The outer ear may be completely normal with a narrow middle ear cavity. The malleus and incus may be present, but the stapes and stapedius muscle may be absent or abnormal. Maternal thalidomide during pregnancy has been associated with this anomaly, and it has been observed in at least one case of Klippel-Feil deformity (McLay and Marar, 1969).

Mondini Aplasia of the Inner Ear. Mondini described a temporal bone in 1791 that showed incomplete development of a flattened cochlea which consisted of only a single basal coil. In 1904 Alexander added more detail to this type of anomaly indicating involvement of auditory nerve and the vestibular canals. Characteristic of this anomaly is that it involves both the bony capsule and membranous labyrinth. This anomaly, which often bears both investigators' names, has been associated with Klippel-Feil and Wildervanck syndromes. It has also been found in cases of mental retardation, hydrocephalus, and hydronephrosis. Middle ear anomalies may be present in these cases and

atresia of the external canal has also been reported. A temporal bone section demonstrating the Mondini-type aplasia is shown in Figure 2.10.

Scheibe Aplasia of the Inner Ear. The Scheibe abnormality of the inner ear, originally described in 1892, is characterized by involvement of only the membranous portion of the cochlea and saccule. This type of dysplasia is the most common of the inner ear aplasias. Histopathology of these inner ears show atrophy of the stria vascularis, degeneration of the organ of Corti, and rolling up of the tectorial membrane, especially in the basal turn of the cochlea. This anomaly has been identified in cases of Waardenburg's syndrome, the cardioauditory syndrome of Jervell and Lange-Nielsen, Usher's syndrome, Refsum's syndrome, and maternal rubella.

Knowledge of these inner ear anomalies are important for accurate diagnosis, proper treatment of the patient, and genetic counseling for the parents of the handicapped child, as well as for the patient when he (or she) is old enough

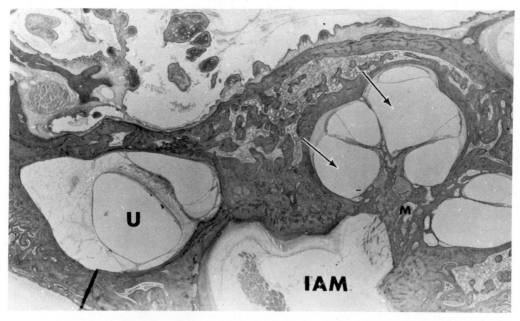

Fig. 2.10. Mondini-type of incomplete development with malformation of the inner ear from a patient with trisomy 13-15 syndrome. Note incompletely developed cochlea with absence of the interscalar osseus septum (arrows), and poorly developed modiolus (M). Utricle (U) and internal auditory meatus (IAM) are also identified. (With permission from I. Sando, B. Baker, F. O. Black, and W. G. Hemenway: Persistence of stapedial artery in trisomy 13-15 syndrome. Arch. Otolaryngol. 96: 441-447, 1972.)

to become a parent. Therefore, differentiation of the above inner ear problems is crucial in the determination of whether the hearing loss in question is of a genetic or an acquired origin.

The degree of abnormal development that is actually involved in any specific patient may vary considerably from other patients with similar inner ear malformations. Diagnostic considerations must include petrous pyramid polytomography of the inner ear, as well as a complete evaluation of the hearing impairment. Malformations in the bone of the otic capsule can be detected by careful x-ray, and differential diagnosis of the Michel and Mondini aplasias are possible. Some of the membranous labyrinth malfunctions may be inferred from audiometric and/or vestibular testing.

Knowledge regarding the residual hearing in children with inner ear anomalies may be of great value in the habilitation of the child so deafened. According to Black et al. (1971), audiometric patterns in the Michel ear should show no hearing since no true inner ear exists. True hearing is impossible and a hearing aid for such a patient can be of limited value. It is theoretically possible for the Mondini malformed inner ear to have some hearing, since the basal coil of the cochlea may be present with intact higher auditory pathways. The Scheibe ear may show residual hearing in the low frequencies, since in this ear the major damage is in the basal coil of the cochlea. The extent of hearing in the Bing-Siebenmann inner ear is dependent upon the area and degree of malformation present in the membranous portion of the cochlea. The Scheibe and Mondini malformations may be unilateral. Black et al. state that asymmetry of malformation is not uncommon, and the patient may demonstrate one type of inner ear anomaly on one side, and another type of inner ear anomaly on the other side. In such cases, x-ray findings and the degree or pattern of the hearing loss may be quite unlike each other.

More information is needed regarding the presence of these inner ear malformations. As of now, the risk of occurrence and the ratio of male-female incidence has not yet been securely determined. The bony inner ear dysplasias may be diagnosed soon after birth by x-ray, but the membranous labyrinth malformations must be inferred or postponed until the temporal bones can be examined. If the defect is an isolated defect, the individual may live a full life as a hard-of-hearing or deaf person. However, these inner ear defects may be associated with other limiting disorders.

Congenital Middle Ear Malformations

Interest in middle ear anomalies has increased with the advent of microscopic surgical techniques and improved diagnostic capabilities of clinicians. Many patients with abnormal middle ears can have the deformity corrected by surgery. Since the middle ear is largely formed during the first trimester of fetal life, gross developmental anomalies of the middle ear are often related to factors that influence the fetus during that time. An excellent description of middle ear anomalies has been presented by Sando and Wood (1971) and Nager (1971).

Malformation of the middle ear may be due to hereditary factors or to disturbances during embryonic development. Failure in the proper development of the first and second branchial arches may result in the absence of the ossicles or a fusion of the ossicles. A malformation of the stapes footplate, however, is related to the development of the otic capsule. A disturbance in the fetal growth of the first branchial pouch may affect the eustachian tube, middle ear cavity, as well as the ultimate pneumatization of the mastoid air spaces.

Isolated anomalies of the middle ear ossicles are not particularly rare. Malleus anomalies include fixation or deformation of the malleus head and bony fusion of the incudomalleolar joint or absence of the malleus. Incus deficiencies may exist in isolation or in conjunction with other middle ear ossicular problems and range from total absence to a deficiency of the lenticular process. The incus may have only a fibrous connection to the malleus or be fused to the lateral semicircular canal wall. Stapes anomalies may involve fusion of the stapes head to the promontory, absence of the head and/or crura, the absence of the entire stapes itself, or the presence of a columellar ossicle. Congenital absence of the oval window or the round window may also exist as a unilateral or bilateral defect.

Middle ear anomalies should be suspected whenever other branchial arch anomalies are observed and are often noted as part of congenital syndromes. Branchial arch disorders include atresia of the external auditory canal, cleft palate, micrognathia, Pierre Robin syndrome, Treacher Collins syndrome, as well as low set auricles. Disorders which feature other skeletal defects may also include middle ear anomalies such as Apert's syndrome, Klippel-Feil syndrome, Crouzon's, Paget's, and van der Hoeve's diseases. Middle ear anomalies have been reported in disorders of connective tissue such as gargolism or Hunter-Hurler syndromes, Möbius syndrome, and dwarfism.

Congenital rubella often creates sensorineural hearing loss with middle ear anomalies as well. Congenital syphilis may also cause middle ear deformations. Maternal thalidomide creates ear anomalies in 20% of the children born. Fortunately, thalidomide was never a major drug in the United States and is now, of course, no longer available for clinical use.

Sando and Wood (1971) offer the following diagnostic clues and suggestions to identify a patient with possible middle ear anomalies:

A. Routine audiometry may, or may not, show conductive hearing loss. Often the middle ear anomaly accompanies profound sensorineural hearing loss so bone conduction audiometry may not be of value. The acoustic impedance test, however, may identify abnormal middle ear systems but will not necessarily reveal the exact nature of the anomaly. The impedance measurement is of value in differentiating ossicular fixation from ossicular discontinuity, and is very valuable in the audiometric assessment of suspect children.

B. Family history of congenital malformations is very important. The clinician should take a careful patient history-taking note of other family members with evidence of hearing loss.

C. Positive maternal history of infectious disease, drug ingestion or ionizing irradiation during pregnancy is important.

D. History of nonprogressive, long standing, unilateral or bilateral conductive hearing loss, present since birth, suggests middle ear ossicular malformation.

E. The presence of other congenital anomalies including branchial arch malformations, skeletal anomalies, or other facial features that may or may not be part of an identifiable syndrome should alert the clinician to suspect a middle ear anomaly.

Malformations of the External Ear and Canal

The auricle develops around the first branchial groove as six knob-like protrusions early in embryonic life. These six hillocks soon lose their identity as they coalesce to form the pinna. With six separate growth centers developing at differing rates, it is not surprising that a wide variation exists in final ear configurations that are within normal limits. The shape of the auricle is so different among individuals that European police forces utilize the configuration of the ear much like American police use fingerprints.

Defects of the external ear and canal may be apparent without damage to the middle or inner ear structures. However, severe middle ear anomalies or aplasia of the middle ear may be associated. Supernumerary hillocks, known as "tags" or preauricular appendages, may remain with an otherwise normal-appearing pinna. However, the presence of tags may suggest anomalies of the external and middle ear systems. In cases of the atretic ear canal, occasionally thick soft tissue is found at surgery where the tympanic membrane should be, or more often a bony atresia plate of varying degrees of thickness is present.

External ear and canal anomalies may be visible at birth, but are often overlooked and the defect is not noted until hearing loss is suspected or discovered. Sometimes the auricle and the opening to the external auditory meatus appear normal, but the meatus may funnel down to complete closure lateral to the tympanic membrane. If the atresia is bilateral, the child should be fitted with a bone conduction hearing aid as soon as possible. If the atresia is unilateral and normal hearing can be established in the opposite ear, treatment or habilitation is generally deferred. Aural atresias may accompany other defects of the cranium, face, skeleton, or mandible. The etiology of the aural atresia may be a chromosomal aberration, heredity, maternal thalidomide, or maternal rubella. Nager (1971) and Linthicum (1971) discussed procedures in problems in the surgical intervention for congenital aural atresia and middle ear ossicular anomalies.

Anomalies of the external ear suggest associated middle ear anomalies. Clinicians should be alerted to identify the malformed pinna during initial observations of children as this clue may lead to identification of associated hearing loss.

The Microtic Ear. The microtic ear has always been a problem to professionals as well as to the unfortunate possessor. Fortunately, it occurs only once in 20,000 births (Holmes, 1949), but this is often enough that we see a number of such cases each year in our clinic. The congenitally microtic ear varies from the mildly deformed ear to the conditions of total absence of pinna with no external auditory meatus, or complete atresia of the canal. Unilateral microtia is about six times more frequent than bilateral occurrence (Dupertius and Musgrave, 1959), is more common in males than females, and is found predominantly on the right side (Brown et al., 1969).

In 1971 the Hearing and Speech Services Program of the Colorado State Health Department had 48 registered children with unilateral or bilateral congenital microtia. The statistics of this group fit very well with the reports summarized above. The Colorado records show that unilateral microtia is about four times more prevalent than bilateral microtia, with 35 males and 13 females registered with this problem. Microtia of the right ear has occurred in 27 cases, left ear only 10 cases, and bilateral microtia exists in 11 registered Colorado children.

When a patient has one normal-hearing ear, obviously the problem of unilateral microtia is not so bad. When hair styles are long, the deformity of the auricle is easily covered. Patients, however, who wish to do something about the microtia have a choice between attempted surgical improvement or the use of a prosthetic-type pinna which is attached to the side of the head by special adhesive material. According to Holmes (1949), and supported by our observations, is the statement that regardless of what surgical techniques are employed, the reconstructed ear can never take the place of a normally developed pinna, and the result will never be inconspicuous. For improved hearing benefit, however, as in the patient who has bilaterally stenosed ear canals, surgical intervention may be successful. Schuchman (1971) has reported the fitting of a special ear level, bone conduction hearing aid for a patient with bilateral atresia.

Team Management of Children with Hearing Impairment

The nature of modern-day hearing losses makes it increasingly imperative that a team of professional people work together to diagnose a hearing loss and chart the management of the child with a loss (Fig. 2.11). The hearing function is not an isolated phenomenon. It lies in an ear which is connected to a brain and a living body, all of which are vital to the development of the child. Medicine is today preserving the lives of children who have multiple problems associated with deafness, and who would not have survived in another age. Whatever the condition, only specialists in the various aspects of the child's health and welfare can put together the total picture of the child's problems and their solution.

We have called such a group of experts the Congenital Deafness Team even though the team will deal with hearing problems that may not literally be congenital. The great majority of hearing losses in our present times will be either present at birth or their later manifestation will be present in the genes at birth. The latter should rightfully be termed congenital. Hearing losses can occur in later life from ear disease, meningitis, encephalitis, measles, mumps, scarlet fever, or high fevers. But these diseases are becoming rarer and rarer, and there is more and more justification for considering "Congenital Deafness" as the main thrust of diagnosis of hearing loss.

Our emphasis on the team approach to diagnosis in no way minimizes the audiologist's art. The role of the audiologist in decisions concerning diagnosis and management is always a vital one. Not only does he contribute essential information on the degree of loss, the auditory behavior and development, and the auditory functioning of the child, but his familiarity with training methods and their

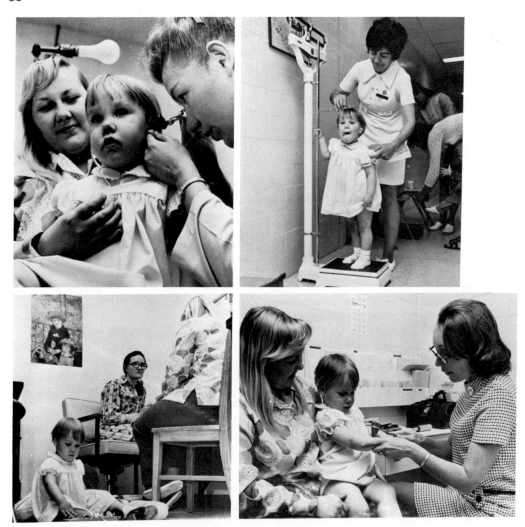

Fig. 2.11. The nature of modern-day hearing losses makes it increasingly imperative that a team of professional people work together for the management of the child with hearing loss. In addition to the audiologist's services, the regularly scheduled check-up should include otologic examination (top left), physical examination (top right), social work interview (bottom left), and pediatric evaluation (bottom right). (Courtesy of The National Foundation—March of Dimes.)

efficacy figures largely in decisions on the placement of the child. Precise audiologic measurements provide the necessary objective data, but the art of audiology weighs strongly in the evaluation. The clinical insight and intuition of the experienced audiologist contribute a much needed element to the decisions that will be made. How does the child relate to the clinician? Is eye contact good? Is the behavior even minimally distractible? Does there seem to be perseveration of auditory behavior? What is the vocal quality and how does he use his voice? How do parent and child relate to each other? These are the questions that can be answered more through intuition than through measurements. They are an integral part of the audiologist's art.

If the audiologist is also a well-trained language clinician—a competence which is most desirable—he can add to his observations the results of tests determining auditory perceptual function.

The ideal team, in addition to the audiologist, will consist basically of a pediatrician, an otolaryngologist, an ophthalmologist, a language clinician, a psychologist, and a social worker. Other consultants should be available from pediatric neurology, renal and endocrine specialties, radiology, genetics, and others where needed. A summary of recommended medical workup for the child with hereditary deafness is shown in Table 2.4.

Once the audiologist has specified that a certain degree of hearing loss exists, and has delineated the status of the auditory development of the child, a standard protocol of examinations is indicated. Any of these studies, if made in isolation, will furnish only a fragment of the total picture of the child and his needs; but when brought together in a team conference, the picture becomes a whole. The team together makes a diagnosis of the etiology, extent, and degree of the problem and decides on the proper management for the child.

After the initial thorough evaluation, it is customary to follow the young child every 6 months to observe his progress and to pick up any loose ends of diagnosis. Not until all facets are put together and the child has stabilized satisfactorily in his program will he be seen only once a year. Such stabilization does not occur until the child is 5 or 6, even if he has been identified in infancy. From then on until adolescence he will be seen once a year, and after that, whenever indicated.

*Table 2.4. Diagnostic Medical Workup of the Child with Hereditary Deafness**

History
    Detailed family pedigree
    Maternal prenatal history
General physical examination
    Generalized congenital bone disorders
    Congenital absence or sparseness of hair and/or nails
    Congenital neurologic deficits
    Ataxia of gait
Concomitant head and neck physical findings
    Atresia of the external auditory canals
    Malformed external ears
    Facial anomalies, especially of mandible
    Congenital facial nerve paralysis
    Branchial anomalies
    Heterochromia of the irises
    Increased intercanthal distance
    White forelock in scalp hair
Routine laboratory tests
    Family audiometry
    Complete blood count
    Urinalysis
Special laboratory tests where appropriate
    (Age 1 year and under)
    Rubella titer
    Cytomegalovirus titer
    Other viral titers
    (Any age)
    Electrocardiogram
    Protein bound iodine
    Syphilis serology
    Serum pyrophosphate and uric acid
    Urine mucopolysaccharide screening

Perinatal and neonatal history
Subsequent medical history

Pigmentary disorders
Congenital heart disease
Hand anomalies

Retinitis pigmentosa
Rubella retinopathy
Congenital cataracts
Dental anomalies
Short neck; neck anomalies
Goiter
Quality of voice and speech

IgM
Viral cultures of urine, throat, and nasopharynx
    for rubella and cytomegalovirus

Dermatoglyphics
Karyotype, buccal smear
X-rays as necessary
Petrous pyramid polytomography
Electroretinography
Vestibular testing

* Courtesy of LaVonne Bergstrom, M.D.

The Congenital Deafness Team should consider itself the monitor of the child's hearing and its function, the advisory group for the family, the judge of the child's potential in relation to his educational program, and the arbiter between the child and the community. Child advocacy is nowhere so effective as when undertaken by a Congenital Deafness Team.

Management of the Child

The identification of the primary problem of the child is the first step in management. Strangely enough, even severe deafness may not always be the chief concern for an infant or child. Physical handicaps, systemic disease, disorders requiring surgery, central motor and perceptual dysfunction, or severe mental retardation often take precedence in the habilitation program. Until proper treatment or placement is made for these difficulties, habilitation for the hearing loss takes a secondary place. The case of an infant or child who requires head surgery for some other defect may suggest postponement of the hearing aid and hearing habilitation until all surgery is completed. The managing physician should guide the team in making the decision as to the sequence of treatment and habilitation.

In the case of very severe mental retardation accompanied by deafness, the judgment of applying a hearing aid may be a difficult one. Some may argue that the limited function that can be expected is not worth the expense of an aid nor the time of therapists. It would be the rare person who would not want to give even such a child the opportunity to see what amplification and therapy can do. One 10-month-old rubella child in our experience who was about to be institutionalized was given such a chance. Although apparently vegetable-like in his development, with severe cataracts and no motor development, he did respond to sounds at 80 to 90 dB. A reprieve from the institution was requested, and binaural hearing aids were applied. His mother, who had totally rejected the infant, was taught to mother him and a home auditory stimulation program was begun. Within a year the child was able to walk unassisted, was babbling nicely, and was beginning to learn elementary hand manipulations. At 8 years of age he is in a program for trainable children. Despite this successful result it is probable that there are many children for whom amplification and training time really cannot be justified. We tend toward giving all children a chance, however over-optimistic that might be.

Once all critical medical treatment or surgery is concluded and the child is cleared for hearing habilitation, the team faces the decision as to program-placement for the child. It is devoutly hoped that the community will have available the variety of training programs that are necessary to a proper placement.

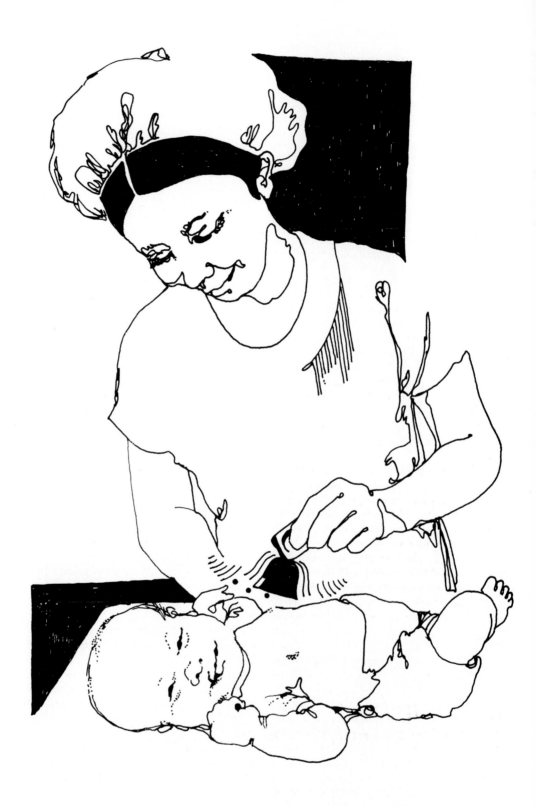

3 DEVELOPMENT OF AUDITORY BEHAVIOR

Auditory Function Development

An understanding of the development of auditory behavior is requisite to the hearing testing of infants and children. Unfortunately this kind of information is not found in audiology textbooks. The audiologist concerned with hearing in children has been so overwhelmed with the immediacy of identifying and managing hearing-impaired children that there has been too little time—and too few workers—for intensive investigation. It is to other disciplines that we must look for insights into the auditory coding abilities of infants and the development of the hearing function.

Experimental psychologists, physiologists, psychiatrists, and occasionally research pediatricians and otolaryngologists have been the chief contributors to our knowledge in this sphere. Most of them have studied auditory behavior strictly in relation to chronologic age, which makes good sense to the clinician who must judge the children's responses at all ages. A review of the literature from many discipline-specific journals begins naturally at the prenatal stage.

Prenatal Hearing

Elliot and Elliot (1964) confirmed physiologically that the human cochlea has normal adult function after the twentieth week of gestation. Johansson and his associates (1964) were among the first to report testing fetal hearing. Using high frequency pure tones presented by means of a microphone placed on the mother's abdomen, fetal heart rate increase response to the tones was recorded after the 20th week of gestation. The demonstration of fetal hearing has value in contradicting the theory that the child is born a tabula rasa insofar as hearing is concerned. The newborn infant has actually been hearing sounds for at least 4 months—fluid-borne sounds, to be sure—but nonetheless, true auditory signals.

It remained for a zealous experimenter,

Bench (1968), to measure the acoustic qualities of the sounds that reach the fetal ear through the specific gravity of the amniotic fluid. With a specially prepared crystal microphone inserted at the cervix of a woman in the 38th week of gestation, Bench measured the noise level of sounds presented through a loudspeaker placed on the abdomen, over the fetal head. The internal background noise was first measured, representing the mother's pulse (80 beats per minute), at a sound level of 72 dB (C-scale). Attenuation of the sound pressure presented at the abdomen was 200 Hz, 19 dB; 500 Hz, 24 dB; 1000 Hz, 38 dB; 2000 Hz, 48 dB; and 4000 Hz, 48 dB. The two highest frequency attenuation levels were not regarded as accurate, since the strength of the applied signal was not sufficient to overcome the masking by the internal sounds of 72 dB.

What is interesting to us in this study is the revelation that the fetus is surrounded by a noise level that many people complain of as being too loud in the environment. Yet the fetus has listened to this noise level for 4 months.

To the research worker in child development, the phenomenon of prenatal hearing is useful in predicting psychologic attributes of later responses to various sound patterns. To the clinician there is little value in determining the presence or absence of hearing function at the fifth month of gestation. Amplification can hardly be applied at this stage—the engineering feat staggers one! Therapeutic abortion is no longer feasible at 5 months. And even a sadist would shrink from burdening a pregnant mother with the knowledge that she is carrying a deaf child. Only one fact would be of value: if it could be well managed, it would be of great interest to know if a fetus that carries known recessive genes for deafness has normal hearing before birth. Geneticists and research otolaryngologists have surmised that often the human infant with recessive deafness genes may develop fetally with normal hearing but at some time before or after birth the hearing degenerates as it does in animals with genetic deafness (Fraser, 1971).

On the whole, at this time there seems to be little clinical purpose for testing prenatal hearing.

Newborn Hearing

Stimulus Properties. It has been hypothesized that because the fetus is accustomed to listening to the heartbeat of the mother, he will be quieted effectively by the same sound in his early days in the outer world. Brackbill et al. (1966) found that a tape-recorded heartbeat is no more effective than any other continuous, low frequency stimulus in lowering the arousal level of the infant. Lowered arousal level means a specific reduction of overt behavior and physiologic patterns: the infants' heart and respiration rates become lower, they cry less, and move about less.

However, lest it be assumed that all babies will be lulled to sleep merely by monotonous low frequency sound, Brackbill and Fitzgerald (1969) investigated neonates' level of arousal under five different conditions: (1) auditory stimulation, using taped heartbeats, played at 85 dB sound pressure level (SPL) with frequencies under 500 Hz attenuated to less than 30 dB; (2) visual stimulation from two 40-watt fluorescent bulbs, 4 feet above the baby; (3) proprioceptive-tactile stimulation from swaddling the infant from neck to toes in long strips of flannel; (4) temperature stimulation of 88°F; and (5) no extra stimulation, in which the sound level was reduced to 62 dB SPL, the visual stimulus was lowered to one 50-watt incandescent bulb in a translucent bowl, the temperature was lowered to 78°, and the infant was not swaddled or covered.

Brackbill et al. (1969) found that the infants cried the least and slept the most when they were continuously stimulated by the light, sound, temperature, and swaddling. Use of three of these stimuli was less effective; even less so were two; and one alone was no more effective than no extra stimulation. In other words, although monotonous low frequency sound is the best auditory pacifier, it would probably not be so unless at least one or two stimuli in other modalities were added.

Brackbill et al. cautioned against the use of keeping a baby for a long time in such a state of high intensity stimulation, unless it is indicated for medical reasons such as occur in prematurity or severe illness. All babies must adjust eventually to the reality of their new world, and to postpone the adjustment should only be done under medical advice.

It should be noted that when anesthetics and analgesics are administered to the mother during delivery, one can expect all central nervous system (CNS)-mediated functions to be depressed in the baby for several hours after birth. Stechler (1964) found that responsiveness to visual stimuli is impaired for as much as 4 days after birth when the mother has been given medication during childbirth. Our clinical observations confirm that the same certainly may be true of the auditory responsiveness of the infant who is only a few hours old. The researcher will do well to keep this fact in mind when observing neonates.

Eisenberg (1970) has demonstrated that most newborns, including those with known CNS abnormalities, can discriminate sound on the basis of frequency, intensity, and stimulus-dimensionality. Thus it is possible that neuronal mechanisms for processing SPL are fully mature at birth.

The processing of frequency differences is described by Eisenberg (1970) as range-dependent. The low frequencies tend to have a soothing, or inhibiting effect on the infant. High frequencies have the property of occasioning distress rather than inhibiting it. However, signals in the range below 4000 Hz are two or three times more response-provoking than those in the very high ranges. The frequency patterns most often used by Eisenberg are matched pairs of ascending and descending tonal sequences. She states that the effectiveness of pure tones or noise bands can be enhanced by increases in one or more, within limits bearing on the characteristics of spoken language.

What is particularly significant to the clinician is Eisenberg's finding that speech-like signals seem remarkably effective in producing responses in newborns. This fact is certainly true of the older infant, as will be described later, but to find that the newborn already responds selectively to the dimensionality of human speech gives us directions for clinical testing.

It is intriguing to speculate whether speech dimensional signals are more attention-getting because of some preadaptive auditory reactivity, or whether the known frequency-dependent sensitivity of the human ear is operating here. That dependency in itself is intriguing: one wonders which came first, the human ears' greater sensitivity to frequencies in the speech range, or the peculiar properties of the human larynx and resonators to produce speech in that particular range of frequencies. In the area of visual behavior, Fantz (1961) has demonstrated that the newborn infant is more attentive to the dimensions of the human face than to any other visual object, a fact which would argue for a preadaptive response to "humanity."

Kagan (1972) suggests that stimulus change is another parameter that should be explored. A 2-day-old infant is more attentive to a moving light than to a steady light. The rate of the light change is also important. In the auditory sphere, Kearsley (1962) found that if an unexpected noise of 70 dB reaches maximal intensity within a few milliseconds, a newborn infant closes his eyes, starts, and shows an increase in heart rate. If the same sound reaches its maximal intensity in 2 seconds, the infant opens his eyes, looks around, and is likely to show a decrease in heart rate. The first reaction is a defensive one; the latter displays interest.

Kagan suggests that the attention-getting power of contrast, so evident in the newborn period, diminishes as early as the second month and is succeeded by a different parameter of the stimulus (to be discussed in the section below on "The Older Child").

We have not been able to find any mention in the literature of research into newborn infants' discrimination of rhythm. It is logical that this line of investigation would be just as fruitful as the others that have been reported. There is no question but what the newborn infant can discriminate all the parameters of an auditory stimulus.

State. Bench (1971) describes the relationship between the infant's state and his response, in terms of the law of initial value (LIV): "The magnitude of response change is influenced by the state of the individual before stimulation in such a way that the lower the initial or prestimulus state, the greater is the increase in level of activity on stimulation; the higher the initial state, the greater is the decrease in level of activity." Bench measured the heart rate of 10 normal newborn babies for 10 seconds before and after stimulation by a 95-dB broad band noise. The results indicated that the heart rate change to auditory stimulation was dependent on the prestimulus heart rate. The implication of this work for infant audiometry is that any given baby may show an increase or decrease in activity, or no change at all, depending entirely on his prestimulus state. Bench recommends that babies be tested at low levels of activities, in order to obtain a positive response change.

In another study Bench and Boscak (1970) applied signal detection theory to infants' responses to three different stimulus levels of 300 Hz (55, 75, and 95 dB). The infants' prestimulus states were rated as 1 (deep sleep), 2 (light sleep), and 3 (limb activity). They found that the signal detection is affected by both the SPL of the stimulus and the state of the baby before stimulation. There was a significant trend for the effect of state in the decreasing order of state 2, state 1, and state 3. A light sleep, then, predisposes to the best response to sound.

Taylor and Mencher (1972) also identified infant state as a significant variable in neonatal testing, reporting that light sleep is the optimal state for evaluating a response to auditory stimuli. They applied single and double presentations of different stimuli at 90 and 100 dB to 225 normal newborn infants. The most common response types which they observed were eye movement and arousal responses. Stronger responses occurred more often in the light sleep than in the awake and quiet state. The sleep state was defined by touching the examiner's finger to the closed eyelid of the infant. If eye or body movement resulted, a light state was judged to be present; if there was no movement, the deep sleep state was judged. So far as the stimulus is concerned, Taylor and Mencher found that a broad band of noise is most effective in predicting a response; second is the narrow band stimulus; and third is the modulated pure tone. Ling et al. (1970) also found that a narrow band stimulus is superior to the modulated pure tones in eliciting responses. Taylor and Mencher recommended using both narrow and broad band stimuli and requiring more than one response for a pass. A completely normal infant thus may be unresponsive to sound as a function only of his state at the time—which may also change momentarily.

Active Response. In addition to responding differentially in a passive way to stimulus patterns and intensity, newborns can be active in regulating auditory events in their environment. Butterfield (1968) reported that babies made bursts of contingent sucking responses that controlled the onset and offset of tape-recorded music: classical, popular, and vocal. An instrumented pacifier nipple operated the musical selections. Four 1-day-old infants were used in his study, and all responded consistently over several tests. This study leaves no doubt but that newborn infants are not passive in their hearing function. Their feedback loop operates actively at as early an age as study is possible. The availability of such an auditory function strengthens the idea of early application of hearing aids to hearing-impaired infants who have sufficient residual hearing to benefit from them. Eimas et al. (1972) used changes in conditioned sucking rates to measure sound differentiation. By 1 month, infants showed, by changes in sucking rates, that they differentiated the onset time distinction between the phonemes "Pah" and "Bah." By 4 months of age the changes were more marked. Differential perception seems to be well established in the first few months of life.

Downs (1967b) has catalogued a variety of neonatal behavioral responses to sound, and has pointed out ways of observing these responses:

Eye Blink or Eyelid Activity: This ranges from a tiny, rapid stricture of the eyelids to a marked closure of the lids in which the eyebrows are also drawn down. This can also be a part of a grimacing response. A slight fluttering of the lids is also seen occasionally. The range of responses includes: 1) a definite eye blink, however small; 2) a fluttering of the eyelids where there has been no such fluttering previously; 3) a contraction of the eyes, including the eyebrows. The eye movement is often accompanied by a grimace.

Moro's Response: This is a violent startle reaction, consisting of a jerking of the entire body, with arms and legs drawn toward the midline. Sometimes a shaking or shuddering of the arms and legs accompanies the response.

Cessation of Activity: This response is most often seen when the baby is crying vigorously and flailing his arms and legs. There is a marked quieting of the crying and limb movement when the sound is heard, sometimes momentarily, sometimes for a longer time. It can also occur when there is merely random movement going on, and the movement ceases when the sound is heard. The range of responses includes: 1) a stopping of crying, even momentarily; 2) a stopping of flailing limb or head movements even for a moment; 3) a "stilling" of mild ongoing activity.

Limb Movements: These are usually seen only when the infant has been resting quietly, and the sound provokes definite movement of hands, arms, or legs. Sometimes shoulder movement is also seen. The range of responses includes: 1) a limb or hand movement—even a flutter—where there has been absolute quiet previously; 2) a movement of any limbs (or shoulders) that is definitely stronger and more sudden than the preceding random activity.

Head Turn Away from Sound or Head Turn Toward Sound: These are commonly seen, either toward the sound or away from it. Both responses are valid. The head may turn directly toward either side or there may be a stretching of the neck and raising of the head upward. The range of responses includes: 1) a movement of the head toward (T) the sound or away (A) from it; 2) any movement, up or down, that involves a stretching of the neck. An arousal from sleep is usually accompanied by head movements.

Grimacing: The face suddenly wrinkles up as if to protest against the sound, and the eyebrows are brought downward. The eyes may open and close for a moment.

Sucking: This can be a slight drawing in of the lower lip or it can be a full sucking activity. Care should be taken to observe whether sucking activity has occurred before the test; in that case it cannot be credited as a response. Sometimes sucking is accompanied by head turn or limb movement.

Arousal: This can only occur when the baby is sleeping quietly or is awake but quiet. There is an awakening of the whole body.

The range of responses includes: 1) some eye opening, with slight to strong movement throughout the body; 2) a slight shudder of the entire body.

Breathing Change: This is difficult to observe, and should not be recorded except by the most experienced observer. A slight catch of the breath, or a momentary cessation of the rhythmic pattern of breathing occurs. The observer must be very certain that the pre-test breathing pattern has been regular.

Widening of the Eyes: When the baby is sleeping, his eyes may open wider than they were before, even momentarily. The range of responses includes: 1) a widening of the eyes from an open state; 2) an opening of the eyes from a closed state; 3) a raising of the eyebrows with an almost imperceptible eye-widening. (With permission from M. P. Downs: Organization and Procedures of a Newborn Infant Screening Program, pp. 11-12, Official publication of the National Assn. of Hearing and Speech Agencies, Washington, D.C., 1969.)

These responses consist of those observed to a 90-dB SPL signal, usually a narrow band centering around 3000 Hz, when presented in a nursery environment. All of them, however, can also be seen in a sound room when the baby is quiet or asleep, and when noisemakers as soft as 35 to 45 dB are presented.

For the investigator, Eisenberg's (1970) more sophisticated observations on the responses of newborns to sound gives substance to the description of responses:

Overt reactions:
  Arousal
  Gross body movements
  Orienting behavior
    Turning of head
    Wide-eyed "what-is-it?" look
    Pupillary dilatation
  Motor reflexes
    Facial grimaces
    Displacement of a single digit
  Crying or cessation of crying
Cardiac reactions:
  Diphasic (deceleration-acceleration or reverse)
  Longer latency than for constant signals
  Associated with "on"-"off" effects, and with the direction of a tonal sequence.

Eisenberg terms many of these selective reactions as representative of higher and more selective levels of neuronal organization. The peculiar effectiveness of speech-dimensional sounds lends weight to the presence of higher processing of sounds stimuli.

To the student of auditory behavior, all of Eisenberg's studies have tremendous significance. It was she who first described differences in habituation to sound as an index of central nervous system integrity. Newborn infants with known CNS involvement failed to extinguish their responses to repeated acoustic signals. Normal infants habituated to the repeated stimuli in a short time. Sometimes called response decrement, this phenomenon is logical for possible use as a screening tool in identifying CNS problems.

Kagan and Lewis (1965) used heart rate deceleration to an auditory stimulus in repeated series as a measure of the speed of model acquisition. When heart rate deceleration no longer occurred after a repeated acoustic signal, the complete response decrement was thought to have taken place. Lewis and Goldberg (1969) hold "that the amount of response decrement to a repeated signal is a measure of the speed of model acquisition and is associated with the efficiency of the model building system." To them, response decrement is not due to sensory fatigue or neural accommodation, but is an indicator of the maturity of the cognitive processing.

In an effort to utilize response decrement in a screening protocol, Brackbill and Downs (1969) attempted to measure normal versus abnormal values for habituation in infants. High risk premature infants and normal infants were compared as to their habituation to white noise at 90 dB SPL at 10 seconds duration. The high risk group averaged 28 responses before extinction; the normal group averaged 17. A later similar study by Downs using a shorter inter-stimulus interval (3 seconds), averaged 8 responses before extinction in 30 normals; 18 in 30 high risk infants. This information has yet to be applied to a practical screening protocol.

The hypothesis that CNS-damaged infants will fail to habituate was tested by Schulman (1970a) using heart rate changes as the measure of response. An 80-dB buzzer for 3 seconds was used at 20-second intervals. Heart rate was recorded from a cardiotachometer. Five high risk premature, five low risk premature, and five normal full term infants were compared. All risk children were matched for gestational age. Significant habituation occurred in all three groups, although latency of response was significantly longer in the high risk subject. Thus Schulman was not able to confirm the lack of response decrement in the AT RISK child that Eisenberg (1970) and Brackbill and Downs (1969) had reported.

It may be that the careful matching for gestational age reduced the differences that others had found in response decrement between the two groups. This fact only points up the hypothesis that response decrement is related to immature central processing.

A case in one of the author's files (M. P. D.) of a child with neurologic deterioration due to cytomegolovirus inclusion disease may confirm this hypothesis. When seen at 2½ years of age, the child already had many neurologic deficits, but was able to give a neck turn response to sounds of 30- to 40-dB SPL level. She gave the usual startle when a speech signal reached 65 dB (re: 0 dB). When seen a year later in the sound room, this child showed hyperreflexes to sounds at 30 to 40 dB, and continued to respond with a Moro-like reflex at every presentation. The large reflex responses and lack of response decrement resembled that of an anencephalic infant. No central processing of the auditory signal was present to inhibit the reflexes. A reverse of the process of auditory maturation seemed to have taken place.

The Older Infant

The maturation of auditory processing proceeds after birth in ways that have been demonstrated in research designs. Already at 4 weeks the infant can distinguish phonemic contrasts in sound signals, as measured by heart rate changes. McCaffrey (1969) presented 4- to 28-week-old infants with standard vowel and consonant stimuli which were then changed to contrasting vowels or consonants. At the point of transition from the standard to the contrasting phoneme, significant heart rate changes were found to occur.

A similar study was made by Moffitt (1969) with 20- to 24 week-old children, utilizing

synthesized speech samples generated by Haskins Laboratories, consisting of the consonants "b" and "g." His 20 infants made significant discriminations of the phonemic transition at the end of the seventh and eighth trials, or after a 30-second exposure to the repeated transitions.

Friedlander (1970) terms these reactions "active, critical evaluative processes characterized by creative model-building and formation of hypotheses as to what is likely to happen next." One can conclude that however simple the paradigm, the responses represent some aspect of learning and cognitive processing. This viewpoint is supported by Neisser (1967) who maintains that choices are made of which parts of the incoming information should be attended to. Attending, even in the infant, becomes a constructive, active process rather than an analytic and passive response.

By the age of 3 months, according to Turnure (1969), babies attend better to mothers' voices on a tape recording than to strangers' voices, even when mothers' voices are modified by filtering. She observed babies' body movements as an indicator of attention in standard time periods during which tape recordings of the mother's natural and distorted voice were played. She also compared their body movements when strangers' voices were played as against mothers' voices in natural and distorted form. Children 3, 6, and 9 months were subjects for the experiment. Turnure reported differences in the way the infants attended to the voices as a function of age level. The 9-month-olds tended to be quieter to the natural mother's voice and progressively less attentive to the distortions.

Further evidence of the selective listening abilities of infants is given by Friedlander (1970). He devised an ingenious PLAY-TEST whereby a large pair of response switches are attached to the baby's crib or play pen. The switches regulate a loudspeaker, an electrical control and response recording unit, and a stereo tape player with a preprogrammed selection of two-channel audio tapes. Whenever the baby operates either switch, a record is made of the frequency and duration of his choice, and he turns on one channel or the other of the audio tape. Thus, a record is made of his listening preferences. Babies 9 to 18 months old were studied over long periods. The findings are summarized as follows:

1. When sounds and voices are placed under the babies' own control, they display phenomenal productivity in listening response productivity, ranging from one 9-month-old girl's 65,000 seconds of responding in 20 days (3000 seconds per day) to the average response record of 1200 to 1500 seconds per day of other children. These data indicate that listening to sounds and voices have a hitherto unsuspected potency as a desirable form of activity to babies whose own speech is still very immature. From this and other investigations, Friedlander suggests that "performance to gain access to recurrent exposure of auditory stimuli can be a major aspect of infants' listening behavior, for which new investigative procedures must be devised."

2. Babies show a great range of discriminative listening to a wide variety of natural, disguised, and synthetic language as well as to other auditory stimuli, as the following examples indicate. (a) A 12-month-old infant preferred to listen to a stranger's voice with bright intonation than to his mother's voice speaking in a flat monotone. (b) A 14-month-old baby couldn't decide for several days whether to select the stranger's voice or the mother's distorted voice. After several days he made an enormous burst of listening to the mother's voice and after that he ignored completely the switch that turned on the stranger's voice. This choice is regarded as an "aha" effect with the child ultimately recognizing the mother's voice despite its distortion. (c) Another baby was offered a choice between two tape recordings of animated family conversations: one edited to run for 240 seconds before it was repeated, the other repeated after 20 seconds. The long cycle was considered to have low redundancy and high information; the short cycle had high redundancy and low information. For the first several days, the baby preferred the short tape with high redundancy and low information. After a week he crossed over into a preference for the low redundancy, high information selection. This redundancy study was replicated on 11 babies, 9 to 18 months, 7 of whom ultimately chose the low-redundancy, high information selection.

It seems inescapable to conclude that these young babies are using some cognitive processes to make their listening selections. They must formulate internal linguistic models against which to compare the recurrent inputs. Such intellectual activity challenges Piaget's idea that cognitive development in the infant begins only after the sensorimotor period ends at 18 months.

Kagan's work (1972) suggests a varied assortment of response parameters for investigation. One of them is the duration of the infant's sustained attention, which Kagan believes is a rough index of how easy or how difficult it is for the infant to understand a new experience. Kagan defines this kind of attention as the duration of sustained orientation that follows the initial orienting response of 2 seconds. He believes that during the period of sustained orientation an infant over 30 days old is trying to build a representation of the event. Further study of this phenomenon may add another parameter to the indices of auditory behavior for infants.

What do these studies mean in terms of differential development in children? A study by Irwin (1952) described the early effects of different kinds of auditory input given to infants. He applied both quantitative and qualitative measures to two groups of infants from the time of birth to the age of 1 year. One group comprised the infants of highly verbal, "white-collar" and professional people; the other comprised a low verbal, "blue collar" working and laborer group. The variable was that the first talked a great deal directly to the infant and in its presence; the second group of parents were less communicative both to each other and to the child. The quantity and quality of their vocalizations showed that at about 3 months, something changed the vocalizations of the two groups. The infants of the highly verbal parents began to increase the number of their vocalizations, as well as the quality of the phonemes used, more rapidly than the infants of the low verbal group. It can be inferred that by 3 months, the amount and the quality of the auditory input to these infants was already being transformed into commensurate output. The more highly stimulated infants had greater opportunity to select acoustic information and to apply it to their own auditory feedback loop. Active participation and expression resulted, but differentially in the two groups. What more pragmatic proof can there be that infants are active, not passive, in their utilization of incoming acoustic stimuli?

Now that the intricate processing that takes place in the first years of life has been described, we can apply this knowledge to the auditory testing of infants. Such testing involves measurements of stimulus parameters under structured conditions that can be repeatable and it also involves the description of observations that any clinician can make. It is therefore a subject quite apart from the investigations that have been described above and will be treated separately in another chapter.

Auditory Behavior as Prelinguistic Activity

Concurrent with the maturation of the auditory function are the developing speech and language skills.

The infant's first use of sounds in a repetitive manner indicates the time at which the auditory feedback loop has become effective. By 2 months he is beginning to put out certain sounds more than others. His selection of which sounds to repeat seems to depend on the nature of the sound. From 2 to 4 months these sounds are vowel-like. The sequence of use of vowels is presumably from middle (the "schwa" sound /ə/) to front and back vowels (Menyuk, 1972). By 5 months the consonant-vowel sequences begin. Irwin (1947) states that back consonants (velars and glottals) predominate at 5 to 6 months, with some of the labial (front) consonants entering in. At 9 to 10 months, the glottal sounds decrease and the alveolar sounds (middle) are frequently used. Menyuk (1972) partially explains this sequence of selection as due to ease of production. It is also possible that the selection is made for them by some differences in the changing vocal mechanism.

Studies of Moffitt (1968, 1969) suggest that the infant responds differentially to acoustic differences between speech sound categories. Perhaps there is a hierarchy of ease of observing distinctions between the acoustic properties of speech sounds. Such a hierarchy might also account for the selection of certain sounds by the auditory feedback loop. Is it related to sound energy? Or to the differential sensitivity

of the human ear to various frequencies? Further research will undoubtedly answer these questions. It seems logical that there is an interplay between selective auditory sensitivity and ease of production of sounds, both of which account for the selection of infants' sounds.

Although the infant is able to differentiate various speech sounds in the first few months of life, his production of the sounds does not develop at the same rate. Berko and Brown (1960) describe the lag between the perception of differences in speech signals and the production of those speech sounds. In the newborn period the infant does not produce phonated sounds, only cries and physiologic sounds. Murai (1960) and Lieberman et al. (1973) postulate that the reason for this early lack of phonation is similar to the reason that primates cannot speak: the larynx is positioned relatively high, almost in line with the roof of the palate, limiting the pharyngeal movement that is necessary to speech. In addition, the infants' large tongues fill the oral cavity and prevent them from changing the shape of their superlaryngeal vocal tract by moving their tongues during phonation.

Menyuk (1972) suggests that experimental results comparing primate vocalizations with those of human infants and adults "indicate that speaking is not simply a learned overlaid function on the muscles and structures of breathing and eating, but that man is pre-programmed to develop a vocal mechanism that is specifically adapted to produce speech."

By 1 month typical cooing and gurgling sounds are made in addition to the crying; by 3 months true babbling begins. True babbling consists of the pleasurable repetition of sounds in the parents' absence, and the increase of these sounds in the presence of the parents.

Up to 5 or 6 months of age, the sounds made by the infant do not seem to be related to the speech sounds he hears. His productive capacity for speech lags significantly behind his demonstrated ability to perceive differences. From our observations of otherwise normal deaf infants, their vocalizations are identical with those of normal infants until 5 or 6 months. Furthermore, the deaf infants increase their vocalizations when the parents speak to them, just as normal infants do (Downs and Akin, 1973). It is obvious that the reason for this increase in vocalizations is not the baby's hearing the parent's voice. We postulate that it is a preadaptive, reflexive response stimulated by the presence of the parent's face, much as is the smile response which appears at the same age. It may be that the increase in vocalization is as necessary a psychic organizer for ultimate communication integrity as the smile response is to ultimate psychic integrity (Spitz, 1965). The phenomenon of increased vocalization may indeed be a milestone that is predictive of eventual communication skills. Certainly the established fact that the auditory feedback loop is present at birth indicates that the elementary babbling sounds have a significant prelinguistic function. How important the lack of auditory feedback is to the deaf child can only be speculated upon.

The invariable presence of the babbling responses in both the deaf and the hearing infant seems to us to represent reflexive, preadaptive behavior unique to the human infant. It can be considered as one of the earliest functions in the preprogrammed schedule of linguistic activities that Lenneberg (1966) describes as being innate processes. Its importance in the prelinguistic sequence of activities may be that it reinforces vocalizations by means of rewards. As Bruner (1968) terms it, a code of mutual expectancy is established between infant and parent when the adult responds to some initiative on the part of the child. Thus the child's behavior is converted into a signal initiating an interaction code. Bruner believes that the language channel is dependent on the growth of such codes.

These self-stimulating sounds strengthen the auditory feedback loop which was earlier demonstrated to be active at birth. The infant begins early to monitor his own speech activity, however primitive. The perception and elementary control of rhythm, intonation, duration, as well as frequency range of sounds is evident by 4 or 5 months of age.

By 5 months Chinese children produce the intonation of the Chinese language. Also, Polish infants' babbling by 5 months can be distinguished from English infants (Weir, 1966). The later skills of linguistic organization are undoubtedly dependent upon these early activities.

Menyuk (1972) describes the beginning of speech from birth on:

Despite the fact that presumably all the possible speech sounds are produced during this stage and that the child merely uses vocalizations to express pleasure or displeasure, all of these studies indicate that the time at which a sound is first uttered and repetitively used depends on the nature of the sound. During the early months of non-cry vocalizations (two to four months) practically all the sounds are vowels or vowel-like, and certain vowels are used earlier and proportionately more frequently than others. Presumably, the sequence of use of vowels is from middle (the schwa sound $/\Lambda/$ or $/\epsilon/$) to front and back vowels. At about five or six months the repetitive production of CV sequences begins, and the consonant of these sequences in terms of frequency of usage varies as the child matures. Irwin (1947) presents data on the proportionate usage of consonants over the age range of one to thirty months and examines the effect of place of articulation on proportionate usage. Back consonants (velars and glottals), and to a lesser extent front consonants (labials), predominate at the five to six months period. At the nine to ten months period there is less use of glottal sounds, and the middle of the mouth sounds (alveolars) are beginning to be used with some frequency. If we examine the distinctive feature characteristics of the sounds that are used predominately and more frequently at the beginning of the babbling period by infants born in American English-speaking environments (as exemplified by Irwin's population) and Japanese-speaking environments (as exemplified by Nakazima's population), we find that consonants that have the features of either +voice, +grave, and +nasal, or some combination of these features, are used first and proportionately more frequently than sounds having the features +diffuse, +strident, and +continuant. If we note that some features appear to be the product of minimal efforts of the vocal mechanism (unmarked features) whereas others require special adjustments of the parts to produce (marked features), then the sequence of proportional usage is partially explained. Thus, for example, sounds produced at the lips (p, b, m) are easier to produce than either alveolar sounds (t, d, n) or velar sounds (k, g, n), because the tongue is in a resting position for lip sounds while it has to be moved to purposefully produce the other sounds. It is, however, also possible that the infant selects for reproduction the speech sounds that have acoustic characteristics he can more easily discriminate. Miller and Nicely (1955) have found that adults preserved best, when given nonsense-syllables in noise, the features of voicing and nasality in reproducing these nonsense syllables. This result is some indication that these characteristics are easier for adults to detect in acoustic signals than are others, but it may not be the case that these characteristics are also easier for infants to detect in the signals they hear. Further, since the relationship between production and perception at this stage of development is not clear, it is possible that infants are producing certain sounds because of the nature of the developing vocal mechanism, while observing distinctions between other and different speech sounds because of the nature of the developing auditory mechanism. (With permission from P. Menyuk: The Development of Speech, pp. 17-18. Indianapolis and New York, Bobbs-Merrill Co., 1972.)

Further research will undoubtedly answer these questions. It seems logical that there is an interplay between selective auditory sensitivity and ease of production of sounds, both of which account for the selection of infants' sounds.

Babbling ceases at about 6 months, and the next few months comprise rather undistinguished progress in vocalizing speech sounds. At this period the mother's feedback of the child's sounds lays the groundwork for his first production of a word. The sounds the child makes are imitated by the mother and additional speech improvisations are added by her. Soon the child imitates the mother's imitations, and speech control is under way. Sometimes the comprehension of the sound sequence precedes the imitation; sometimes imitation precedes understanding of the meaning of the sound sequence according to Murai (1963, 1964).

This latter observation has great significance for aural rehabilitation of the deaf child. One often sees, in a severely deafened child who has been trained to speak through audition, that he is able to produce words without recognizing the meaning of the word. In the normal hearing child, first the sound sequence is made (imitated) by the child; then the parent repeats it for him and indicates in some way what the sound represents, by pointing to an object or showing it. But it may be that by the time the child first imitates the sound, he has already absorbed the meaning of it through past listening experiences. Or he may have heard it so often in the past that his curiosity is piqued to the extent that a readiness to learn the meaning of it is present. Is it the lack of many previous experiences in hearing the sound that causes a longer period between production of a sound sequence and the learning of its meaning? If so, then the limited hearing child should be given a long period of input before any attempt is made to stimulate speech activity. However the normal hearing child learns meanings, the production and understanding must be in a closely related time sequence that is dependent upon a large number of past experiences with the sound. Aural rehabilitationists should take note of this developmental sequence.

Kaplan (1969) measured the heart rate and orienting responses of 4 to 8-month-old babies to a string of morphemes with changing frequency contour and the same morphemes in both declarative and interrogative sentences. No changes were noted until 8 months, when there were significant differences in responses to the second series of morphemes. The infants appeared to be able, by 8 months, to differentiate between the intonation of questions versus statements. This skill takes its place as one of the significant prelinguistic functions.

Of such stuff is language made. The long period of reception of auditory language symbols is the prerequisite to later language formulation. By the time speech and language emerge, there have been 12 to 18 months of receiving complex adult spoken language and distilling it into the matrix of the child language structure. This act of refining out of a complex language structure the basic one- and two-word sentences that are the baby's first speech language utterances must rank as creation's noblest day. Chomsky (1966) proposes that the ability to decode and organize these grammatical structures is an innate function, unique to human infants. Lenneberg (1966) prefers to rely on biological functioning to explain language development. Whichever theory one supports, the important fact is the primacy of reception in the language acquisition of children. Listening to language for a long period of time is essential to the ultimate usage of language. From the studies described above, it is evident that this listening is not a passive process, but one in which the infant participates by acting upon the incoming signals.

Exploring the reasons for the lag between language reception and its production is an academic exercise that does not seem to be useful to us. What is important is the fact that there is an early maturing receptive system which appears to establish a readiness for the later maturing expressive system to be employed at the proper time.

By the time the child's first meaningful word is uttered, miraculously full-blown at around 1 year, a whole world of listening activity has taken place. Nothing he will ever achieve is as intellectually complex as what has preceded his first utterance. Lenneberg states, "By the time language begins to make its appearance about 60% of the adult values of maturation are reached."

Critical Periods

How early is it necessary for the hearing-deprived child to receive language input, if he is to avoid language retardation? The answer to this question is based on whether there exist critical periods for the development of various functions. The theory of critical periods states that there are certain periods in development when the organism is programmed to receive and utilize particular types of stimuli, and that subsequently the stimuli will have gradually diminishing potency in affecting the organism's development in the function represented. In the case of audition it means that at a certain developmental stage auditory signals will be optimally received and utilized for important prelinguistic activities, but that once this stage has passed the effective utilization of these signals gradually declines. An analogous theory for language development holds that language input must be experienced at a certain stage, or it becomes decreasingly effective for utilization in emergent language skills.

The most vociferous opponent of this theory has been Bench (1971) who claims that the concept has no more than heuristic value, and that its importance in the field of diagnostic audiology has been greatly over-emphasized. Bench requires of the critical period theory that to be thorough, it would demand an irreversibility of the effects. "If a method can be found to change the effects back to normal ('reversing the apparently irreversible'), it is clear that the so-called critical period is not critical after all." He cites the animal studies of Denenberg and Morton (1964), who were able partially to reverse heightened emotional activity in animals caused by deprivation of extrinsic stimulation in infancy, by exposing them to a free environment after weaning.

It is evident that there is a semantic difference between Bench's concept of the critical period theory as demanding a totally irreversible effect, and our interpretation of it as implying an effect becoming more and more devastating with the duration of deprivation following the onset of the period. It can be demonstrated that in the field of auditory perception, total sensory deprivation over a period of time eventually results in an irreversible inability to perceive differences in speech sounds. Downs (1954) undertook a vocational rehabilitation project to determine whether applying hearing aids to deaf graduates of a manual school system could be justified. Four young adults (17 to 19 years old) with normal or above normal performance IQ's who had never worn hearing aids were selected for the study. All had measurable hearing through 2000 Hz, with average losses in the speech range of 75 to 95 dB (ASA, 1954). This amount of hearing, it should be noted, has permitted children who were given early amplification, to achieve quite adequate speech discrimination. For 2 months the subjects were given 4 hours a day of auditory training and corresponding speech training, on elementary words and sounds. At the end of the period, test results showed that their recognition of simple speech sounds had not developed beyond random chance. They were able neither to repeat speech sounds accurately nor to identify differences between them. It was concluded that the value of hearing aids to such young people was limited to hearing the difference between noise and non-noise.

It may be argued that the 2-month period

was insufficient to demonstrate learning of auditory perceptions, or that another therapy approach may have been more effective. The fact remains that these young people were given every chance to develop gross perception of sound, and did not. It is possible that in their cases, a lifetime would not be long enough to develop the skills necessary to understanding elementary speech. By postpuberty it appears that the inability to perceive the complex auditory signals of speech is irreversible.

Lenneberg (1966) is of the opinion that puberty marks the last milestone for acquisition of language. In regard to the effects of early deprivation, he cites the difference between the congenitally deaf child and the child who acquires deafness through meningitis after a brief exposure to language. He states that those who lose hearing after having been exposed to the experience of speech, even for as short a period as 1 year, can be trained much more easily in all language arts, even if formal training begins some years after they had become deaf. According to Lenneberg (1967), "It seems as if even a short exposure to language, a brief moment during which the curtain has been lifted and oral communication established, is sufficient to give a child some foundation on which much later language may be based."

A classic case in point is that of Miss Helen Keller, whose great achievements in mastering language skills are rightly admired. However, it must be remembered that Miss Keller acquired her deafness and blindness from meningitis at age 2. One cannot expect equal language achievements from a congenitally deaf and blind child and indeed, one does not see them develop.

Lenneberg (1966) describes in detail the case for the time-locked nature of language learning, and concludes:

The inferences we may draw from this material (animal studies on critical periods) is that many animal forms traverse periods of peculiar sensitivities, response-propensities, or learning potentials. Insofar as we have made such a claim for language acquisition, we have postulated nothing that would be extraordinary in the realm of animal behavior. But at the same time we must sound a

warning. Merely the fact that there are critical periods for the acquisition of certain types of behavior among a number of species *does not imply* any phylogenetic relationship between them. Age-linked emergence of behavior may be due to such a variety of factors that this phenomenon by itself is of limited heuristic value when it comes to tracing evolutionary origins of behavior. In the case of language, the limiting factors postulated are cerebral immaturity on the one end and termination of a state of organizational plasticity linked with lateralization of function at the other end of the critical period. (With permission from E. H. Lenneberg: Biological Foundations of Language, pp. 175-176. New York, John Wiley & Sons, Inc., 1966.)

By the time language begins to make its appearance, Lenneberg states that about 60% of the adult values of maturation are reached. He assigns the reason for this rapid achievement to the very rapid brain maturation rate during this period.

In the area of language for the sighted deaf, where intensive training has been given the deaf in an attempt to remedy the language lag, only partial reversibility can be demonstrated when training is begun even as early as 2 years. But partial reversibility does not confer on the individual language functioning adequate to our complex life and its demands.

The "Survey of Hearing Impaired Children and Youth" taken in the Spring of 1971 by the Gallaudet College Office of Demographic Studies (Series D, No. 9) reports the results of the administration of the Stanford Achievement Test Series to all students in schools for the deaf and hard-of-hearing in the United States. The highest average reading competence level (paragraph meaning), attained at age 19, was equivalent to grade 4.36. As might be expected, academic reading areas were lowest for those with the most severe degree of hearing loss. Related to the low reading levels of all the students are poor vocabularies and knowledge of word meanings—skills upon which reading ability is built. However, in the nonverbal area of arithmetic computation, the more profoundly deaf students score higher than their better hearing contemporaries. This fact demonstrates that the lowered degree of language and reading skills of these very profoundly deaf students is not caused by lowered intellectual function in this group.

The Gallaudet Survey makes this cautionary statement in reference to the results: "They should not be used to compare the general academic achievement of hearing impaired students to the achievement level of hearing students. More appropriately the results should be considered as relative values that show relationships between sub-groups of the population that participated in the testing program." This statement is an extraordinary reflection of the general attitude of hearing people toward the deaf: although the normal hearing expect the deaf to compete with hearing people in a hearing world, they are willing to compare their academic achievement with something other than that of the normal hearing population. What should the achievement of the deaf be compared with? A norm for the deaf? A norm for the blind or the brain-injured? To think of the deaf as a separate population is to consign them to a second-class citizenship which they do not merit. The goal should be for the deaf to achieve skills that will allow them to compete on the same basis as the normal hearing population. Therefore, their language competence should be compared with normals. Otherwise we will continue to be satisfied with lower goals than the deaf are capable of achieving.

In an expertly designed study, Templin (1966) compares the language skills of deaf children with the skills of matched groups of normal children. In some of the language areas the deaf showed no systematic improvement in their performance beyond 11 years. At that point such skills as understanding of word meanings, sentence construction, and analogies, hit a plateau and remained there without further insights or improvements. The normal hearing went on to achieve to the 14-year language level that was the upper limits of the study. It should be emphasized that there was no substantial difference in intellectual abilities between the deaf and the normal hearing group and that the deaf had had intensive language training in their schools. Their rate of learning up to 11 years was comparable with that of the normal hearing group. But an irreversible language deficit appeared at this age level and precluded further development. The complexity of language forms and of abstract language symbols takes a great leap about this age and leaves the deaf helplessly behind. The blame can only be ascribed to early language deprivation covering many periods critical for language learning.

Reisen (1947) reported that a chimpanzee raised in total darkness for the first 3 months of life never developed adequate vision. But if chimpanzees are raised in light for the first 3 months and subjected to total darkness for the next 6 months, they quickly regain perfect vision when exposed to light. The analogous situation in humans is found in the child born with strabismus of one eye (thrown to a side focus). Ophthalmologists report that unless that eye is forced to be used, through patching the other eye, by the age of 4 no useful perceptions can ever be developed in it despite the fact that organically it is a perfect organ of vision. It is the central perception of vision which, untrained during critical periods, can never regain function. There seems to be no demonstrated reason why auditory perceptions do not fall into the same category as the visual modality. Whether the auditory irreversibility also occurs by age 4 is difficult to prove, but we feel it is probably fairly comparable with vision.

The reports of animal research supporting a critical period theory of development are numerous. Reisen (1960) reported that chimpanzees showed a reduction in the efficiency of auditory learning following early sensory deprivation of hearing. In addition he found, in cats deprived of visual sensation, three concomitant manifestations: hyperexcitability, increased susceptibility to convulsive disorder, and localized motor dysfunction. This latter experiment has profound implications for the student of deafness. What are the effects on the central nervous system of early hearing deprivation? Many clinicians have described symbolic language disorder, minimal cerebral dysfunction, or other kinds of central involvement in the deaf. Can these disorders be a direct result of the auditory deprivation? If sensory deprivation in animals produces central nervous system disorders, can deprivation have the same result on the human central nervous system?

What has not been considered is the effect of the language deprivation on the deaf infant. If biological theories of language acquisition are correct, then the human infant is just as preprogrammed to develop language skills as he is to develop motor skills. The effect of early sensory deprivation could then be expected to have far-reaching consequences on central nervous system functioning in integrative areas of the brain. The concept of language as a biologically predetermined function thus extends the speculation of early sensory deprivation in humans to another plane where animal research cannot apply. It opens up a whole new area of investigation.

Edwards (1968) has summarized concisely the state of the educator's attitude toward critical periods:

> The supremely difficult feat of building language recognition and response which takes place during the first years of life can occur because there is a built-in neurological mechanism for language learning present in every normal human organism. But like the image on the sensitized negative, this potential will not appear as reality unless the proper circumstances develop it. Experience—the right experience—is essential.
>
> Heredity and environment interact. Hereditary possibilities are shaped by the influence that only human culture can provide; they are potentialities that must be developed while the young neurological organism is still rapidly growing, malleable, open to stimulus. If the "critical periods in learning" hypothesis applies to human beings (as we know it does to other creatures—dogs, for instance—and as evidence increasingly indicates it does to us), then the right experience must come at the right time, or the potential must remain forever unrealized (p. 70).

Edwards' solution to this problem is well worth detailing:

> We are going to have to make educational stimulation available from babyhood on for the children whose families cannot provide it for them. Whether tutors should go into the homes, whether children should be brought into carefully planned, well staffed *educational* (as distinct from baby-sitting day-care) programs, we do not now know. Experiments going on in several places in the country should help us decide. But however we do it, intervention by the age of eighteen months should be the rule for the children of deprived inner-city or poor rural families. (With permission from E. P. Edwards: Kindergarten is too late. Saturday Review, p. 77, 1968.)

Fortunately, since Edwards wrote the above, studies such as those by Heber and Garber (1970), cited in Chapter 4, have confirmed her premise. In addition Herber and Garber have developed the program and materials to implement the early training Edwards proposed.

Although it is difficult to pinpoint the exact age at which it is critical that infants be given language stimulation, a report by Dennis (1973) gives some definitive guidelines. In an institution for homeless children in Lebanon, he tested the foundlings at all ages, before and after their adoption into homes. Those who were adopted by or before age 2 soon reached normal intellectual functioning, with a mean IQ jump of 50 points postadoptively. But those adopted after age 2 never overcame their preadoptive experiential retardation. Dennis concludes that there is a period near the second birthday that is critical for complete recovery from the effects of experiential deprivation.

The beginnings of language learning occur at birth and—who knows?—possibly before birth. Condon and Sander (1974) have shown that the human neonate moves in precise and sustained segments of movements that are synchronous with the articulated structure of adult speech. He is a participant in the rhythm of many repetitive speech structures long before he uses them for communication. These rhythms comprise a prelinguistic activity of the human infant even at birth.

In summary, we are entirely in accord with these theories of the importance of critical periods. Any denial of their importance must be solely a semantic one. The entire section on language as the goal in the selection of the appropriate rehabilitation program is based on the proposition that the best potential language development can be secured only by applying the proper training procedures at an age which will take advantage of critical periods for prelinguistic and linguistic skills.

Disorders in Auditory Learning

Part of the audiologist's task is to determine whether in addition to a peripheral hearing loss there may be another disorder of the auditory system. Chapter 5 details the behavioral clues that should alert the clinician to a possible central auditory problem. In order to understand the central disorders which may produce deviant behavior, it is pertinent to review what is known about the involved pathways and their breakdowns.

The peripheral auditory mechanism extends from the outer ear to the termination of the acoustic nerve in the cochlear nucleus of the brain stem (Goldstein et al., 1972). The neurons leading into the synapse in the nuclei are the auditory input stations for the central nervous system, and we include them functionally in the peripheral system. A lesion at any point along this system results in reduced auditory sensitivity, represented by decreased thresholds for pure tones and speech.

Beyond the cochlear nuclei in the brain stem lie the neurons of the central auditory system, which transmit the auditory information to the brain. Several synapses along the way to the brain begin the coding and analyzing of the information. For example, the neck-turning reflex of the infant to a loud sound is presumed to be mediated at the level of the superior olive. Even at this level and in newborn infants, the reflex can be inhibited by central processing: the normal infant will cease to give a neck turn after several repetitions of the arousing stimulus. The known brain-injured child, on the other hand, once having given this neck-turn response, will be unable to inhibit it on successive presentations of the stimulus (Eisenberg et al., 1966). Even the simple coding system required for inhibiting the reflex will be disrupted by CNS damage.

The complexity of the mechanism involved in merely inhibiting further neck-turn reflexes at the level of the midbrain is awesome. Is it any wonder that we have difficulty understanding what happens to complex auditory information when it finally reaches the brain? The temporal lobe of the brain receives the incoming auditory impulses, in a sequence of increasing complexity. "Wernicke's" area is the primary receiving area for gross interpretation of sound; beyond that lie areas of increasingly complex perception and integration. For example, a primary area perceives "sound or no sound." The next area may perceive "low or high" or "loud or soft"; the next may perceive quality relationships that would distinguish a barking dog from a human voice. And only at the highest level does perception of verbal speech occur and become integrated into cognitive processing.

An example of the higher level of processing was brought home to the author in a unique human instance: a 57-year-old man was referred for auditory testing following brain surgery for removal of a small tumor in the lower part of the left temporal lobe. Preoperatively his speech, hearing, and language were completely normal. The neurologist referred him for testing of "deafness secondary to brain surgery." In the audiologic laboratory it soon became evident that the gentleman was quite able to hear gross sounds, and in a short time learned to raise his hand to the pure tone signals. A perfectly normal, consistent pure tone audiogram was obtained, but no speech tests could be obtained other than as detection thresholds. He neither understood nor could he repeat any sounds accurately. Yet his speech was completely normal, and he was able to read and write without any impairment. When asked in writing what it sounded like when others spoke, he said "When you talk, it sounds as if you are saying 'wurr-wurr-wurr-wurr'." (This is the closest transcription I can make of his description.) Unfortunately the man was lost to follow-up, and we do not know whether he ever recovered any meaningful understanding of speech.

The only hypothesis that can be made in this case is that the small tumor was located in an area of the brain that takes care of auditory verbal integration at the highest level. The surgery damaged vital brain tissue in this area, and resulted in a specific auditory verbal agnosia for speech. It is rare that such a specific diagnosis can be made of a central auditory disorder, and particularly rare in someone who had developed all functions of speech, language, reading, and writing. When such CNS dysfunction is present in a child who has yet to learn all these functions, how can the clinician arrive at a meaningful understanding of the problem?

An example of how long it may take to understand such dysfunction is illustrated by another case history: Brent, a 3-year-old male, the third of eight siblings, presented with a 60-dB sensorineural loss in the right ear, 85 dB in the left. He conditioned very well, and retests over many years showed the same hearing levels. Mother's pregnancy, labor, and delivery history were uneventful. Brent sat alone at 6 months but at 7 months developed meningitis. He was treated with cholomycetin, sulfa, and penicillin. At discharge he was alert, happy, and had no evidence of neurologic disorder. After this disease he did not sit again until 9 months of age, and walked at 11 months. He walks with his left toe turned in and drags it slightly.

At 3 years Brent was fitted with binaural hearing aids and started on an exclusively auditory program. After 6 months he was babbling spontaneously and could localize sounds, but day after day was noted as being "unresponsive to auditory therapy." A Merrill Palmer performance test at this time gave an IQ of 116, and the psychologist noted that although he was visually alert to signs, he had no word comprehension. She felt that there was a specific "auditory comprehension deficit," and noted that "one should not be fooled by his perceptiveness of motor cues and by his perceptiveness of voice inflection into thinking that he understands words."

Six months later the therapist made exactly the same report as before—no meaningful auditory perceptions had been developed in 1 year's time. A psychometric test at that time showed average intelligence on a Leiter scale, and "organic brain damage indications" on a Bender Gestalt test. He could not make simple visual discrimination of forms or perceive and reproduce simple designs.

Brent was then placed in a program emphasizing lip reading and oral training. His teachers reported that he was unable to discriminate any words through lip reading, nor to relate them to reading forms. He mimicked and mouthed words, but only singly. At age 7 he was given an

EEG, which was normal, and another psychometric test. "There were indications that mild neurological dysfunction was interfering with his perceptual motor performance. His nonverbal abilities were good, but his lack of language was the main difficulty." At this time the only method of communication he had was by gesture.

At age 9 Brent was finally sent to the state school to learn signing and finger-spelling, where he has had his only success at learning language—but only through signs and reading. He is still at age 16 not able to finger-spell. He still cannot speak more than single words. Auditory communication is so unrewarding to him that he has not worn an aid for several years. His reading is at the 11-year-old level, and it gives him pleasure, which television listening does not.

This case illustrates one of the fundamental principles in differential diagnosis: that peripheral hearing loss and central disorders are two separate entities, but that they both may exist in the same individual. If tests for auditory acuity show reduced hearing, it is due to a true peripheral lesion, not to a central one. Brent's final diagnosis was "auditory verbal agnosia and visual agnosia for any rapid denotational movements"—all this in addition to a peripheral hearing loss. Each problem must be treated for its own needs, and the combination of problems should, in this case, have been identified sooner.

Goldstein et al. (1972) state, "It is now well established that unilateral, upper level, central nervous system lesions, regardless of their severity, produce no impairment in auditory sensitivity as long as the peripheral auditory mechanism remains intact." The authors cite the electrocochleograms on Rh children reported by Aran (1971) and by Portmann and Aran (1971). The action potentials recorded were clearly from the cochlea, and showed reduced auditory thresholds commensurate with the behavioral audiometry, in contradiction to the long-held view that the hearing loss in Rh incompatibility is due to central lesions. Goldstein et al. point out that even bilateral CNS lesions do not produce reduced auditory acuity, and they conclude, "We know of no clinical instance in which a confirmed central nervous system lesion, at any level, in the presence of a normal peripheral auditory mechanism has led to a reliably measured impairment of auditory sensitivity."

Lindsay (1971b) reported an extraordinary finding on a temporal bone of a man known to be deaf from anoxia at birth. The audiometric findings were typical of hearing loss due to anoxia: normal hearing range at 250 and 500 Hz, with a sudden drop to 95 dB at 2000 Hz. The histopathologic sections of the cochlea showed absolutely no damage to any of the cochlear structures, the spiral ganglia, or the eighth nerve. Lindsay concluded that the damage represented by the audiogram must have been in the cochlear nuclei. Subsequently he has suggested the possibility that the lesion may have been on the input side of the cochlear nuclei synapse (personal communication, 1973). Such a suggestion gives a clearer picture of the delineation between peripheral and central lesions.

Once this separation between central and peripheral lesions is made clear, one can proceed to test for each problem individually, without confusing the two. In the section on auditory testing we will describe auditory tests on children with central problems, based on this premise.

The evaluation and therapy for central auditory disorders is a discipline in itself, and it is not our province to describe this subject in detail. Experts have written extensively on the subject. If we can demonstrate the differentiation between peripheral and central disorders, we will have fulfilled the requirements of clinical audiology. It is difficult enough to understand all that needs to be known about peripheral hearing loss without attempting another monumental task.

However, in order to understand the abnormal we must be familiar with the normal. We have described the infant's auditory behavior development as manifested under experimental conditions. One of the significant factors is the early emergence of auditory reception and the late development of expression. These activities are paced by maturation. The time clock for development is similar in all

children. As Lenneberg (1966) states: "We are, therefore, suggesting as a working hypothesis that the general, non-specific states of maturation of the brain constitute prerequisites and limiting factors for language development. They are not its specific cause."

By 4 months the localization of sounds begins. This is a primary skill, and need not be affected by subtle cerebral dysfunction. When localization does not appear at 4 months of age, it may mean a general retardation of the time schedule. It has been our experience that the infant with auditory central dysfunction is more apt to give a localization response at this age than he will at a later age. As such a child grows older, speech becomes meaningless and his responses to it unproductive. He will eventually cease to respond as there is no survival value in his response to speech. Most often, however, he cannot inhibit his reflexive responses to sound, and these responses will be similar to the child with normal hearing. It is extremely rare that both localization ability and auditory reflexes will be absent in a very young, centrally disordered child. Even an anencephalic infant will give large startle reflexes to loud sound. In fact, he will continue to give them ad infinitum as he is not able to inhibit his response because of lack of cerebral control. So testing proceeds much the same for the brain-damaged child as for the normal child, and if a lack of response is seen, one must believe that it is due to a peripheral lesion. Too many brain-damaged children have had amplification denied because of the erroneous belief that their audiometric loss was due to a central lesion.

By 6 months the infant localizes to very soft speech; by 8 months he imitates some sounds and intonations. To do this, he must have a long period of auditory differentiation, and we know that this skill has been present since birth. Any disruption in the processing of the information disrupts the development of the imitations and of the child's ability to differentiate voice intonations. Usually the 8-month-old child understands the meaning of "no-no" or at least the intonation that accompanies it. When a child is not able to make this differentiation, there begins in his mother the subtle bewilderment that is so often reported by the mothers of centrally-involved children. There is a similarity here between the deaf and the centrally-involved child: neither shows the milestones of prespeech and prelinguistic skills. The lack of integrity in responding to human communication puzzles the mothers of both such children. The mother-child relationship depends upon an interplay between the two. When this becomes a one-way street, with the child's responses to mother subtly lacking in meaningfulness, a deterioration of the relationship begins. If a problem of peripheral deafness is discovered early, understanding soon reverses the interpersonal breakdown. Once the mother recognizes that the child has a sensory loss, but no other deficit, she is able again to "mother" the child appropriately. Such mothering is difficult for the mother of a perceptually disordered child. Often hyperactive to some degree, these are the children whom nobody understands.

In the hierarchy of auditory function, disruption can occur anywhere from the primary receptive areas (auditory agnosia) to higher levels such as inability to integrate the sounds into meaningful units (verbal integration disorder). Auditory signals cannot be coded, interpreted, and carried in memory except for short periods. If the child cannot store the meaning of a sound in his brain, he must forever reinvestigate the sound whenever it is heard. This compulsive behavior of attending to any and all sounds in his environment causes the hyperactivity of this type of child.

But more than discrimination of speech sounds is necessary to language learning. Temporal patterns of speech may be even more significant than frequency formants in perceiving language. It has been demonstrated that if one isolates discrete words on a tape of rapid ordinary conversation, a normal-hearing listener is not able to identify any word in isolation. We do not speak in carefully articulated phonemes; we slur over many sounds, sometimes reducing others to inaudibility. Speech in any language is a Gestalt consisting of distinctive rhythms, durations, intonations, interconnecting transients and almost incidentally specific frequency formants. If one listens to a completely unfamiliar foreign language spoken rapidly, one

appreciates the impossibility of isolating its speech phonemes into recognizable units. Long listening experience with an intact auditory system is necessary to process this information into meaning.

Where it is that a breakdown comes in the listening function is only vaguely understood. Some researchers are painstakingly producing bits of evidence. Friedlander (1970) has demonstrated the kinds of information that will give us insights into the breakdowns in auditory processing. He and DeLara (1973) presented 44 children, 5 to 8 years old, with a choice between the natural sound of a Sesame Street recording and a degraded sound track taped with various levels of distortion. Choices of one or the other were made every 15 seconds. Thirty-three of the children consistently chose the natural, undistorted sound track. The other 11 chose the natural sound slightly more than half the time, or almost at random. All the children were given the Cooperative Primary Tests, developed by the Educational Testing Service. A significant correlation was shown between the listening selections and the score on the listening subtest of the examination, with the nonselective listeners scoring lower. In addition, all of the 11 nonselective listeners were reported by their schools to have a variety of reading and language dysfunctions. The 33 selective listeners were not regarded as having any problems in these learning areas. The authors report that further studies of larger numbers of children show that 25% of the students have similar defective listening functions.

A study such as this reminds us that we have not begun to tap the specific disabilities of auditory learning. Traditionally these dysfunctions have been given names, orders, or hierarchies, and discrete perceptual categories. Traditionally they have also been categorized and defined, almost operationally, by the tests that distinguish them. Lerner (1971) describes these functions and their operations as fourfold:

Auditory discrimination is referred to as the ability to distinguish a difference between phonemes and between words. The Wepman Test of Auditory Discrimination (1958) delineates the understanding of the contrast between two phonemes. The child is asked whether two words presented auditorally (without lip reading) are the same or different: "mit-mat"; "big-pig." The STAP (Screening Test for Auditory Perception) (1969) tests the ability to distinguish between long and short vowels and between initial consonants and consonant blends.

Auditory memory is defined by the ability to store and recall auditory material. In the Detroit Tests of Learning Aptitude—Oral Directions and Oral Commissions (1935), a sequence of three commands is given the child to determine whether he can keep in his memory the three stages of directions. A STAP subtest evaluates a child's ability to remember rhymes.

Auditory sequencing describes the child's ability to remember the order of items in a sequence. "Monday, Tuesday, Wednesday . . .", "ABCD . . ." are sequences whose exact order must be retained in memory. Subtests for this ability include: the Auditory Sequential Memorial Test of the ITPA, the Digit Span Test of the WISC, the Auditory Attention Span for Unrelated Words of the Detroit Test, and the rhythmic pattern tests of the STAP.

Auditory blending (or closure) is defined by the ability to put together isolated phonemic elements into a word: "m . . . a . . . n" to form the word "man." The subtest on Sound Blending and Auditory Closure of the ITPA and the Roswell-Choll Auditory Blending Test describe these operations.

Other workers have further divided the subskills that make up auditory perception, and have formulated various sequential hierarchies of these skills. Messing (1969) describes eight such categories: auditory awareness, auditory focus, auditory figure-background, auditory discrimination, auditory memory, auditory scanning, auditory integration and synthesis, and auditory feedback.

The hierarchy of increasing complexity of listening levels according to Lerner (1971) are (1) auditory perception of nonlanguage sounds; (2) auditory perception and discrimination of isolated single language sounds; (3) understanding of words and concepts, and building of a listening vocabulary; (4) understanding sentences and other linguistic elements of language; (5) auditory memory; and (6) listening comprehension composed of (a) following directions, (b) understanding a sequence of events through listening, (c) recalling details, (d) getting the main idea, (e) making inferences and drawing conclusions, and (f) critical listening.

Lerner further delineates these listening levels by means of the teaching strategies employed. Her descriptions of the range of listening disorders found in children are the most comprehensive to be found.

Tests that are available to evaluate listening skills include: *Peabody Picture Vocabulary Test,* the *Ammons Full Range Picture Vocabulary Test, Van Wagenen Listening Vocabulary Scales, Listening Comprehension Test* (a portion of the *Sequential Tests of Educational Progress*), *Brown-Carlsen Listening Comprehension Test, Durrell Listening-Reading Test,* the *Auditory Reception and Auditory Memory* tests (subtests of the *Illinois Test of Psycholinguistic Abilities*), and the receptive language portion of the *Northwestern Syntax Screening Test.*

Chalfant and Scheffelin (1969) describe various levels of auditory perceiving in an operational manner:

1. Attention to auditory stimuli. A dysfunction in this area results in distractibility, hyperactivity, and attention difficulties.
2. Sound versus no sound. Lowered activity for acoustic signals reduces discrimination and detection abilities.
3. Sound localization. Inability to localize the sound source results in confusion in differentiating people's voices.
4. Discriminating sounds varying in one acoustic dimension. Discrimination is defined as indicating whether two acoustic stimuli are the same or different. Tests which identify this function are the Wepman Test of Auditory Discrimination (1958) and the PERC Test (Drake, 1965).
5. Discriminating sound sequences varying on several acoustic dimensions. Here, groups or patterns of auditory stimuli cannot be reproduced or differentiated.

Tapping tests will show the inability to reproduce rhythmic patterns accurately. Lesions of the premotor region result in such disorders. Familiarity to the taps can give success, so the task must be varied to rule out counting.

6. Auditory figure-ground selection. The child may be unable to attend to a stimulus that is deemed to be significant in the presence of competing insignificant stimuli.

7. Associating sounds with sound sources. This dysfunction is termed "auditory agnosia" and results in the inability to recognize sound patterns such as speech or to establish associations between sounds and their situations and sources.

The above descriptions of the functional hierarchies of auditory processing are useful to the language clinician who must suit the therapy to the specific disorder. For the clinical audiologist whose first task is to distinguish between peripheral and central disorders in a young child or infant—and to apply numerical measures to these functions, another delineation of levels of function must be made.

For the purposes of audiologic testing of these children, the most useful description of auditory processing is a physiologic one. In Chapter 5 we are proposing the use of various auditory reflexes in measuring the hearing of the disordered child (mental retardation, autism, perceptual disorder). To this end it is most useful to relate the specific disorder to a level of neural activity and to see what auditory reflexes occur at the various levels. If we can then distinguish at what levels perceptual auditory disorders occur, we will approach an understanding of the application and limitation of auditory reflexive response measures in the centrally disordered child. Such understanding may also lead toward the development of strategies that will be useful to the clinician in the therapeutic situation.

Relevant Research

We have described the operational definitions of various auditory disorders as they are currently employed in the field. Friedlander and DeLara (1973), previously cited, is one of many provocative investigations from other disciplines that may eventually shed light on the mechanisms involved in auditory dysfunction. Perhaps the greatest contribution in this field has been made by Berlin and Lowe, whose chapter on "Temporal and Dichotic Factors in Central Auditory Testing" in Katz's *Handbook of Clinical Audiology* (1972) presents the scientific data that are available. Their approach to these problems, plus a review of some of the salient information from various discipline-specific publications, permits us to make a gross correlation between the operationally-defined auditory disorders and their underlying brain mechanisms. From this review, we find that certain facts have been established in the literature.

Primacy of Left Hemisphere in Speech and Language, Particularly of the Left Temporal Lobe. Wernicke's area (behind Heschl's gyrus) has been shown anatomically to be larger on the left side in 65% of brains and larger on the right side in only 7% (Geschwind and Levitzky, 1968). The planum temporale is, on the average, one-third longer on the left than the right lobe. This finding correlates with the known specialization of speech and language in the left hemisphere (Penfield and Roberts, 1959; Kimura, 1961; Studdert-Kennedy and Shankweiler, 1970). Right-handedness and right-earedness in most people show the critical nature of the cross-over of sensory messages to the opposite side.

Milner et al. (1968) demonstrated in a dramatic experiment that speech processing in both hemispheres is bound to the left hemisphere. Seven patients with midline section of the cerebral commissures, including the corpus callosum, were given dichotic and monotic competing number tasks. (In dichotic stimulation each ear receives simultaneously a different message, usually speech, from a separate channel of a tape recorder, via earphones. In monotic listening one ear is stimulated at a time by any number of related or unrelated signals.) Milner et al. showed that when each ear of their patients was tested individually on the monotic task with competing numbers, the scores were 100% for both ears. However, when the dichotic mode was presented, there was essentially no perception of speech in the left ear. In other words, the right hemisphere has the ability to perceive speech on a rudimentary acoustic level, but when the right hemisphere is disconnected from the dominant left, the messages that are essential to speech interpretation are not transmitted on to the left hemisphere, resulting in an inability to identify and classify the speech material. Speech information transmission seems to be a one-way street, from the right to the left hemisphere, but not in the opposite direction.

A second task was given to these patients, that of retrieving objects through touch alone, when competing messages were given simultaneously in each ear. In this task, the scores for left-handed retrieval were higher for the objects named through the left ear, while through the right ear there was little success in identifying objects. Moreover, when asked to name the left ear items, the subjects commonly gave the names of the items that had been given through the right ear. The specialization of the left temporal lobe for speech in particular, and of the right temporal lobe for tactile identification, seems well demonstrated here.

In an article aptly entitled "Is Speech Special?" Berlin et al. (1972b) offer experimental corroboration of our contention in this chapter that speech and language facility is preprogrammed in humans. Their normal subjects were given dichotic listening tasks with intensity differences generated between ears. One ear received nonsense syllables at 80 dB SPL, and the other ear received them at as low as 30 dB. As the intensity was varied in one or the other ear, a gradual increase occurred in the scores for the unattenuated ear, and a reciprocal decrease in scores was seen for the attenuated ear, to about 20 dB. Beyond that point the unattenuated ear improved sharply, reaching 100% at a 50-dB difference between ears. A right ear superiority was seen when the intensity condition was equal, and was maintained even with a 10-dB attenuation. However, when the patients with temporal lesions were given these tasks, the results changed.

On three patients with unilateral temporal lobectomies, Berlin et al. then presented the dichotic speech tasks at equal intensities. As expected, the ear contralateral to the lesion gave poorer scores than the ipsilateral ear. However, as the intensity of the ipsilateral signal was increased from threshold in the dichotic task, the intelligibility function of the contralateral ear dropped almost reciprocally. The same decrement was not seen in the presence of an ipsilateral noise signal, when noise was used instead of speech. Berlin hypothesizes that the contralateral ear was signalling its recognition of speech in the ipsilateral ear by gradually reducing its articulation score as the speech elements in the ipsilateral ear became more intelligible. As we have indicated heretofore, it seems evident that speech dimensionality is perceived and attended to by man in a way different from his perception of other acoustic material.

Berlin and his colleagues (1973a, b) have thrown further light on the cerebral dominance of the left temporal lobe in children. Nonsense consonant-vowel (CV) combinations (/pa/, /ta/, /ka/, /ba/, /da/, and /ga/) were used in dichotic speech tests on 150 right-handed children 5 to 13 years old. Precise alignment was made for the simultaneous presentation of a different CV to each ear at the same intensity levels. The results showed that an advantage for the right ear in giving correct responses was already evident in the 5-year-olds, and did not vary with increasing age. Right-earedness for speech and left temporal-lobedness seem definitely established by age 5, lending strength to Lenneberg's (1967) hypothesis on the age of development of handedness as critical to language learning.

Berlin et al. did find that the number of CV's correctly identified increased with age, a factor which they term a reflection of the increasing channel capacity for the children studied.

Nagafuchi (1970) also gave dichotic speech tests to young children and found that by 6 years the adult right-earedness was established. At age 3 a sex difference was found: girls were superior to boys in both dichotic and monotic listening tasks. This finding is in line with known earlier development of speech and language skills in girls.

Tests utilizing speech material show even

more clearly the breakdown of the auditory system and have more clinical applicability to children. Kimura (1961) presented different digits dichotically to both ears of temporal lobectomy patients. When the left temporal lobe was the involved site, the total number of digits reported from the contralateral ear, as well as from both ears, was greatly reduced; whereas in the case of right temporal lobectomy the scores were higher. Kimura concludes from this finding that the crossed pathways are the stronger, and that the left temporal lobe is more important in the perception of spoken material. This perceptive disruption seems analagous to short term memory dysfunction, but is perhaps dependent upon perception rather than on temporal memory.

In interpreting the data on right ear advantages, it should be noted that in normals the advantages are probably related to a combination of acoustic, linguistic, semantic, and possibly procedural variables. However, in patients with lobectomies, the contralateral ear deficit is most likely due to the suppression of the neural homologue of the acoustic event only, not to the encoded linguistic event.

Contralateral Strength of the Auditory System and Its Sensitivity to Temporal Sequence. Auditory encephalographic studies have shown objectively the strength of the contralateral temporal lobe in processing auditory stimuli. Rosenzweig and Rosenblith (1953) stimulated observers' ears with single or paired clicks through earphones. When only one ear was stimulated, the observer localized the sound accurately, and his cortical-evoked responses were larger in the contralateral hemisphere. A similar study by Hirsch (1969) used delays between the two signals, and showed that at some frequencies when the contralateral ear receives the leading signal, the amplitude of the evoked response is larger.

Temporal sequencing takes place in the temporal lobe, and is manifested when breakdowns occur due to lesions in the temporal lobe. Sequencing appears to be critical in auditory processing, and has pertinence to children's auditory dysfunction. Efron (1963) tested aphasic patients with high and low tones, and with red and green lights. The task was to determine the order in which the tones or the lights were presented. The intervals between the two tones were varied, as they were for the lights. The aphasics required as much as 500 msec between the two stimuli to make judgments on the order of presentation both for the tones and the lights. Normal subjects require only a few milliseconds to make the same judgment. Normal central processing thus is shown to be crucial in temporal sequencing.

A breakdown of temporal sequencing in the auditory system occurs uniquely when bilateral temporal lobe lesions are present. Jerger et al. (1969) described specific auditory precedence problems in such a patient on the basis of identifying the order of auditory stimuli as in Efron's study. However, this patient had no difficulty in identifying the visual sequence of red and green lights. Such an experiment differentiates a specific auditory disorder from a generalized aphasic disorder.

Cat studies confirm the sequencing function specific to the temporal lobe. Neff (1961) and Masterton and Diamond (1964) removed the auditory cortex of cats and found that the cats were then unable to judge sequence and order of clicks; all auditory sequence tasks previously learned could not be retrained. Yet the cats could learn simple frequency difference limen and intensity threshold tasks, and could localize a signal to the correct ear.

Dichotic and monotic speech tests using time lags between presentations of two phonemes (time-staggering listening) demonstrate other parameters of the perceptual process. Lowe et al. (1970) systematically separated their CV nonsense syllables by 15, 30, 60, and 90 msec and presented them to normal listeners. In monotic tests, the lead stimulus was more easily perceived by both ears equally at all time intervals, indicating that the precedence of the first signal suppresses the awareness of the second when one ear is stimulated. However, when a dichotic presentation was given, the right ears' scores for both the lead and the lag signals were consistently better than for the left ear, although the lag syllable was more easily perceived by both ears. Improvement of the lag scores was noted as the time interval increased to 90 msec. By that point the left ears' lag scores approximated the right ears' scores.

In an extension of the above study, Berlin and Lowe (1972) separated the syllables from 90 out to 500 msec, and found that they became equally intelligible by 180 msec, with no enhancement of the perception of the lag syllable out to 500 msec. They postulate that a short term memory model would have predicted greater lag effects as time separations increased. If this is true, then what we have traditionally termed defects in short term memory, may actually be defects in signal perception rather than in storage capacity.

The use of time-staggered tests in clinical assessment of recovery after a temporal lobe lesion has been reported by Berlin and Lowe (1972). A patient with a gunshot wound to the superior convolution of the left temporal area was given time-staggered dichotic speech tests. Two months post-trauma there was no lag effect, and the left ear gave the higher scores for both lead and lag positions. One month later the left ear scores were even higher, and the right, lower. Later tests showed further accentuation of the left ear's superiority and the right ear's lowered perception of the speech signals in any position and at any time-staggered intervals up to 500 msec. Berlin and Lowe (1972) identify this progression as demonstrating a growth in perceptual capacity for auditory sequence perception in the left ear, and suggest the use of such tests in monitoring the growth of the right temporal lobe in perceptual capacity. These authors also point out that if this patient's memory for words past 250 msec was impaired, he should have more easily recalled the lagging than the leading signal, and should have had an even greater lag effect than normals. However, as the time-staggers increased he continued to retain a leading left ear stimulus 250 msec longer than the trailing right ear signal.

These studies have demonstrated that the ability of temporal auditory sequencing is specific to the temporal lobe, and that it has primacy in the left temporal lobe. They also cast some doubts on our traditional definition of short term memory. Instead of being related to disruption of storage of signals, it may be that it is perceptual breakdowns related to temporal lobe functioning that create what we have called defective short term memory problems.

Specialization of Left Temporal Lobe in Extraction of Linguistic Features of Speech. A group of research reports in which the dichotic listening performance was assessed, indicate in detail the further specialization of the auditory temporal lobe. Studdert-Kennedy and Shankweiler (1970) presented consonant-vowel-consonant nonsense syllables dichotically to their subjects, manipulating only one of the sounds of the CVC, the initial or final consonant, or the vowel. They found that the right ears of their subjects perceived all consonants better than the left ear, but that the right and left ears perceived the vowels equally.

Differences in perception of consonants based on the manner of their production have been reported in several studies. Lowe et al. (1970) and Thompson et al. (1972) found in dichotic speech tests a marked advantage for the unvoiced consonant over the voiced consonant. In an effort to determine whether this advantage is based on some unknown process of selection in the auditory cortex or on an artifact of the test condition, Berlin et al. (1972a) revised the test condition. They hypothesized that when both bursts of the CV's are initiated simultaneously, the boundary of the unvoiced CV's occurs later in time than that of the voiced onset CV's. They were able, using an electromechanical delay line, to align the onset of the large amplitude vocalic portion of two syllables. When a voiced syllable competed against an unvoiced syllable, the alignment gave the voiced syllable a lag in comparison to the initial plosion of the unvoiced syllable. The results of this test on normal subjects showed that the advantage of voiceless over voiced consonants was markedly reduced.

Berlin et al. (1972a) explain the differences engendered by the alignment change in terms of some switching-sensitive mechanism in the auditory nervous system which must coordinate the two ears into one listening world. They propose that when the voiceless CV's onset is simultaneous with the voiced CV, the central "processor" would view a voiceless CV as coming later because of its long burst duration.

When the onset of the voiced consonant was moved over in time so that the vocalic onsets of both CV's coincided, the voiced CV's were more equally intelligible with the unvoiced. Berlin et al. (1972a) explain this phenomenon as demonstrating the time-limited nature of the auditory analyzer as it processes the incoming CV's: "If it is interrupted in its analysis, it is 'switched,' perhaps by a large amplitude periodicity cue, to analyze the new signal coming in, thus enhancing the lag signal's intelligibility independent of the ear from which the CV arrived."

From early infancy, the child is stimulated by the acoustic signals generated by vocal tract movement, and Berlin et al. (1972a) believe the child may be organizing his nervous system around this stimulation. An experiment by Sussman (1971) is cited to support this hypothesis. He gave subjects the task of tracking target tones in the right or left ear using either tongue or right hand as controllers. He found that the tongue functioned better when working with the right ear than with the left ear, but there were no differences when the right hand was used.

Even semantic and syntactical levels of information can be subjected to fine research analysis. Lewis (1970) used as his dichotic speech material pairings of words having low associative strength, high associative strength (nonsynonyms) and also low associative strength (synonyms). Lewis' results indicated that the unattended message (low associative strength) is perceptually analyzed and can interfere with the perception of the attended message (high associative strength). He did not report whether there was a right ear advantage, as might be expected.

A dichotic study by Zurif and Sait (1970) did show right-eared laterality effect with nonsense sentences which were either structured or unstructured. The structured sentences were modified from a primary reader, and the connective words were included. These sentences were read with normal intonation. The unstructured list was read without intonation, "like a laundry list." The results showed that the structured material produced the larger laterality effect. Whether this effect demonstrates that it is syntax that is better perceived

in the right ear, or that rhythm and intonation are crucial elements in the learning of speech and language, is a moot question. We prefer the latter explanation. Language learned through auditory signals must be inseparable from the signals produced by changes in inflection, loudness, and rhythm. When these features are tasked in a fine test such as dichotic listening, they would logically be associated with the language area in the left temporal lobe. Perhaps the task tests both these features and syntax as well, but it is difficult to see how they can be separated.

The bold experiments of Penfield and Rasmussen (1968) of stimulating the exposed cortex with electrical probes give us an idea of the localization of various auditory functions. Their studies show that only the temporal lobe close to the fissure of Sylvius will produce auditory sensory responses. The patients report hearing simple sounds (motor sound, crickets, knocking, buzzing, etc.). The points of stimulation from which responses were obtained are shown in Figure 3.1. Penfield and Rasmussen state that the majority of the responses were found in Brodmann areas 42 and 22, the "auditopsychic" area. When stimulation was given at point "A" in Figure 3.1, the patient reported that he felt as if he were singing. At

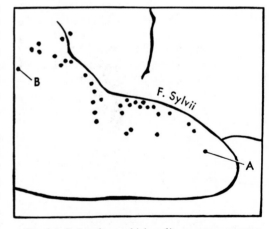

Fig. 3.1. Points from which auditory responses were obtained by stimulation of right and left hemisphere shown above as though all stimulation was done on the right side. (With permission from W. Penfield and T. Rasmussen: The Cerebral Cortex of Man. New York, Hafner Publishing Co., 1968.)

point "B" another patient heard a quiet buzzing. These points are considered out of the primary auditory area. The "audiosensory" area (41 of Brodmann) lying within the fissure of Sylvius on Heschl's convolution, could be stimulated only once, resulting in a ringing sensation. Whenever sound was produced at any point, it was heard in the contralateral ear in most instances. In general, Penfield and Rasmussen felt that stimulation close to the fissure of Sylvius was more apt to produce simple tones, ringing, etc., whereas stimulation at a distance on the first temporal convolution tended to produce some interpretation of sound. Thus he concluded that interpretive elements are seen in the secondary auditory area rather than the primary area.

Penfield and Rasmussen feel that their studies indicate that there is some degree of intellectual function localized to the temporal cortex. Only in the temporal regions will electrical stimulation (as well as epileptic discharge) activate acquired synaptic patterns, not in other brain areas. Therefore they postulate that the organization of the temporal cortex is evidently different from that of other areas of the brain. For the reader's information, Penfield and Rasmussen's chart of the areas of the brain where various functions are considered to be localized is shown in Figure 3.2.

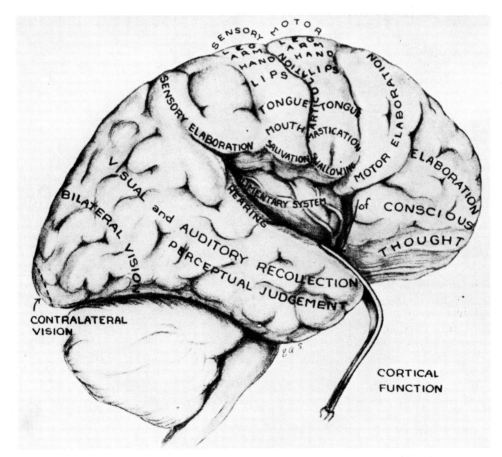

Fig. 3.2. Cortical function. This illustration will serve as a summary restatement of conclusions, some hypothetical (e.g., the elaboration zones), others firmly established. The suggestion that the anterior portion of the occipital cortex is related to both fields of vision rather than to one alone is derived from the results of stimulation. (With permission from W. Penfield and T. Rasmussen: The Cerebral Cortex of Man. New York, Hafner Publishing Co., 1968.)

Midbrain's Function as a Binaural Integration Mechanism and the Mediator of Lateralization Phenomena. Two-ear fusion was first demonstrated by Matzker (1959) by means of a dichotic integration test. In one ear of normal listeners he presented a speech signal through a 500- to 800-Hz band-pass filter and in the other ear the same speech signal through an 1815- to 2500-Hz filter. Neither band could be discriminated alone, but when both were presented dichotically, frequency fusion occurred and speech sounded normal. When patients with later-demonstrated, postmortem degeneration of ganglion cells through the olivary regions were given these tests, they made many errors. It appears that integration of binaural signals occurs at a low level in the olivary complex.

The psychophysical judgment of sidedness, or localization of auditory stimuli, is mediated at the level of the accessory superior olivary complex, according to Hall (1965). In terms of a model suggested originally by von Bekesy and later by Van Bergeijk (1962), Hall considers that the superior olivary nucleus can be regarded as a transducer that converts differences of interaural time and intensity into differences of the number of cells excited in the left and right accessory nuclei. On anesthetized cats, he measured the spike discharges in the nucleus as related to click stimuli that were presented in various time and intensity configurations. He found that time and intensity configurations did indeed affect the number of cells excited in the superior nucleus. The manner of excitation was consistent with results from psychophysical experiments in humans on binaural localization (Deatherage and Hirsh, 1959). Further confirmation was given by Galambos et al. (1959) of the site in the superior olivary nucleus as the mediator of localization.

However, it appears that in man the interaction of the auditory temporal lobe is requisite to localization-lateralization ability—or that the transaction required in reporting the sidedness sensation depends on an intact temporal lobe. In the previously cited studies of Neff (1961) and Masterton and Diamond (1964), decorticated cats were able to localize a signal to the correct ear. Yet Sanchez-Longo and Forster (1958) showed that patients with diseased temporal lobes had poor abilities in localizing sound in sound field when it arrived first to the ear contralateral to the lesion. Matzker (1959) demonstrated that accurate lateralization of sine wave pulses, presented dichotically under earphones with time leads, occurred in normal listeners when the time delays were as small as .018 msec. But in patients with temporal lobe lesions, the lateralization reports were greatly reduced in accuracy.

The ability of decorticated cats to localize a signal may represent the same level of functioning as the head-turn reflex in newborn infants. Both are mediated at the brain stem level. But when a semantic transaction is involved in both lateralization and localization, the picture may be clouded by the necessity of cognitive functioning, which occurs in the temporal lobe. Whether the localization of the 4-month-old infant involves a cognitive transaction or is a residual of the head-turn reflex, is an interesting point.

Another experimental procedure has been used to confirm the function of the midbrain in certain integration and cancellation mechanisms. Feldmann (1965) utilized the "release from masking" phenomenon which has been used to compare normals with patients who had temporal lobe lesions. In this task, speech material is given to an ear along with a masking noise sufficient to reduce the intelligibility of the speech. When the same masking is introduced into the opposite ear but 180° out of phase, there is an improvement in intelligibility scores, indicating that the out-of-phase masking in the opposite ear has released the tested ear from some of the masking effects. This test is presumed to rely on midbrain mechanisms.

Cullen and Thompson (1973) confirmed the site-of-function operative in this test by comparing normal test scores with those of temporal lobectomized patients. They used CNC lists (Peterson and Lehiste, 1962) at 60 dB SPL and filtered noise at 63 dB SPL in the test ear. This combination reduced the normals' discrimination to 40%, and that of the patients to about 33%. (The patients with lesions had poorer discrimination scores in all tests.) But when out-of-phase masking was introduced into the ear contralateral to the test ear, both normals and lobectomized patients showed almost equal gains in discrimination of the CNC words (20% to 31% in the normals, 20% to 29%

in the patients). Cullen and Thompson propose that this experiment indicates that release phenomena are mediated by two-ear interaction at the subthalamic level, subserved by the same neural mechanisms which play a role in the lateralization-localization phenomena described above. If the auditory cortex were active in suppressing signal pathways for speech, it would be expected that much poorer release scores would be obtained.

Bocca and Calearo (1963) have presented classic studies on the use of distorted speech tests in identifying the level of interruption in the auditory pathway. They applied the following tests to normals and to patients with unilateral temporal lobe tumors.

1. Low pass filtered speech tests using PB lists of 10 disyllabic meaningful words sent through a low pass filter that eliminated the frequencies above 800 Hz. The temporal lobe patients showed markedly reduced discrimination scores in the ear contralateral to the lesion. Normals elicit scores of 70% to 80% whereas the patients with tumors gave scores of 50% in the contralateral ear, 65% to 75% in the ipsilateral ear. Hodgson (1967) confirmed these findings on a patient with left hemispherectomy after temporal lobe damage. The scores for filtered speech tests were consistently lower in the right ear than the left, both pre- and postoperatively.

2. Time-compressed speech in which speech is speeded up on a tape recorder, leaving the acoustic spectrum intact. Although Bocca and Colearo found reduced discrimination scores on this test in ears contralateral to temporal lobe lesions, the results were not as significant as those for frequency-distorted speech.

3. Interrupted speech, in which the speech signal is either electronically chopped or blank pieces of tape are interposed between segments of the recorded speech. Bocca and Calearo found no reduction of discrimination scores on temporal lobe patients who were given this task, indicating that the test assesses brain stem function rather than cortical integration. Berlin et al. (1972a) indicate that in patients with brain stem lesion, periodic interruption of the speech signal does produce lowered discrimination scores.

It is therefore evident that interrupted speech tests provide another tool for assessing brain stem function, but that frequency distorted speech and time-compressed speech stress the cortical level of the auditory pathways.

Note that we have not included the cochlear nuclei in our discussion of brain stem lesions. This is because no evidence is available showing that cochlear nuclei damage results in symptoms any different from that of the usual peripheral findings. Reduced pure tone speech thresholds and speech discrimination commensurate with the configuration of the audiogram have been our findings in cases with implied cochlear nuclei damage due to hypoxia and kernicterus. Lindsay's previously discussed observations (1971b) of the normal cochlear findings in a case of hypoxia with a markedly dropping, high frequency audiogram confirm that damage to the cochlear nuclei was in all probability responsible for the hearing loss. In cases of Rh incompatibility with reduced audiograms, it has been our experience that in the absence of marked central damage, children who are given intensive auditory training from an early age have adequate discrimination for speech—as good as that of any peripheral hearing loss with similar audiometric configurations.

We must constantly reiterate the fact that any lesion higher than the cochlear nuclei does not result in a reduction of hearing acuity. All of the studies cited show that temporal lobe lesions, and even hemispherectomies, demonstrate normal acuity on pure tone audiometric tests. The auditory dysfunctions which are present in such cases are more subtle, and can only be demonstrated by the kinds of tests we have described.

Discussion. We have spent a great deal of time reviewing the above literature because we feel it has relevancy to diagnosis and to therapies for central auditory dysfunctions. A wide range of possible strategies has not yet been touched, when one considers the complexity of the auditory nervous system exemplified in the research reports described. If we relate the categories of auditory dysfunction described by Lerner (1971) to the studies reported, some provocative questions emerge.

Auditory Discrimination. The analysis of the features of speech phonemes, particularly the consonants, is shown to be predominately a function of the left temporal lobe (Studdert-Kennedy and Shankweiler, 1970). Right-earedness is demonstrated in many studies referred to above. Speech information transmission was shown by Milner et al. (1968) as proceeding only from the right to the left hemisphere, not in the opposite direction. Binaural fusion, on the other hand, was shown to take place at the midbrain (Matzker, 1959).

Can we determine in children whether there are breakdowns in their right-earedness— whether consideration should be given to concentrating training on one ear or the other? Berlin et al. (1973b) were able to give dichotic speech tests on children as young as 5 years old, Nagafuchi (1970) on 3-year-olds.

Can we determine in children whether there is a breakdown in binaural fusion due to a midbrain disruption? Matzker's frequency-fusion tests seem simple enough to give to young children, and would offer direction to earedness therapy.

Auditory Memory. The hypothesis of Berlin and Lowe (1972) that in temporal lobectomies apparent defects in short term memory may really be defects in signal perception rather than in memory storage may have some relevance to therapies for children assumed to have central auditory dysfunction.

Can it be demonstrated that proper training of perception and discrimination for speech as suggested above, will accomplish improvement in auditory memory dysfunctions? If so, strategies for therapy could be revised accordingly.

Auditory Sequencing. If a relation can be made between the operations defining auditory sequencing disorders and the studies described by Efron (1963) and Jerger et al. (1969), diagnostic and therapeutic methods take on new dimensions. Jerger and associates demonstrated that tests of different sensory modalities distinguished a specific auditory disorder from a generalized aphasic disorder.

Can the temporal sequencing tests, described by Efron and Jerger et al. be applied to children to determine the specific nature of their dysfunction? If a specific auditory sequencing problem is identified, may it be related to earedness, and what kinds of therapeutic strategies might be evolved?

Auditory Blending (or Closure). The time-staggered dichotic tests of Lowe et al. (1970) and Berlin et al. (1972a) may have relevance to the child's inability to perceive isolated speech sounds as a whole. They showed that in one ear listening, the lead stimulus is more easily perceived, the first signal suppressing the awareness of the second. However, in dichotic listening the right ear scores for both lead and lag signals were better than the left, although the lag syllable was perceived better by both ears than the lead. Berlin et al. postulate that this result should probably be interpreted as a perceptual interference function rather than a disruption of short term memory function.

Can auditory blending problems be related to earedness in children, or to a breakdown in perception? If so, then therapeutic strategies would be best directed toward these avenues.

The presentation of such possible correlations between behavioral phenomena in children and the lesion localization demonstrated by the studies cited requires a great deal of temerity—something possessed in full measure by the authors. We are quite aware of the simplistic nature of our attempted correlation and its vulnerability to attack. The point we are making is that so long as clinicians continue to look at the child with central auditory problems only in terms of his behavior on standard speech and auditory tests, no progress will be made in developing strategies to ameliorate the problems.

Dyslexia

Problems in reading skills seem to be mounting in direct ratio with the escalating demands of our culture for higher learning abilities. Normally-functioning children in every other respect are emerging in increasing numbers with deficiencies in reading abilities. An assortment of therapies for reading disorders has proliferated throughout the country, all reporting improvements on the basis of various strategies. None has come forth with the panacea—a permanent cure for the problem.

Few people have made any relation between reading dysfunction and auditory skills, yet the two may be more closely dependent than has been thought. Zigmund (1966, 1973) was able to show that dyslexia may be related specifically to auditory problems. She compared paired associate learning of normal children with that of children with reading disabilities. Her evidence showed that the dyslexic children organized and used psychologic processes in a different way, on the basis of differences in auditory integration abilities.

Can one predict reading dysfunction on the basis of any known auditory tests? Some research suggests that it can be done. DeHirsch et al. (1966) found two auditory perception tasks that made a significant contribution to her predictive reading index: the Wepman Auditory Discrimination Test and the Imitation of Tapped-out Patterns Test. Dykstra (1966) found five measures that contribute 'to a predictive reading index: (1) discrimination between the difference between initial sounds of words (pat-bat); (2) identification of the rhyming elements in the final sounds of words; (3) identification of correct pronounciation of words; (4) use of auditory clues with context clues to identify unfamiliar words; and (5) discrimination between the differences in final consonants and rhymes.

The Illinois Test of Psycholinguistic Abilities (Kirk et al., 1968) subtests on auditory short-term memory and grammatic closure have been shown to identify reading disabilities.

One must appreciate the direct relationship between previous language experience and the learning of reading. When children come to the reading-learning task with inadequate previous language, as many of the hearing-impaired do, reading becomes a laborious process. As Lenneberg (1967) points out, ". . . the deaf come in contact with language at an age when other children have fully mastered this skill and when perhaps the most important formative period for language establishment is already on the decline."

How to teach reading to a child who has not had adequate previous language experience? The solution in many schools has been to teach reading through theoretical grammar—the use of sentences learned through the drilling of nouns, verbs, adjectives, and their place in the language structure. Lenneberg calls this "a situation in which the children are on the one hand quantitatively deprived of a large body of examples, and on the other hand are immedi-

ately given a meta-language, a language about the language which they do not have." Although we •know the extent of language retardation in the deaf population at large, the wonder is that their level of achievement is as high as it is (Fig. 3.3).

No one has yet devised a man-made system as effective for teaching language rules either to the deaf or to the normal child, as was provided by biological evolution. In our struggle to reproduce the process, we have created intellectual dead ends. Language develops naturally through hearing endless repetitions of sounds, words, inter-relationships between words, and corresponding meanings. It will be our contention that if such endless repetitions bombard the deaf child in early infancy, whether through signs or acoustic signals, language will be learned as it has been programmed to be learned. Reading follows as the natural cultural accretion of the fundamental skill of language.

In the neural mechanisms previously discussed that are involved in auditory dysfunction, we may yet find a link with reading disorders. Evidence in the literature on acquired dyslexia points to a relationship between the two.

For example, Geschwind (1962) notes that

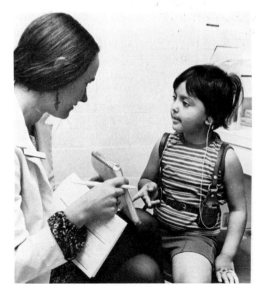

Fig. 3.3. Language and speech development is a life-long task for the profoundly deaf child.

the brain lesion producing alexia usually destroys color-naming ability, but does not affect the ability to name objects and numbers. He suggests that the reason is that objects are learned through multisensory associations including tactile, auditory, kinesthetic, and olfactory sensations. Numbers are learned originally by using our fingers. But both letter-naming and color-naming involve purely arbitrary connections between the auditioned name and the visualized letter configuration. Objects exist as separate entities in the world; letters do not. In order to make the connection between letters and a name (auditoralized), one must proceed from the purely visual configuration directly to the name—a fairly tenuous pathway from one section of the brain to another. Any slight disruption of this connection could result in dyslexia. But even if the visual-language connections are destroyed, objects can be named because the large number of other sensory modes that have been trained allow alternate anatomic routes to be taken.

Confirmation of this theory is found in reports of a few individuals with brain lesions who had formerly been able to read both English and Chinese ideographic language. These individuals, post-trauma, lost the ability to read phonetic English but were able to read the ideographic language. The latter uses symbols related to objects and apparently stimulates more learned sensory and motor associations (Gardner, 1973).

Recently, Rozin et al. (1971) applied this theory to therapeutic procedures for severely dyslexic children. They gave English meanings to 30 different Chinese ideograms and were successful in teaching eight second grade children to read them in a few hours. They recommend that these children initially be given characters that represent words rather than sounds, and that a transition be made through a system of syllables each representing a phoneme in one configuration.

When one recalls the subtle auditory breakdowns described by Milner et al. (1968) in patients with commissural section—patients who had already learned speech and language—and the effects of other neurologic lesions in the perception of speech and language, it can be understood that the disruption of delicate pathways may result in various degrees of dysfunction in the visual-auditory realm. Research designs such as those described for auditory disorders may shed light on the relationships between the visual and the auditory connections in dyslexia.

Final Note

If the point of view we have taken in this chapter appears strange to speech pathologists, language therapists, and reading therapists, it must be remembered that it is the point of view of clinical audiologists. In order to fulfill our task of identifying hearing impairment, we must look at the child in a different way—as a basic, reactive organism rather than as a presently behavior-specific child. We must move into the broad stream of investigating disorders as developmental phenomena. We must identify what has occurred in the maturational sequence as well as what the status quo presents. The two approaches are not inseparable, and with time it is hoped that they may become one.

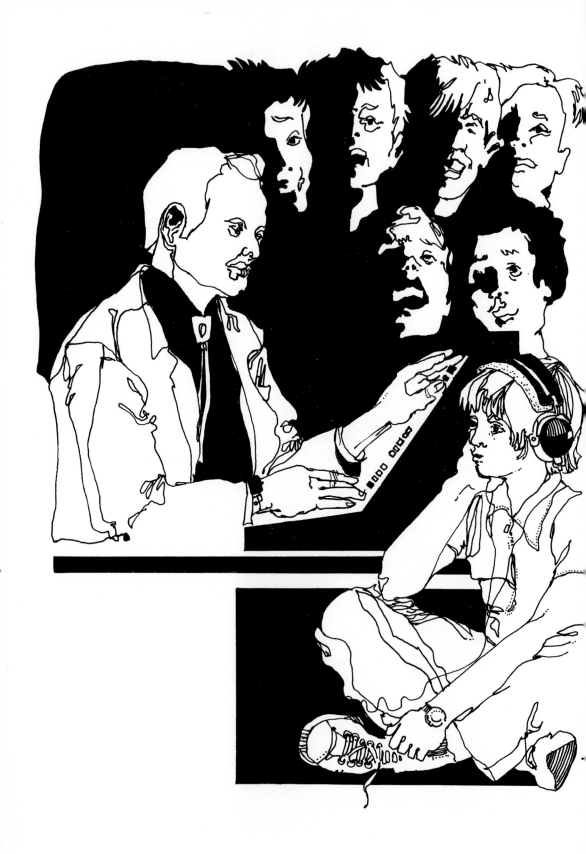

4 IDENTIFICATION AUDIOMETRY WITH CHILDREN

Screening is the process of applying to large numbers of individuals certain rapid, simple measurements that will identify those individuals with a high probability of disorders in the function tested. A criterion measurement point is always involved, below or above which the individuals are suspects. Screening is not intended as a diagnostic procedure; it merely surveys large populations of asymptomatic individuals in order to identify those suspected of having the disorder, who require more elaborate diagnostic procedures.

Screening for hearing loss in the public schools has been an acceptable practice since 1927. It has been judged to identify successfully the child with a hearing loss that is educationally handicapping (Downs et al., 1965). The literature abounds with descriptions of the progress of audiometric screening dating from the introduction in 1927 of the Western Electric 4-C group speech test (McFarlan, 1927), up to the designation in recent years of the individual pure tone sweep test as the most acceptable tool for hearing screening in the schools (Darley, 1961).

One also sees reports in the literature concerning a series of attempts that have been made to screen the hearing of 2- to 5-year-olds in as acceptable a way as the hearing of the school child (Downs, 1954; Mencher and McCulloch, 1970). Programs for screening newborns are only now being recommended and have not yet been implemented universally (Downs and Silver, 1972). It seems that screening of the school-aged child is the only entrenched hearing screening program in the child sphere.

Inasmuch as in this book we are suggesting some innovational approaches to screening methodology at all ages, it might be well to look at the philosophy of screening as viewed, not from the limited view of hearing screening alone but from the vantage point of all the health sciences. A great many Public Health agencies have taken a long, hard look at the theoretical framework of screening. Discussion

of such a framework may help us to re-evaluate the entire structure of our previous approaches to hearing screening. From this discussion will derive a new set of goals for screening that lead in turn to some suggested changes in the methodology of screening.

Public Health Aspects of Screening

Screening for disease as early as possible in the child's life is now an accepted Public Health mandate. It has been recognized that the status of health and the delivery of health care in the United States is considerably lower than that of many other countries of the world. As of 1970, among the nations of the world, the United States ranked 18th in male life expectancy at birth and 13th in infant mortality at birth. The latter is among the commonly accepted indices of the status of health care.

Another accepted indicator of health system functioning is the prevalence of otitis media in a population. The most thorough epidemiologic study of this disease was reported by Eagles et al. in Pittsburgh (1967). They found 15.2% of the entire school population to have otologic abnormalities in one or both ears, indicative of past or present ear disease. In a 5-year follow-up study, 1,200 of these children—almost 30% of the original population screened—either had otoscopic abnormalities prior to the study or developed such during the 5-year period.

Few reports are available that compare our otitis media statistics with those of other countries, but if one can use perforated eardrums as an index, Hinchcliffe (1972) reports the following:

Finland	7	per	1000
Guam	8	per	1000
Denmark	10	per	1000
USA	20	per	1000
USR	41	per	1000
Navajo	53	per	1000
India	62	per	1000
Alaskan (Eskimo)	300	per	1000

93

Audiologic screening for hearing loss has identified similar differences in populations. For example, Fay (1972) has found that among disadvantaged, "inner city" children in New York, 19% failed screening tests and were found to have abnormal hearing. Compare this figure with other similarly conducted screening programs of the total school population. Such programs may produce only 2½% abnormal hearing (Doster, 1972), 90% of which is due to medically remediable ear problems.

Wood (1972) in a preliminary study of Navajo Indian school children found 5% with ear disease requiring surgery. This does not include nontreatable conditions or evidence of previous ear disease, which numbered an additional 20%.

A perspective on the causes of a high prevalence of otitis is provided by an anecdote concerning an Alaskan village which had originally reported an unusually high rate of otitis media. Oil was discovered near the village. This discovery resulted in a much improved standard of living, and chronic otitis media all but disappeared, without any change in direct state or federal health services (Beal, 1972).

These are grim facts, but even grimmer is the direct relationship of handicaps and diseases of all sorts to the condition of poverty. Data from the *Statistical Abstract of the United States*, 1967, showed that states with the highest per capita income have the lowest infant mortality, and those at the bottom of the economic ladder have the highest infant mortality (Gold, 1970). The development of the child beyond infancy is also affected by poverty conditions and the health of the mother. Charles Lowe, Scientific Director of the National Institute of Child Health and Human Development, stated in 1970 before the Senate Select Committee on Nutrition and Human Needs: "Malnutrition, high infant mortality and prematurity rates and high levels of mental deficiency co-exist as the constellation of abnormalities that are most frequent among families living in poverty" (Gold, 1970). The fact that maternal deprivation during pregnancy, and infant deprivation during the neonatal period, can seriously endanger the mental and physical development of the child is reported by Richard Masland (Gold, 1970):

"Mothers whose diets during pregnancy were deficient in proteins had children whose IQ's at age four were, on the average, 16 points below children born to women who were on more normal diets during pregnancy. Negroes outnumbered whites more than four to one among women whose diets were deficient in protein. This finding suggests some slow learning responses observed among children who live in poverty could be accounted for by the malnourished state of their mothers during pregnancy.

Most neurological problems resulted from prematurity (frequently caused by malnutrition of the expectant mother). At three years of age, children who had survived severe hypoxia during birth showed only minor neurological defects." (From E. M. Gold: Prevention of mental retardation. In Earlier Recognition of Handicapping Conditions in Childhood: Proceedings of a Bi-Regional Institute, p. 69. University of California, Berkeley, School of Public Health, 1970.)

Approximately 30 to 50 million Americans are poor; of these, perhaps 15 million are children (Powell, 1970). Not only do these children suffer physiologic deficits because of poverty, but they are also blighted in their intellectual capacities as a result of other deprivations. Wherever both high quality language stimulation and a variety of experiences are not available to the infant, irreversible cognitive deficits result.

The effect of a poor environment on intellectual function has been dramatically demonstrated by the studies of Heber and Garber in Milwaukee (1970). These authors conducted a survey on the IQ's of slum-dwelling children, revealing that the children of mothers with IQ's below 80 show a progressive decline in mean intelligence as age increases. Furthermore, the survey data showed that the lower the maternal IQ, the lower the child's IQ tended to be. Heber and Garber hypothesized that the mentally retarded mother in the slums creates a social deprivation which predetermines the child's IQ.

To test their hypothesis Heber and Garber instituted a longitudinal investigation on 40 slum-dwelling mothers with IQ's of 70 or less. A random number of these mothers and children were assigned to an experimental group for comprehensive intervention. Soon after these mothers returned from the hospital, their infants were given a precisely structured program of stimulation at an Infant Education Center. The mothers were given a program of homemaking, baby care, and occupational training.

A variety of measures were applied at different age levels to the experimental group as well as to the control group. The most dramatic of the results were the mean IQ levels of the two groups, as shown in Figure 4.1. These data represent Cattel and Binet IQ scores obtained at intervals between 24 and 42 months, on both groups. A contrast group is also shown, representing the mean IQ's of the offspring of mothers with IQ's below 75, taken from the original population survey. The difference between the mean IQ's of the experimental group and those of the control group was 33 IQ points. On all language measures, the experimental group was also markedly superior to the control group at every age level that measures were applied. The similarity between the control group and the contrast group substanti-

ates the validity of the differences between them and the experimental group. It is also depressing to see the fall-off in IQ scores of the contrast group during later years. Unfortunately this decline is what can be predicted for the control group because no intervention has occurred.

Heber and Garber's study is a classic reference for all disciplines. It points the way not only to preventive measures for mental retardation but to possible massive intervention in other areas. What would be the effects on ultimate ear disease if large scale medical treatment were applied to all slum children in infancy? What would be the result if the mothers were taught to apply good aural hygiene to their infants? What effect would good nutrition have on these children?

Whatever the implications of this study, it is abundantly clear that something happened to separate the children with 130 IQ's from the children with 80 IQ's. It follows that making something happen in all areas of handicapping conditions is a good thing, devoutly to be sought.

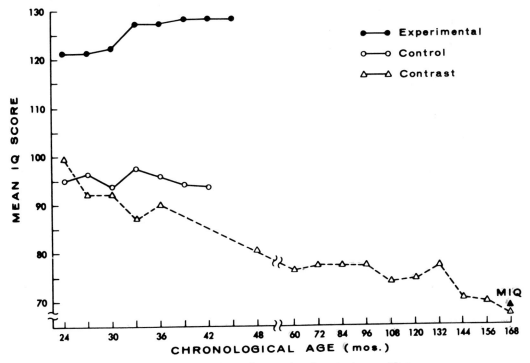

Fig. 4.1. Experimental, control, and contrast group IQ scores.

Particularly poignant in the examination of these statistics is the evident fact that the most humanitarian and effective solution for most of the problems would be the improvement of the quality of life in these United States. There is no need to regard poverty as a crime—to sustain the notion that there is a class of people who are shiftless and should be forced to work or be denied help. HEW's own statistics show that able-bodied men comprise less than 1% of the people on welfare; that half of those on welfare are children; and that the rest are mothers, the blind, the disabled, or those too old to work. Furthermore, many poor people do work, but their low-paying jobs do not provide adequate income to support their families. This is the quality of life for too many Americans.

Belle Dubnoff has pointed up further problems in the psychologic and psycholinguistic area related to early deprivation (1970):

"We have found learning disabilities at a very early age in children who come from unfavorable backgrounds, in which they have been exposed to inconsistency of treatment and lack of stimulation to the point where trust in the mother or caretaker could not be built up. These children are restless, have short attention spans, and are unable to perform in a preschool situation. They are deprived in the language area because no one has taken the time to talk with them and to listen to them. Because they have received no gratification from successful participation in tasks and in social situations, they are easily frustrated and disappointed; and they are fearful or unmotivated in attempting other tasks. They have not learned to discharge frustration, tension, and aggression except in very primitive ways. They have been unable to substitute words for action; and all their conflicts, disappointments, and disturbances are usually transferred from the home directly to the nursery school." (From B. Dubnoff: Early detection and remediation of learning disabilities. In Earlier Recognition of Handicapping Conditions in Childhood: Proceedings of a Bi-Regional Institute, pp. 132-133. University of California, Berkeley, School of Public Health, 1970.)

Dubnoff also reports that it is now generally accepted that learning patterns are set by 2 years of age and cognitive patterns by age 4. It seems that the target year for prevention of intellectual deficits of any sort is the first year of life.

The relevance of all these facts to the child deprived of hearing from birth is inescapable. No language deprivation is so complete as that resulting from deafness; none requires greater efforts to overcome. But steps are being taken in many areas to remedy these situations. One of the steps is the development of screening programs for all the conditions that are amenable to early treatment or prevention. The Department of Health, Education, and Welfare has sponsored meetings in recent years directed at evaluating both the needs for screening of various diseases and the state of the screening art in those areas. The concensus has been that our knowledge in such fields as biochemistry, cytogenetics, and immunology reached a high state in the 1960's, but that these and other bodies of knowledge have far outstripped the action that has been taken to use them. Where has the action been, if any? We can point with pride in some areas.

A number of simple and accurate tests have been developed for the screening of newborns for hereditary metabolic defects. Legislation requiring compulsory screening at birth for phenylketonuria has been enacted in many states. Further efforts are being made to develop tests that will identify the asymptomatic carriers of hereditary metabolic defects. A mass attack on preventable or treatable mental retardation may see a real decrease in this handicap in the next few years (Hsia, 1970).

Whether a similar attack on experiential deprivation can be successfully launched remains to be seen. The target population is certainly well defined, but the means are not so clear. Early child care programs offer the most promising solutions, provided they can be instituted with due respect to the dignity of the individual. The involvement of the parents and their right to freedom of choice in a program must be respected. The social stakes are high enough to warrant giving a high priority to solving these problems. When one considers that of the 7% of the gross natural product that was spent in 1970 on Health, only 10¢ was spent for child health as against every dollar for geriatric care (Richmond, 1972), it becomes apparent that a shifting of priorities is in order.

Where does the state of the art of hearing screening stand in relation to that of the physical and mental deficits outlined above? It compares very well indeed, despite the fact that there is still much to be done, and some of us tend to lose patience at the delays. We have in our hands highly developed tools, well researched methodology, and a trained professional cadre knowledgeable in both screening and rehabilitation.

Let us look first at some theories of screening and how they relate to hearing conservation programs. Then we will describe what appear at present to be the most efficacious methods for accomplishing the identification of hearing defects. Two aspects of screening philosophy are relevant to us: (1) the selection of the disorder or disease which should be screened and (2) the evaluation of the screening procedures.

Which Diseases Should Be Screened?

The first question that must be asked is whether a certain disease should be screened. Certain criteria should be applied to the selection of disorders to screen.

Occurrence Frequent Enough or Consequence Serious Enough to Warrant Mass Screening. How prevalent is the disease in the population to be screened? Some balancing of cost with the numbers of children who have the disease must be made. We estimate that only one in 2000 children will have severe congenital deafness at birth, but at the age of 2 years, one in 25 children will have mild to moderate hearing losses from ear disease. To the disparity between these figures must be applied Dr. George Cunningham's statement (1970): "From the point of view of a public health program, in order to justify a mass screening program, the condition must be reasonably frequent or if rare it must have serious consequences if not detected."

In the case of hearing, screening for congenital deafness can be justified on the basis of its severity and resultant disastrous consequences;

the screening of the older child can be justified on the basis of numbers alone, if not on consequences.

The screening of hearing appears in an even more favorable light when one compares the figures of one in 2000 at birth and one in 25 after 2 years of age, with the prevalence of one in 14,000 or more that is found in phenylketonuria, which is routinely tested for at birth.

Amenability to Treatment or Prevention That Will Forestall or Change the Expected Outcome. What would be the prognosis for the individual if treatment is instituted, and also if it is not instituted? It perhaps matters little if such a disorder as color blindness is detected early, as no treatment will change it. But the tragic consequences of untreated hearing loss are all too commonly seen: the complete lack of speech or language development at ages when these functions should be well implanted; the deterioration of the parent-child relationship into subtle rejection or bewildered overprotection; and personality deviations of a wide variety, ranging from autistic-like withdrawal to hyperactivity and acting out.

So long as a disease state can be accurately identified, its severity should at the very least be lessened by treatment if we are to regard screening for the state as a profitable endeavor. The detection and treatment of phenylketonuria may result in the amelioration of the resultant mental retardation; but treatment may be harmful if applied to a child inaccurately designated as symptomatic (Cooper, 1967). Treatment is not always an unmixed blessing.

There is no question but that the sequellae of a true hearing loss can be ameliorated if the disorder is given proper treatment. Note, however, the words *true* hearing loss and *proper* treatment, for herein lies the essence of accountability for the audiologist. If a child were falsely labeled as having a hearing loss and were treated with a hearing aid, there is a possibility that noise-induced damage to the ear would result. There perhaps would be little chance of damage, and only slight damage would result, but we cannot evade the possibility.

It is well to point out this area of accountability for the audiologist, but once having done so, we must assume the competence of the professional to do his job. Not to do so would require questioning of a multitude of health programs.

In the case of hearing screening, then, we can be assured that the prognosis, if treatment is applied, is highly favorable and that the alternative is untenable.

Availability of Facilities for Diagnosis and Treatment. If a child is identified as being a suspect for a disorder, can he be properly assessed and treated, without too much expenditure of cost and effort? This question largely concerns the state of the art and the number of trained professionals that can be depended upon to produce accurate evaluations and remediation for the child. If 1-year-old Johnny is found in Podunk Center to have profound deafness, there may not be a facility for his diagnosis and training for hundreds of miles. Or, it can be argued, even in a big city the facilities available may be viewed with a jaundiced eye by critical fellow professionals. When these situations occur—and they doubtless do—can we justify screening for the disorder in that location? The concerned professional must answer YES to that question. Yes, we should screen in Podunk Center and, when a child is suspect, insist that some agency provide the necessary funds for his travel and follow-up in a larger city center. Yes, we should screen in the poorly staffed Big City, and with a suspect child we should challenge the professionals to attain the requisite skills. Unless we invoke the law of supply and demand, we will never have enough professionals to fill these supremely urgent needs. The skills are known; they need only to be transmitted to more people.

Cost of Screening Reasonably Commensurate with Benefits to the Individual. Is the screening equipment costly to purchase and to keep up? Do the personnel administering the screening tests require expensive training or high level salaries? We are hard-put to designate any costs as excessive where the health and welfare of many individuals are at stake, but there are sometimes limitations to the funds available in any area. Fortunately, most of the audiometric equipment necessary to screen at any age ranges

from $350.00 to $1500.00. Such equipment can continue to be used for long periods of time and for many thousands of tests before any repair or calibration is required. And, as the trend toward nonprofessional aides continues, the cost of screeners continues to decrease. Take, for example, a public school where the school nurse trains volunteer mothers to do the screening. With this kind of arrangement, the cost of screening one student could be a few cents per child. Included in this cost is the nurses' time to train a number of volunteers, plus the individual audiometer's cost of $400.00, plus all other incidental costs of records, reports, etc., in screening several thousand children.

A more extensive program is illustrated in the public school system of Denver. There, Dr. Mildred Doster of the School Health Service estimates a cost of approximately 84c per child for personnel to carry out comprehensive school audiometry. This program consists of screening tests in certain grades, screening the new enrollees at all other grades, individual rechecks, evaluations of all those entering special education and speech classes, follow-up reports on all pupils, and additional evaluations for speech discrimination and the adequacy of hearing aids.

In this case, one full-time audiologist and one full-time and one half-time audiometrist do all the screening tests as well as the follow-up threshold tests and audiograms prior to referral for further care. Ninety percent of the time of these three individuals is devoted to work on students; the rest is spent on adult employees. The 90% time is required to screen and follow-up over 30,000 pupils per year. The kindergarten, first, third, and seventh grades plus all new enrollees are tested annually.

For the Denver school program three audiometers at $350.00 each are used, plus a clinical audiometer costing $1500.00. A permanent sound room costs an additional $2500.00. With upkeep, these equipment costs prorated over 5 years are estimated to amount to about 3¢ per pupil. When the total outlay of about $27,000.00 per year for equipment and salaries in this comprehensive audiometric program is compared with the cost of about $1000.00 per student to repeat a grade, then this expenditure for an audiometric program seems warranted to the school district. If about 25 pupils were saved from repeating grades, the program cost is balanced by the educational budget savings each year.

The cost analysis of screening the infant and preschool population also varies, but in no case would it be considered to be unfeasible when compared with the benefits accrued, even expressed in terms of man-hour economics.

A Screening Tool That Validly Differentiates the Disease from Nondisease. Many authors have addressed themselves to the question of the most dependable method for evaluating a screening tool. A discussion of this question follows in the next section. The conclusion is that screening techniques for hearing have reached a higher statistical adequacy than many of the health screening procedures.

Acceptance by the Public. Once the adequacy has been established, the only remaining problem is to obtain professional and lay acceptance of the procedure. If the procedure is worthy of support, the first requirement is to obtain the approval and endorsement of the medical community. When that has been secured, a program of educating the public can be instituted. Only when widespread acceptance is obtained can the screening program be initiated.

Selection and Evaluation of the Screening Procedure

The success of a screening program depends largely on the effectiveness of the measures used to identify a suspect. The validity of a screening process is poor if it misses many of those who ultimately turn out to have abnormal findings in the function studied. If the process tags as abnormal large numbers of individuals who are actually normal, it is not economical as to time and effort and may cause anxiety to many. It is therefore necessary to set up rigid criteria for the screening procedure in order to select the one which is most feasible. The following criteria compiled from reports by a number of public health physicians (Thorner and Remein, 1967) and others interested in screening (Frankenburg, 1970) refer no less to the health problems in the public health sphere than to auditory screening.

Reliability. Reliability refers to the reproducibility of the results obtained. Can the procedure be replicated by anyone else who follows the same directions? Several types of reliability may be considered.

Intertest Reliability. The procedure used must be subjected to repeated tests on the same individual and on different samples of individuals. Does it give the same results when the same individual is tested several times? Does it give comparable results on different groups when the individuals are tested separately? If we test the hearing of a number of school children in the same way three times on three different occasions and obtain significantly different results each time, the instrument used has no test-retest reliability. If we divide our school children into two groups and test each separately, the test results should not vary significantly between groups. Any test instrument should be subjected to this kind of scrutiny, basic as it may sound.

Tester Reliability. The personnel administering the test should be uniformly expert so that two people administering the same test to the same child will obtain similar scores. This requirement is quite different from that of co-positivity and negativity, discussed below, which pits the trained technician against an acknowledged expert. Tester reliability in newborn testing means that two people can look at a baby who is given a sound stimulus, and score the response in the same way. In audiometric screening it means that two testers can screen the same child independently and report similar responses. Brooks (1973) has demonstrated that great discrepancies can exist between two testers' results on the same child.

Function Reliability. All characteristics or functions that are being measured, and their dependent states, should be consistently normal or abnormal, and should not change from moment-to-moment or day-to-day. The presence of the rubella virus in an infant, for example, will not vary over fairly long periods of time, so that the titer test for this virus can be depended upon to measure the real presence or absence of the virus. On the other hand, when one tests the hearing of newborn infants, the state of the infant, on which a response directly depends, can vary from moment-to-moment. It was shown in Chapter 3 that the level of arousal in an infant affects both his physiologic and his behavioral responses. Some stages of sleep, for example, are so deep that no response of any sort can be seen. Yet the infant may be perfectly normal. For this reason, modifications have to be made of the testing protocol so that it is possible to test babies at several different spaced intervals, in order to catch them in a good arousal state at some time.

Co-positivity and Co-negativity in Tester and Test. Often a screening test is evaluated by comparing it with a criterion test considered to be, but not known to be, infallible. Or a tester may be evaluated by comparing his screening results with those of a presumed expert. Co-positivity is the extent to which the test agrees with the criterion test in identifying positives; co-negativity is the agreement in identifying negatives. We might, for example, compare the efficiency of a criterion test for hearing that uses speech signals, with the efficiency of a fixed intensity pure tone screening test for which accuracy in identifying hearing loss is not known. An expert tester may be selected to conduct the criterion test. Unfortunately, both the criterion speech test and the expert tester may be in error in determining who is abnormal and who is not. On the other hand, however, if the results of the criterion test and those of the expert testing have been validated against a standard diagnostic test conducted by a professional, then we must assume they can be utilized in comparing results with those of the screening test and testers. The ideal would be to compare both the screening tests and the tester's results directly with the diagnostic tests by the professional, thus avoiding the intermediate stage.

Sensitivity and Specificity. The validity of an audiometric screening test for hearing is determined first by the agreement between the rating of a child as positive (abnormal) on the screening test and his rating as positive on the diagnostic threshold test, and second by the agreement between the screening test's classification of a child as negative (normal) and the threshold diagnostic test's designation of him as normal. According to public health terminology (Thorner and Remein, 1967), the accuracy of a screening test in correctly identifying the positive (abnormal) subjects is called sensitivity; its accuracy in classifying correctly the negative, or normal, subjects is called specificity. Inasmuch as formulations around these terms are in widespread use for the general health areas, we should apply them to our field of screening hearing.

The method of formulating sensitivity and specificity is shown in Table 4.1. Dr. William Frankenburg, co-author of the Denver Developmental Screening Test describes the use of this table:

"Perfect agreement between the screening test in the identification of all of the diseased is achieved if a or (a + b) equals (a + c). In such a situation, no diseased subjects would be classified as negative with the screening test, thus c would equal 0. The accuracy of a screening test in correctly identifying all of the diseased subjects is termed sensitivity and is calculated as a percentage by utilizing the formula a/(a + c) × 100. Since it is possible to correctly identify all of the diseased subjects by classifying all of the subjects with positive results as diseased, one must also determine the accuracy of the test in correctly identifying the non-diseased subjects. A perfect agreement between a test and the diagnosis also exists if use of the test makes it possible to classify all non-diseased subjects as negative. To meet this situation, d or (c + d) would have to equal (b + d). Specificity, the second type of test validity, is the agreement between the test in classifying subjects negative and the diagnosis in classifying the same subjects as non-diseased. Specificity is calculated by the formula d/(b + d) × 100." (From Frankenburg, W.: Evaluation of screening procedures. In Earlier Recognition of Handicapping Conditions in Childhood. University of California School of Public Health, Berkeley, pp. 45-46, 1970.)

Relationship between Sensitivity and Specificity. "The relationship between sensitivity and specificity can be represented by two curves, as shown in Figure 4.2. Unfortunately, most biological phenomena have considerable overlap between the non-diseased and diseased subjects. The oversimplified diagram would suggest that designating all subjects to the right of cutting point A as abnormal would achieve 100 percent sensitivity but less than 100 percent specificity, because the non-diseased subjects with levels between cutting point A and cutting point B would mistakenly be classified as diseased. Similarly the use of cutting point B would result in 100 percent specificity since the diseased subjects in the

Table 4.1. Calculation of Sensitivity and Specificity *

Screen Test	Diseased	Nondiseased	
Positive	a	b	
Negative	c	d	
	a + c	b + d	a + b + c + d

* Sensitivity: Percent of diseased designated positive with screen test a/(a + c).
Specificity: Percent of nondiseased designated negative with screen test d/(b + d).
False positive = b; false negative = c.
Results are random if sensitivity= % positive a/(a + c) = (a + b)/(a + b + c + d).
Results are random if sensitivity + specificity = 100%.
Note: The same computations are made for co-positivity and co-negativity.

area between the two curves would incorrectly be classified as negative. Thus, when the diseased and non-diseased subjects overlap on a scale it will be impossible to achieve both 100 percent sensitivity and 100 percent specificity. Furthermore, the movement of the cutting point to achieve greater sensitivity will invariably result in less specificity; the reverse also holds true. In addition, as the sensitivity is increased there will generally be more over-diagnosis and as the specificity is increased there will be a greater amount of under-diagnosis." (From Frankenburg, W., source as above, p. 47.)

It is valuable to elaborate on these details sensitivity and specificity, not only because they represent currently acceptable public health criteria, but because they should be useful to the audiologist in evaluating hearing screening tests and the testing of nonprofessionals. For example, they have been relevant to Downs in assessing newborn screening tests and the use of a high risk register in identifying congenital deafness. The most extensive study in this area was one reported by Feinmesser and Bauberger-Tell in Israel (1971, 1972). Newborn

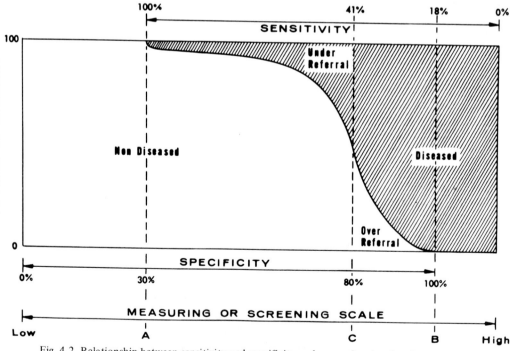

Fig. 4.2. Relationship between sensitivity and specificity and over-referral and under-referral.

infants numbering 17,000 were given hearing screening tests at birth and a high risk register was applied. Of these, 85% were followed periodically until the age of 3 in state well-baby clinics, where they were given hearing tests and developmental screening tests. These successive follow-up tests can be considered the diagnostic criterion evaluation against which the hearing screening tests and the risk register can be compared. Two comparisons can be made so far as high risk categories are concerned: an all inclusive high risk register, which included 20% of the newborn population, and a simplified register (described under "Goals at Birth" below), which included 7% of the population. The hearing screening tests resulted in 3% positives. The comparison between the high risk register as a screening test and the ultimate hearing losses is shown in Table 4.2.

Applying the sensitivity and specificity formula, described in Table 4.1, we see that there is 72% sensitivity and 93% specificity for the high risk register. Over-referrals are only .01% and under-referrals only .003%. These figures place the high risk register as an acceptable tool for the purposes of identifying congenital deafness. On the other hand, when compared in this manner the hearing screening tests showed a sensitivity of 27% and a specificity of 97%. The low sensitivity causes one to reject the hearing screen as a sole identifier of deafness.

We can also evaluate some preschool tests that have been reported in the same way. A study of the VASC (Verbal-Auditory Screening Test for Children) test proposed by Griffing et al. (1967) was done by Mencher and McCulloch (1970). They compared the VASC test with a

Table 4.3. Pure Tone Screen*

VASC	Diseased	Nondiseased	Total
Positive	1	0	1
Negative	9	43	52
Total	10	43	53

* Co-positivity: 1 ÷ 10 = 10%; co-negativity: 43 ÷ 43 = 100%. (These terms are used because we are comparing two tests for hearing loss, either of which may be in error when we are looking for hearing loss.)

pure tone screening test, with the results shown in Table 4.3. The co-positivity of 10%, even with a co-negativity of 100% for the VASC test in this study would cause us to reject the test as a valid screening instrument.

The presumption in school hearing screening in the past has been that the goal is to search out the deviations in hearing level, not the ear disease. Only Melnick et al. (1964) have subjected an entire population to a standard criterion test such as clinical threshold audiometry or otoscopic examination. Some studies have compared screening tests with random samples of the population who were tested on criterion threshold audiometry (Griffing et al., 1967). Others have compared the efficiency of various group hearing tests with that of the individual pure tone screening test (DiCarlo and Gardner, 1953), which is not a criterion test.

When the public health approach to evaluating screening tests is applied to such reports of studies of audiometric screening, the studies seem wanting. In our subsequent discussions on hearing screening, these facts will be taken into consideration. Furthermore, the new look we are taking at screening will re-evaluate the goals of screening and suggest a revision of the entire philosophy of screening at various age levels.

So far as school hearing screening is concerned, the evaluation of the test depends on the selection of the disorder to screen. Melnick et al. (1964) infer that we should screen for evidence of past or present ear disease, and they demonstrate that the pure tone screening test, and even threshold audiometry, are inadequate. On the other hand, if we set as our goal the identification of educationally handicapping hearing loss, as Downs et al. (1965) suggest, then the pure tone screening test is acceptable.

Table 4.2. Ultimate Hearing Level at 3 Years*

Screening (High Risk)	Diseased	Nondiseased	Total
Positive	13	1,190	1,204
Negative	5	15,792	15,796
Total	18	16,982	17,000

* Sensitivity: 13 ÷ 18 = 72% (over-referrals = 13/1190 = .01%).

Specificity: 15,792 ÷ 16,982 = 93% (under-referrals = 5/15792 = .003%).

An examination of the study by Melnick et al. shows a meticulous survey of pure tone screening, otoscopic examinations, and threshold audiometric tests on all of 860 school children. It is important to look first at the agreement that was found between the pure tone screening test and the diagnostic threshold pure tone test. Keeping in mind that when we use a hearing screening test, our logical goal is to find a hearing disorder for which a threshold test is diagnostic, Table 4.4 shows the calculated specificity and sensitivity.

The sensitivity of 85% indicates that there is reasonable agreement between the screening test and the threshold test in classifying abnormal hearing, but 21 of 143 children with reduced hearing were not properly identified. Although this is not an ideal situation, it may be satisfactory when one considers cost efficiency factors. This study represents the only one that has compared both threshold and pure tone screening on a large group of children who have also been given otoscopic examinations, and it causes us to examine more closely the routine tests we have so long taken for granted. All that we can say for the screening test is that it has fairly reasonable threshold correspondence with the diagnostic test.

However, when we compare the otoscopic findings in this study with the threshold audiometric tests, a great discrepancy appears, as shown in Table 4.5. It is evident that although the specificity is high for the threshold test, the sensitivity is too low to be acceptable: 90 of 127 otoscopically abnormal children were passed by the threshold test. Such under-referral completely obviates the usefulness of the test if what we are looking for is past or present ear disease.

Table 4.4. Threshold Hearing Test*

Screen Test	Diseased	Nondiseased	Total
Positive	122	13	135
Negative	21	704	725
Total	143	717	860

* Sensitivity: 122 ÷ 143 = 85% (over-referrals = 122/13 = 10%).
Specificity: 704 ÷ 717 = 98% (under-referrals = 21/704 = .03%).

Table 4.5. Otoscopic Findings*

Threshold	Diseased	Nondiseased	Total
Positive	37	78	115
Negative	90	532	622
Total	127	610	737

* Sensitivity: 37 ÷ 127 = 29%; Specificity: 532 ÷ 610 = 87%.

The obverse of the coin is to treat the threshold audiometric tests as the validation tests—which they well can be considered if we agree that we are looking for hearing loss. When we compare these tests in the study by Melnick et al. against the otoscopic findings, a different picture emerges, as seen in Table 4.6. It is completely valid to do this in order to discover whether otoscopic exams may miss sensorineural losses, which are a significant objective in any screening program.

These results, of course, approach randomness, indicating that otoscopic examinations in no way identify the important sensorineural losses; 78 children with significant hearing losses were not identified by the otoscopic examinations. This aspect of the otoscopic examination versus audiometry has not often been looked at, but it is essential to the over-all picture.

We will belabor this point a bit more because of the importance of the new look we are taking at screening. Studies like Melnick et al. (1964) are rare in that they submit the entire population studied to both the screening test and the validation test. Most studies have only applied the validation test to the cases that were positive (abnormal) on the screening test, leaving the entire negative (presumed normal) population untested. There is no way that this approach can demonstrate the validity of a

Table 4.6. Threshold Tests (as Validation)*

Otoscopic (as Screen)	Abnormal	Normal	Total
Positive	37	90	127
Negative	78	532	610
Total	115	622	737

* Sensitivity: 37 ÷ 115 = 32%; specificity: 532 ÷ 622 = 86%.

screening test. Unless we begin to apply as rigorous criteria to audiometric tests as have been applied to other health field disciplines, we can make no claims for the screening techniques.

Goals of Hearing Screening

Let us make it very clear at the outset just what it is that hearing screening programs can accomplish. An important question is: To what degree can the devastation caused by ear disease be prevented? We make a grave error in assuming that we can identify even a mild hearing loss in an older child, put a hearing aid on him, give him speech therapy, auditory training, and preferential seating, and that he will always live happily ever after. Not so. Usually by the time he is identified he has had the sensory deprivation over a period that includes optimal times for the development of language, of various auditory perceptions, and of speech skills. We cannot assume that the resultant dysfunctions can be overcome easily— or that they may ever be overcome. And, here we are not talking solely about severe or even moderate sensorineural deafness. We are talking about slight to mild hearing loss caused by otitis media at various times during infancy and early childhood.

In our clinic we first became aware of these conditions in testing the hearing and examining the ears of children who came in for delayed speech problems, minor language disorders, auditory perceptual difficulties, and learning problems. Most of these children would pass a 15-, 20-, or 25-dB screening test, and an air conduction audiogram would show what we usually consider normal hearing range. However, comparison between air conduction and bone conduction would often reveal very slight air-bone gaps—and, more important, the oto-logic examination under an examining micro-scope would show evidence of past ear disease. Confirmation of this clinical observation was found in the literature as early as 1935. Bond (1935) studied a sample of 128 children in New York schools and noted that among those retarded in reading, slight loss from otitis media was 15 times more common than among those whose reading skills were normal. However, a causal relationship was not established by this survey.

In 1956 a study by the Scottish Council for Research in Education of 310 school transfer children aged 10 to 12, with a history of otitis media, showed significant language retardation relative to children with normal histories. What is notable here is that achievement declined in relation to the severity and duration of hearing loss, establishing a more than casual relation-ship with the history. Further proof was given by Ling (1959), who matched 38 children having a history of otitis media with children who had no history of ear disease. He con-trolled all factors: IQ, social maturity, environ-ment, etc. The hearing levels ranged from 15 to 45 dB. He found that the hearing-impaired group was significantly retarded in reading and arithmetic over the nonhearing-impaired group, and the greater the impairment, the greater the retardation. Other studies show the same inexorable results (Holm and Kunze, 1969; Luke, 1965) and allow us to formulate certain principles regarding the effect of ear disease in infancy and early childhood.

In a hearing conservation program we must be careful to specify what it is we are looking for. The goals of screening determine not only what screening tools or measures will be used, but what ratios of specificity to sensitivity we will settle for. For example, although we would like to find medically remediable hearing problems at all ages, we may have to sacrifice this goal as a primary objective at some ages because of the reduced practicability and economy of the effort involved. The objectives of hearing screening and their relationship to the methods selected are summarized in Table 4.7.

Goals at Birth

At birth, it is practical at this time to screen primarily for severe to profound hearing losses.

The ear pathologies associated with hearing losses that are present at birth result chiefly in severe sensorineural losses, although middle ear anomalies occur frequently. The pathologies include ear anomalies related to embryologic development, genetic ear pathologies, and con-genitally acquired ear pathologies.

Table 4.7. Relationship of Screening Techniques to Developmental Ear Pathology

Time of Identification	Pathology	Chief Identification Factors	Most Representative Type of Loss	Objectives	Logical Technique for Screening
Newborn period	I. Congenital ear disease 1. The embryologic-related pathologies 2. The genetic pathologies 3. The congenital, acquired pathologies	1. Overt physical defects, family history 2. Family history 3. Prenatal and neonatal history	1. Severe sensorineural loss, severe conductive anomalies 2. Severe sensorineural loss 3. Same as 2	Primary: Detecting severe hearing loss for early habilitation Secondary: Middle ear anomalies and otitis media	Mandatory at birth: Establishment of minimal high risk register and in-depth testing in sound room of all high risk babies Optional: Behavioral screening
4–24 mo.	II. Congenital ear disease 1. The embryologic-related pathologies 2. The genetic pathologies 3. The congenital, acquired pathologies 4. Otitis media	1. Overt physical defects, family history 2. Family history 3. Prenatal and neonatal history 4. Altered tympanum and middle ear impedance	1. Severe sensorineural loss, severe conductive anomalies 2. Severe sensorineural loss 3. Same as 2 4. Mild conductive hearing loss	Primary: Detecting severe hearing loss for early habilitation Secondary: Middle ear anomalies and otitis media	Mandatory follow-up of high risk plus all others: 1. Orienting test using calibrated noisemakers 2. Query of mother 3. Communication and developmental scales 4. Acoustic bridge test
2–5 yr.	III. Later acquired ear diseases 1. The middle ear pathologies 2. Viral diseases 3. Late developing sensorineural loss 4. Sensorineural loss related to otitis media	1. Altered middle ear impedance 2. Altered tympanic membrane 3. Hearing loss 4. Hearing loss	Mild to moderate conductive loss	Primary: Detecting medically remediable ear disease Secondary: Detecting sensorineural hearing losses	2–3 years: 1. Acoustic bridge test 2. Pneumatic otoscopy 4–5 years: 1. Acoustic bridge test 2. Pneumatic otoscopy 3. Pure tone sweep audiometry (play-conditioned)
5–18 yr.	IV. School age acquired loss Same as above	Same as above	Same as above	Primary: Educationally adequate hearing Secondary: Detecting remediable ear disease	Pure tone sweep audiometry; consideration of acoustic bridge and of pneumatic otoscopy

Two methods that have emerged as feasible for screening at birth are the high risk register and behavioral testing.

High Risk Register. Each newborn infant is examined for history or physical findings that are known to be concomitant with deafness. The categories of historical or physical findings must be preselected for their high probability of being related to hearing loss. Richards and Roberts (1967) report that a high risk register, to be efficient, should identify a disease that is 14 times more prevalent in the register than it is in the general population. It will be shown that for hearing loss the prevalence in a small high risk register is at least 35 times more than in the general population. The size of the register that will be advocated has been reduced to cover about 7% of the population.

Behavioral Testing. Observations can be made of the infant's behavioral response to sound in the newborn nursery, as described in the "Guidelines for Infant Hearing Screening Program" below. Or more definitive observations can be made of the infant's responses to sound in a sound room. Either, of course, depend on subjective judgments but can be relied upon under the structured situations described.

In a unique attempt to quantify objectively these behavioral responses, Dr. Blair Simmons (1973), of the Stanford Medical School, reports:

> *CRIB-O-GRAM.* An automated method for detecting hearing loss in newborns is under development at Stanford Medical Center. Each baby's motor and respiratory activity is automatically recorded on a multi-channel strip chart recorder at 20 pre-determined intervals per 24 hours by a motion transducer on each bassinet in the nursery. A test sound is delivered half-way through 15-second recording periods. Changes in activity states, pulse, or respirations immediately following the sound are scored daily, in about 45 minutes, for an average of 25 babies. The average newborn receives 30 exposures and responds to 44% of narrow-band noise test sounds during his nursery stay. At this time, approximately 4,000 babies have been tested and a probable severe hearing loss has either been confirmed or is strongly suspected in six.

The method offers considerable promise, inasmuch as there is no interference with nursery routine, no subjective response criteria, and no technically trained personnel required for scoring. Testing can be done 7 days per week at times of low ambient noise, late at night and in early morning hours, automatically and inexpensively. However, the sample of babies and length of follow-up are still inadequate to determine the reliability and accuracy of this technique.

Goals, 4 to 24 Months

In the period of 4 to 24 months, the goals and pathologies are identical with those at birth. However, in addition, we can and should identify babies who have mild to moderate hearing losses that might impair their language function. This is the critical age for speech and language development and all efforts should be made to detect even the milder impairments. Fortunately, by 4 months the infant begins to show consistent responses to certain sound levels.

There are several techniques available to fit the expanded goals.

Orienting Tests. Sir Alexander and Lady Ewing (1944), in Manchester, England, first described using noisemakers to obtain orienting responses in infants. Their rather large armamentarium of noises included such things as a toy xylophone, a china cup and metal spoon, tissue paper, a rattle, and voice and unvoiced consonants. The responses they described are those which have withstood the test of time: eye-shifts and head-turns toward the sound, becoming more definite with increased maturation. Dr. Kevin Murphy (1962b), of Reading, England, made detailed observations of the orienting responses and reported refinements. He was able to identify the exact direction of the head and eye movements in relation to chronologic age, thus opening up a valuable line of inquiry.

Hardy et al. (1959) reported further on the use of the Ewing technique and illustrated their procedures in a movie, "Auditory Screening for Infants" (1959). Feinmesser and Bauberger-Tell (1971), utilized similar procedures (Sheridan, 1957) in their Jerusalem study and found them to be the best single test for hearing loss in infancy. These techniques and modifications of them are described in the "Manual on Infant Testing" which follows later.

Structured Questions of the Mother. It is assumed that the mother has information about the child that can be brought out by proper questioning. Bergstrom et al. (1971) has shown that on the average, mothers of deaf children were aware by 11 months that the child was not responding auditorally. Yet the average time of diagnosis was 2 years, 3 months. It follows that the question "Have you been concerned about your child's hearing?" is one whose answer should be acted upon if it is affirmative. A deaf child is often unusually alert visually, so one must structure carefully any question about his orientation to sound. It is probably best to eliminate vision entirely by asking about the baby's waking to sounds when he is sleeping.

Communication and Developmental Scales. Frankenburg and Dodds (1967) have established normative data on the Denver Developmental Scale Test, in which questions of the mother play a large part. Dr. Margaret Giannini (1972) and her Committee on Children with Handicaps of the American Academy of Pediatrics have developed an even shorter check list for developmental screening. These can be incorporated into a communication and developmental questionnaire that is especially structured to find hearing problems. The questions have been modified on the basis of certain findings that we have made on a deaf child. These questions are listed in the "Guidelines for Infant Hearing Screening" in the next section.

In 1964 a profoundly deaf infant was identified in the newborn nursery of Colorado General Hospital on the basis of lack of responses to newborn screening. The cooperative parents agreed to set up a tape recorder next to the baby's crib and to tape the sounds she made at random intervals. The samples covered the first 6 months of the baby's life. At 6 months her vocalizations became very infrequent. Some 12 hours of the earlier recordings were carefully reviewed by the author and by Dr. Johnnye Akin, an expert phonetician and Professor of Speech at the University of Denver. Sample recordings of a normal infant were also made and reviewed. Two significant conclusions emerged.

1. The average listener is not able to hear a difference between the vocalizations of the deaf child and the normal child at any point in the first 6 months of life. Both the quantity and the quality of the noises were similar in both infants. However, on the basis of careful phonetic analysis, Doctor Akin was able to delineate differences in the deaf child's phonemic content by the age of 3 months, but not before.

2. When it was obvious on the tape that the deaf child's mother had entered the room and was bending over her and talking, the baby's vocalizations increased. Just as in the normal child, the deaf baby appeared to be "talking back" to the mother as if she heard the mother speaking. This means that one cannot assume that a child can hear, even if a mother reports this kind of babbling response. Any communication scale must be structured accordingly, so that cooing in response to mother's voice is not taken as a sign of hearing.

Goals, 2 to 5 Years

The period of 2 to 5 years gives us real problems in identification. These children are not seen often at well-baby clinics or at doctors' offices. Although Head Start programs are making many children available, there are large numbers who are not seen for health visits unless special efforts are made to reach them. Nursery schools, play schools, and child care centers should be entered for hearing screening programs.

At this age we look primarily for medically remediable hearing losses, on the assumption that the more severely handicapping losses will have been found by 2 years. The chief pathology we are looking for is otitis media—the disease that can result at this age in subtle auditory disorders or permanent middle ear damage. The disorders that should be screened for at this age include middle ear pathologies, viral diseases, and sensorineural hearing loss. The tests that are adequate to identify these disorders are hearing screening, plus acoustic impedance audiometry and/or otoscopic examination.

Goals, School Age

At school age, the primary goal again changes. Now we assume that we are looking for educational problems—hearing losses that keep the child from functioning to his potential in the classroom. It would be nice to identify even the minor medical problems of the school age group, but the public schools at this time may not be able to afford to do so (Downs et al., 1965), nor do they feel at this time that they are in the business of identifying minor ear problems that do not reduce effectiveness in the classroom. It may be that this outlook will change in the future. Certainly it would be greatly desirable to identify all ear disease in school-aged children. Such a philosophical change does not seem to be in the immediate offing. If a change is made, it should be in the direction of acoustic impedance audiometry testing or otoscopic examination, or both, as adjuncts to pure tone screening.

Screening the Infant, Birth to 2 Years

Background

Dr. Eric Wedenberg in Stockholm first reported screening the hearing of 100 newborn babies in 1956. He used 100 dB (re: audiometric zero) at various frequencies as the signal, and categorized the responses as "auro-palpebral," meaning reflexive eye-blinks. The term was later used to cover any response to sound. More recently Wedenberg (1971) reported using only arousal from sleep as the criterion for a hearing response. As we will see later, this response has been the one most generally accepted in current usage.

In 1964, Downs and Sterritt reported the first study of newborn screening in this country. Their study determined that high interobserver reliability could be obtained in reporting infants' responses to sound. In other words, they found that two or more people could look at a baby and see the same thing. With this assurance they felt that large scale application of sound signals to newborns could be attempted, and that the observations of the infants' responses could be deemed reliable.

Screening programs were instituted in all Denver hospitals, using volunteers from the local Junior League or from the hospitals' auxiliaries.

The first year's study showed that nine deaf infants out of 17,000 newborns screened had been identified by the screening (Downs and Hemenway, 1969). However, as the program progressed and was scrutinized from many viewpoints, two things became evident. First, a number of "false-negatives" were showing up regularly—those babies who had been passed at birth, but who were found at a later age to have hearing impairment. Of six in this category, two were suspected of having developed the hearing loss later. Second, all but one of the babies identified at the primary research hospital fell into high risk categories for deafness.

These findings tended to destroy confidence in the behavioral screening. If the test missed a large number of eventually deaf children, it could not be considered a valid procedure. Furthermore, if the majority of deaf children would be found on a high risk register, why waste time in testing the entire population?

Further questioning of the Downs' techniques came from Goldstein and Tait (1971) and Ling et al. (1970). These superb researchers demonstrated rightly that there were many flaws in the techniques. They proposed that other means of identifying hearing losses be considered. In general their philosophies are incorporated into the current recommendations.

Several groups took a hard look at screening as a result of these questions. A National Joint Committee on Newborn Screening was formed which issued the following statement:

STATEMENT ON NEONATAL
SCREENING FOR HEARING
IMPAIRMENT
September 16, 1970

A common concern with the current status of screening procedures for hearing impairment among newborn infants has led to the formation of a Joint Committee comprising representatives of the American Academy of Ophthalmology and Otolaryngology, the American Academy of Pediatrics, and the American Speech and Hearing Association.

A majority of the committee agreed on the following statement, with the minority opinion endorsing the conclusions but not the preamble:

In recognition of the need to identify hearing impairment as early in life as possible, auditory screening programs have been implemented in newborn nurseries throughout the country. Review of data from the limited number of controlled studies which have been reported to date has convinced this committee that results of mass screening programs are inconsistent and misleading.

To determine whether mass screening programs for newborn infants should indeed be instituted, intensive study of a number of variables is essential. These should include stimuli, response patterns, environmental factors, status at the time testing, and behavior of observers. Furthermore, confirmation of results obtained in the nursery must await data derived from extended follow-up studies which involve quantitative assessment of hearing status.

In view of the above considerations, and despite the committee's recognition of the urgent need for early detection of hearing impairment, we urge increased research efforts but cannot recommend routine screening of newborn infants for hearing impairment.

However, the urgency of some action that would foster new approaches to identify hearing loss in early infancy spurred further efforts. In February 1971, the State Public Health Department of California, funded by the Maternal and Child Health Bureau of Health, Education, and Welfare, held a conference of multidisciplinary experts, co-sponsored by the Joint Committee (Cunningham, 1971). As a result, in April of 1973 the Joint Committee issued a supplementary statement as follows:

SUPPLEMENTARY STATEMENT
JOINT COMMITTEE ON INFANT
HEARING SCREENING

In light of the urgent need to detect Hearing Impairment as early as possible, a 1970 statement of the Joint Committee urged further investigation of screening methods but discouraged routine hearing screening which is not research oriented. In consonance with that statement, and in view of the information that application of high risk data can increase the detectability of congenital hearing impairment perhaps as much as ten-fold, the committee considers it appropriate to make additions to the 1970 statement.

The committee recommends that, since no satisfactory technique is yet established that will permit hearing screening of all newborns, infants AT RISK for hearing impairment should be identified by means of history and physical examination. These children should be tested and followed-up as hereafter described:

I. The criterion for identifying a newborn as AT RISK for Hearing Impairment is the presence of one or more of the following:

   A. History of hereditary childhood hearing impairment.
   B. Rubella or other non-bacterial intrauterine fetal infection (e.g., cytomegalovirus infections, Herpes infection).
   C. Defects of ear, nose, or throat. Malformed, low-set or absent pinnae; cleft lip or palate (including submucous cleft); any residual abnormality of the otorhinolaryngeal system.
   D. Birthweight less than 1500 grams.
   E. Bilirubin level greater than 20 mg./100 ml. serum.

II. Infants falling in this category should be referred for an in-depth audiological evaluation of hearing during their first two months of life and, even if hearing appears to be normal, should receive regular hearing evaluations thereafter at office or well-baby clinics. Regular evaluation is important since familial hearing impairment is not necessarily present at birth but may develop at an uncertain period of time later.

The effectiveness of the limited high risk register has been documented by several studies. One, already referred to, took place in Jerusalem. Feinmesser and Bauberger-Tell (1971) reported that an all-inclusive register of 20% of the population identified 14 of the 18 ultimately deaf children, whereas the simplified register recommended in the Joint Committee's statement incorporated only 7% of the population and identified 13 out of the 18. The authors felt that one, and possibly two of the non-high risk infants had developed their hearing losses after birth.

Dr. M. Altman of Rambam Hospital in Haifa, Israel, reported in 1968 a study differing slightly in design from the Jerusalem report. Altman reported his findings for two groups separately, one from the hearing screening aspect and the other from the high risk register. Although Altman's population was not all followed in a consistent way, his results point up essentially the same conclusion that Feinmesser and Bauberger-Tell reached. Of the ultimately deaf children, 75% would have been on a small high risk register.

In 1971, Dr. LaVonne Bergstrom of the University of Colorado Medical Center compiled the high risk factors that were present in the then 262 limited-hearing children currently managed by the Congenital Deafness Clinic of the hospital (Table 4.8). Approximately 70% of this group would have been on the simplified high risk register. Bergstrom emphasizes that this retrospective survey is of questionable accuracy, but it does lend weight to the choice of the few high risk categories which were chosen by the San Francisco Conference and the Joint Committee. A comprehensive look at newborn screening has been taken by Mencher

Table 4.8. *High Risk Factors in 262 Deaf Children**

Factor	No.	%
Near family history	60	22
Rubella or questionable rubella	60	22
ENT deformity	30	11
Syndromes associated with deafness	25	10
EBF with transfusion	5	2
Far family history	12	5
Ototoxicity (Kanamycin)	1	.2
Prematurity	9	3
Other defects (Non-ENT)	7	3
Failed in a newborn screening test; also had ABO blood incompatibility	1	.2
Unknown	52	20

*From L. Bergstrom: Personal communication, 1971.

(1972), who studied 10,000 newborn infants and was able to follow-up 80% of this number for 2 years at intervals of 1, 3, 6, 12, 18, and 24 months. He applied both the simplified high risk register and behavioral screening to the newborn population. Nine babies were found to have confirmed auditory impairment. Two of these infants had been cleared at birth, both by behavioral screening and by high risk classification. Mencher reports that one of these has a sensorineural loss of 50 dB with a family history of congenital origin. The other has "normal end organ function," but has a "central hearing deficit."

Only five eventually impaired babies had been on Mencher's simplified high risk register; seven were identified by behavioral screening. Mencher's conclusions are important enough to report in detail:

1. Infants in light sleep are more likely to respond to auditory stimuli than those in any other state—particularly when narrow band noise is the stimulus.

2. Use of broad band signal as sensitizers to alert the child to a narrow band or warble tone following, does not work to increase either the number or intensity of the responses (Kushner and Mencher, 1971).

3. Five of the nine children would have been placed on a high risk register for hearing loss suggested by the Joint Committee for Infant Hearing Screening, 1971, which includes the following factors:

   a. history of hereditary hearing impairment
   b. rubella or other non-bacterial intrauterine fetal infection during pregnancy
   c. defect of ear, nose, or throat
   d. birth weight less than 1500 grams
   e. bilirubin level greater than 20 milligram per 100 millileters of serum

4. Of the children tested in a sleep state, that we have identified as totally deaf, not one has responded with an arousal response. Apparently, children with a loss of 75 dB or less in the speech range will respond to the arousal test. Those with a loss greater than 75 dB will not.

5. Our results lead to the tentative conclusion that the high risk register, coupled with the use of the arousal response in mass hearing screening will result in optimal identification procedures, *and, we*

recommend implementation of that combination on a large scale experimental basis. (From G. T. Mencher: Screening infants for auditory deficits: University of Nebraska Neonatal Hearing Project. Presented at the XIth International Congress of Audiology, Budapest, Hungary, October 1972.)

Mencher's conclusions support the authors' feeling that behavioral screening should not be abandoned. Ideally, both techniques, the simplified high risk register and behavioral screening, should be applied. They can be accomplished economically if trained nonprofessional aides are trained to do a great deal of the testing and to apply the register. A modification of the behavioral testing originally described by the author (Downs, 1968) is being recommended in the following. This modification is based on a suggestion by Dr. Aram Glorig to the Joint Committee and on Mencher's findings. It consists of a simple arousal response during sleep, as described by Mencher (1974).

A 20-month investigation at the University of Colorado Medical Center, 1972-1973, under the direction of Janet Stewart, M.D. (1974), demonstrates the effectiveness of applying a high risk register in conjunction with the simple arousal response during sleep. A total of 3681 newborn infants were studied for high risk factors; 8.8% of them were found to be on the short high risk register. This number is higher than would be found in the usual private hospital because it included a number of sick infants who were transferred to the high risk nursery from other hospitals. In a private hospital where a similar high risk register was applied, a 6% figure was found.

The 288 high risk infants in this study, as well as 23 failing the screening test, were called back for audiologic testing within a few weeks after leaving the nursery. Five infants were found to have severe hearing losses; seven presented with conductive hearing losses. Five of the conductive hearing losses were due to serous otitis media; two are considered to have possible middle ear anomalies as well. Tables 4.9 and 4.10 show the summary of the results. This study demonstrates that in a high risk group there is a prevalence of deafness 35 times that found in the total population.

The finding of seven infants with serous otitis is not considered a high prevalence for babies under a year of age. The prevalence of this ear disease may be a great deal higher than has been supposed. McClellan et al. (1967) reported otoscopic signs of otitis media in 21 of 84 babies examined in a newborn nursery. Jaffee (1971b) found 18 newborn Navajo Indian babies with poorly mobile drums out of

Table 4.9. Statistics of Newborn Screening (University of Colorado Medical Center May 1972 to January 1974)*

Number Screened: 3681
  High Risk: 288 (8.8%)
  Screening Failures: 23 (.6%)

Confirmed Deafness

High Risk Factors	Degree of Loss	Type of Loss	Hearing Screening Results
1 Low birth weight	Severe	Sensorineural	Failed
1 Maternal rubella	Severe	Sensorineural	Failed
1 Low birth weight	Severe	Sensorineural	Failed
1 Family history plus cleft palate	Moderate	Sensorineural	Failed
1 High bilirubin (lost to follow-up)	Moderate	Sensorineural	Failed
1 High bilirubin (reported by doctor)	?	?	Failed

Yield for High Risk Register: 1 in 57
Yield for Hearing Screening: 1 in 736

Table 4.10. Results of High Risk and Auditory Screening.

Confirmed Losses	High Risk Factor	Diagnosis	Auditory Screen
Mild or conductive (7)	High bilirubin	Serous otitis	Failed
	Cleft palate	Serous otitis	Passed
	Rubella exposure	Serous otitis	Passed
	5-min. Apgar	Serous otitis	Passed
	Positive family history	Serous otitis and middle ear anomaly	Passed
	Maternal rubella	Serous otitis	Passed
	None	Serous otitis	Passed (referred by doctor)

* From J. Stewart: Personal communication, 1974.

101 he examined. Suppurative otitis media occurred in 17% of the premature infants but in only 8% of those full-term. It is our clinical observation that serous otitis media in the first year of life may certainly be at least as high as 10% in any population.

Stewart's study (1974) demonstrated that the high risk register and the auditory screening could be accomplished by a group of intelligent volunteers from the women's auxiliary, providing they were well trained and very closely supervised by pediatricians, otolaryngologists, and audiologists. A coordinator of the program is necessary to the organization and follow-up of the program. Where such constant supervision is not possible, it may be more effective to involve nurses—certainly where the establishment of the high risk register is concerned. There is no question but what any hospital, large or small, can apply the simplified register to its newborn population. Where physicians elect to utilize this procedure it should become self-supporting, with an automatic laboratory fee of $2.00 to $5.00 charged each patient. The income can be used to pay a coordinator, to purchase instruments and supplies, and to provide further paid personnel in larger hospitals.

The following Guidelines represent a workbook for instituting a comprehensive newborn screening program. A large part of the Guidelines for infant and preschool screening, and most of the Guidelines for school screening, have been modified with permission from an unpublished manuscript being developed by a Sub-Committee on Identification Audiometry of the American Academy of Ophthalmology and Otolaryngology, Dr. Francis Catlin, Chairman.

Guidelines for Infant Hearing Screening Programs

The purpose of these guidelines is to secure for all deaf children their fundamental right to acquire the best language skills possible for them. The ultimate language abilities of the deaf are dependent upon the age at which their deafness was identified and, therefore, early detection of the hearing loss is vital. Whether the habilitation of the deaf child involves auditory, oral, or manual language training, it will be most effective if begun in the first year of life.

Not everything is known about how and why congenital deafness occurs, and no one has yet developed foolproof procedures for identifying the disorder. Nevertheless, experience has shown that a large number of deaf infants can be identified utilizing the skills and knowledge presently available.

This guide will delineate the procedures that are recommended in conducting a program of screening infants for hearing problems. It is proposed that these directions be utilized by the pediatrician or otolaryngologist directing the program to help him organize it and to train the personnel who will conduct it.

The recommended program attacks the problem of identifying deafness in infants from three aspects: (1) the application of a simple register of infants at risk for deafness; (2) the conducting of audiologic evaluations on the newborns on this list, or, if desired, hearing screening of all the newborn population in addition (optional, recommended by the authors); and, (3) the follow-up screening of infants on the list at each office and clinic visit.

This three-fold attack on congenital deafness will be described in detail in the following pages.

WHY Should Hearing Screening Programs Be Instituted for Infants?

The Problem. There are 42,000 severely deafened children attending special schools or classes in the United States at the present time. At least one child in every 2000 births is deaf or severely hard-of-hearing. In addition, 15 to 30 per 1000 school children who attend regular school classes have hearing loss of some degree, numbering almost 500,000 (U.S. Department of HEW, 1964). It is the 560,000 children who will be born deaf or hard-of-hearing in the next 18 years that are the target population for this guide.

Studies of children in schools for the deaf have shown that the primary handicap of these children is lack of adequate language skills (Templin, 1966). The language deficiency is not due to lack of dedicated teaching during the school years, but to the failure to institute language learning until after the age of 2, 3, 4, 5, or 6 years old. Language acquisition has been shown to be a time-locked function, locked to early maturational periods in an infant's life. The longer language stimulation is delayed, the less efficient will be the language facility (Tervoort, 1964).

The existence of critical periods for language learning is postulated as the cause of language retardation in the deaf child just as it is for the experientially deprived child. The most crucial of the critical periods for language are thought to occur during the first 2 years of life, when the organism is biologically programmed for language learning (Tervoort, 1964; Lenneberg, 1966; Edwards, 1968). It has been erroneously assumed that language could be introduced at 3, 4, or 5 years of age to the deaf child with competely successful results. A great loss of manpower and human satisfaction results from such assumptions.

Even a 1-month-old deaf infant can receive language input through a hearing aid if he has sufficient residual hearing, or through visual and manual language inputs if he is totally deaf (Downs, 1971d). Placement in an appropriate therapy program is mandatory for the deaf infant just as soon as his problem is identified. Many centers throughout the country carry on active home-training programs for the deaf infant aged birth to 3 years (American Speech and Hearing Association, 1969), and there is available a home correspondence course in auditory, visual, and manual language training procedures (Alpiner, 1971). This kind of early training will ensure for the deaf child the development of his potential language skills to their optimal level.

When one considers that there are 235,000 individuals in this country with severe hearing loss and a total number of over 8 million with bilateral hearing impairment of some degree (Health Information Series, 1971), both the economic implications of early training and the value in human happiness become staggering.

The Yield. An incidence of deafness of 1.2 per 1000 school children has been reported in this country and abroad, (U.S. Department of HEW, 1964). These figures do not mean that one can expect such a high detection rate in screening the newborn population. On the contrary, the most ideal identification program will probably yield no more than one in 1000 or 2000 (Transactions of the National Conference on Newborn Hearing Screening, 1971). Two factors are operating here: first, that no screening procedure can be expected to identify 100% of the affected individuals; and second, that many severe deafnesses occur at some time after birth in both the genetic and exogenous categories (Fraser, 1971; Bergstrom et al., 1971). The fact that even inherited deafness can occur at some time after birth makes it necessary to screen vigilantly for hearing problems during all the early months and years of life.

The physician who is familiar with programs that screen newborns for other defects will recognize from the above that the yield from hearing screening is far greater than that reported for phenylketonuria and for several other neonatal screening procedures. Economically, hearing screening may cost no more than many of these tests, and the yield is greater in terms of both numbers and ultimate benefits

The kind of program that is being recommended rests on the principle that most deafness will occur in those infants who are AT RISK for deafness. Actual figures from infant screening programs have found that 75% to 90% of the infants ultimately shown to be deaf would have been listed on a high risk register (Transactions of the National Conference on Newborn Hearing Screening, 1971; Bergstrom et al., 1971). Supposedly the cases of deafness which would not be on a register are those caused by recessive deafness for which the family history is too remote to recall. A certain number of these cases may develop deafness at some time after birth rather than being born with the disorder (Fraser, 1971). The actual numbers of this type of deafness are not yet fully known.

WHO Should Conduct Infant Hearing Screening? Hearing screening is a task for a team of professionals: pediatricians, otolaryngologists, audiologists, nurses, and house staff. Each has his role in the program, but it should be remembered that data collection is a vital part of a project, and therefore the Public Health Agency in the area should be a partner in the activity.

Although each community has different needs and solutions, it is probable that the professional roles will follow the outline below.

The Pediatrician directs the over-all program in the hospital. His specific responsibilities are: (1) to plan for personnel and their training; (2) to direct the organization, scheduling, and reporting of the screening; (3) to help train those who will apply the high risk register; and (4) to be personally responsible for the kinds of examinations required for the high risk identification.

The Otolaryngologist consults with the pediatrician in the direction of those aspects pertaining to the ear and vestibular apparatus. Specifically, his responsibilities are: (1) to help to train those who will examine the infants' ears and do the vestibular tests; (2) to train personnel in high risk categories for deafness; (3) to help in the planning for reporting and follow-up of the positives found in the program; and (4) to consult with the pediatrician and audiologist on the follow-up of the high risk infants.

The Audiologist supervises the conduction of the screening tests. He should have clinical certification in audiology with the American Speech and and Hearing Association. Specifically, his responsibilities are: (1) to organize the scheduling of the program; (2) to see to all instrumentation and calibration; (3) to find an appropriate testing room by making sound level measurements; (4) to conduct or to train those who will conduct the screening tests on newborns and older infants; (5) to arrange for follow-up testing of positives in his hospital and for referrals to other facilities; and (6) to assure the continuance of a high level of competence in screening and in the follow-up.

The Nurse (or trained volunteers) may conduct both the screening tests and the application of the high risk register. If so, their duties specifically will be: (1) to learn to conduct the oral or written interview of the mother; (2) to learn to search the medical records for the high risk categories described; (3) to conduct the hearing test (where approved); and (4) to report the results.

The House Staff may have the same duties as the nurses, above. In addition, residents may be assigned to assume some of the responsibilities outlined for the pediatrician and for the otolaryngologist.

HOW Should Infant Screening Be Done?

For the Newborn Infant. There are two basic steps to follow in identifying deafness in the newborn infant. First, the application of the high risk register, and second, the actual hearing screening tests.

I. Application of the High Risk Register

The high risk categories that are recommended for a register are ones which have been culled from exhaustive lists. Although only a few categories are listed for inclusion in this program, it is recommended that all participants in a program should study the longer list and become familiar with all the syndromes associated with deafness (Transactions of the National Conference on Newborn Hearing, 1971; Bergstrom et al., 1971; Black et al., 1971a). As a mnemonic aid, the categories can be remembered as the a, b, c, d's (Downs and Silver, 1972):

a. Affected family. The presence of any form of hearing loss (other than presbycusis—hearing loss that begins in older age) in a family member.

b. Serum bilirubin level greater than 20 mg/100 ml. Hyperbilirubinemia due to blood group incompatibility in the newborn period.

c. Congenital rubella syndrome. Rubella at any time during pregnancy. Sometimes the hearing loss is the sole symptom.

d. Defects of the ears, nose, or throat. A malformed, low-set, or absent pinna; a cleft palate or lip (including submucous cleft); any residual abnormalities of the first arch; any other anatomic abnormality of the otorhinolaryngeal system.

s. Small at birth. Infants weighing less than 1500 grams at birth·have an appreciably greater risk of having hearing defects.

Functionally, the high risk categories are divided into three sections: those identifiable by query of mothers, those identifiable by visual examination, and those identifiable by physical examination in medical records.

The detailed procedures in each of these sections that will be used in identifying the infants in the high risk categories are as follows:

A. Identification through query of the mother (history of deafness in family member; history of rubella in mother at any time during pregnancy)

1. Written questionnaire (following are the questions as they appear on the form; translations in Spanish and other languages should be made)

1. Do you know anyone of the baby's relatives who couldn't hear well before they were 50 years of age? Think hard about all of your family and your husband's family.
YES___ NO___
a. If NO, proceed to question 2.
b. If YES, answer these questions:
1. Who were they? (relationship to baby)_____
2. How old are they now?_____
3. How old were they when loss occurred?_____

2. Did you have a rash with fever during pregnancy? YES___ NO___ At what time in your pregnancy? _____ Did the doctor call it German Measles? YES___ NO ___

3. Do you have any reason to worry that your child may have a hearing loss?_____

_____ _____

This questionnaire should be given to all new mothers in the hospital at some time after the baby is born. It should be prefaced with an explanation that "We are conducting a survey of all the babies born in this hospital, to see how many families have certain hearing problems. We would appreciate your help in this survey. There is nothing to worry about if you answer yes to any of the questions, so do the best you can with them."

2. Interview following the questionnaire

When the forms are collected, each should be looked at, and a brief confirmation obtained on the negative responses: "You don't know of anyone in your two families who couldn't hear well before they were older?" and "You had no illness during pregnancy?"

If there has been a YES answer to the first question, check on the three sub-questions. The age of the beginning of the loss should be queried further: "Does this relative speak clearly and distinctly?"; "Did he always speak clearly?" (If he was never able to speak well, it is a sign that a profound hearing loss was present very early in life or at birth.); "Did he go to regular schools or to special schools?"; "Did he ever wear a hearing aid?"; "Did he ever have surgery for his ear problem?"; "When?" (Surgery when a child can indicate that the loss was caused by otitis media, which may not be inherited; surgery after 20 years of age can point to otosclerosis, which is inherited.)

The cause of the loss can be queried further: "Was the cause diagnosed and identified by a doctor?"; "What exactly did he say about it?"; "From whom did you get the information about the loss?" (If second or third-hand, the information may be faulty.)

3. Oral query

If writing is a problem for the mother, the same questionnaire can be administered orally and the answers recorded.

B. Identification through visual observations of the infant

1. Cleft lip or palate, including submucous cleft

The cleft lip is an immediately observable malformation, but cleft palate—and particularly submucous clefts—will be searched for by a physician. Submucous cleft has been found to be associated with congenital middle ear anomalies, so it is important that the palate be carefully examined.

A bifid uvula always accompanies submucous cleft, but the cleft may be present without this symptom. Palpation of the juncture between the soft and hard palate will reveal a notch in the bony part.

2. Malformations of the ears

Abnormal pinnae may be obvious, but they also can be very subtle. Atresia, with partial formation of the pinna, or a small tab of skin where the pinna should be, are easily observed. Often, however, the ears are merely low-set, or they may not have complete formation of helix, antihelix, tragus, or antitragus. A small tab of skin may occur in front of the pinna, on the cheek, with an otherwise normal-looking ear. Sometimes these symptoms are accompanied by cranial malformations of the nose, eye orbits, maxillae, or cranial bones, so any old-looking feature may be a clue (Black et al., 1971a).

Do not be misled if one ear looks perfectly normal, but there is some abnormality of the other ear. The apparently normal ear does not necessarily have normal hearing; the incidence of congenital middle ear anomalies in the "good" ears opposite malformed ones is extremely high.

C. Identification through search of the medical records and physical examinations

Whoever is assigned to examine the mothers' and infants' medical records must be well trained in interpreting doctors' abbreviations and terminology (as well as their handwriting). The following items should be searched for:

1. Birthweight less than 1500 grams

2. Bilirubin titer greater than 20, or if early transfusion of blood was given

D. Proposed additional test findings

The application of the following examinations was suggested at the National Conference on Newborn Screening. Neither have been validated on large numbers of infants, but are considered useful in the hands of the knowledgeable physician.

1. Abnormal otoscopic examination

The ear of the newborn is difficult to examine properly, and experience is required to become skillful at it. A detailed description of this special technique and the findings to look for are found in the "Transactions of the National Conference on Newborn Hearing Screening" by Dr. Burt Jaffee (1971).

2. Abnormal vestibular tests (courtesy of Dr. Isabelle Rapin, Albert Einstein College of Medicine, 1972)

"The child is held at a 30 degree angle with his head facing down toward the observer's head. The observer then rotates holding the child aloft and looking at his eyes. When the observer rotates to his left (counter clockwise) he will note that the child's eyes will deviate in tonic fashion to the child's right. When rotation is stopped the child's eyes will move over to the child's left in tonic fashion and coarse nystagmic oscillations will be seen with the slow component toward the midline and the midline and the fast component toward the child's left. It is, of course, important that the child have his eyes opened at least a slit, but I have noticed that when you hold a child up in this position the children who may have had their eyes closed when they were supine will frequently open them. After a minute or two, the test is then repeated in the opposite direction, i.e. with the examiner turning to his right, clockwise. There will then be a tonic deviation of the eyes toward the child's left during turning, then nystagmus with fast component to the right in the post-rotational period.

"There are no special precautions to be taken other than not dropping the child! The response is usually very obvious because it is in no way subtle owing to the fact that the newborn does not have visual fixation to inhibit the response. It is most important to hold the infant with his head 30 degrees up from the prone horizontal position which places the horizontal canal in the horizontal plane and at right angles to the axis of rotation" (see also

Lawrence and Feind, 1953).

II. Application of the Hearing Screening Test (recommended by the authors) (Fig. 4.3)

A. Instrumentation

It is recommended that a signal of 90 dB (SPL) or less be the criterion level for the test. A high frequency, narrow band signal is preferable, with an available white noise source of 90 dB. The instrument should be calibrated with a sound level meter so that the intensity at a given distance is known. Some form of calibration check should be available at least once a week.

B. Environment

A study should be made of the noise level of the nursery area, with a sound level meter. If the usual level in the nursery at the time testing will occur is greater than 60 dB, a quieter room should be found. The cribs can then be wheeled into this room one by one, and the babies tested.

C. Pre-testing observation of the infants' state

The baby should not be tested until he is sleeping quietly. There are varying stages of the depth of sleep in babies this age, and some of the stages may not permit any response at all. The best state of sleep for testing purposes is a light sleep state, and this is the one most commonly seen. To test for this state, flip the eyelid slightly or touch the eyelid lightly with

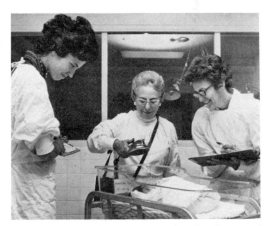

Fig. 4.3. Trained volunteers performing the arousal test with sleeping newborns.

finger or a tongue blade; if there is a quiver of the eyelid, however small, the infant is in a light sleep state. Any other small movement of the body to this stimulus also indicates the light state. This fact should be recorded before testing proceeds.

A deep level of sleep is indicated if there is no movement of the eyelid or any part of the body in response to the flicking of the lash. This state is the second best for testing purposes, but the fact should be noted on the record form.

If the child appears to remain in one of the these two stages of sleep, the testing can continue.

D. The criteria for responses

The loudspeaker of the testing instrument should be placed at the predetermined distance from the infant's ear. The most accessible ear should be tested. A length of string or a stick attached to the loudspeaker can serve as a measuring device.

The signal button should be depressed for a 2-second signal duration. The infant should be observed for no more than 3 seconds following the end of the signal. Any activity after this length of time must be considered random, and cannot be recorded as a response.

THE ONLY RESPONSE THAT CAN BE ACCEPTED IS AN AROUSAL FROM SLEEP. The acceptable criteria for an arousal response are: (1) opening of the eyes; (2) a stirring movement of the whole body, indicating arousal from sleep; and (3) a strong and immediate eye-blink, followed by one of the above responses.

After the infant has quieted again, the signal should be presented two more times and the response (or lack of it) should be recorded.

Two credible responses must be seen and agreed upon by the observers before the infant is passed. If only one response out of the initial three trials can be observed to the high frequency signal, a broad band signal (white noise) at 90 dB can be used three times to obtain one more response that will confirm the first observed response. If a broad band signal is not available, the narrow band level can be increased to 100 dB.

E. Reporting of the findings

One member of the team should have the responsibility of making up the list of high risk infants, of referring the critical high risk categories to an otoaudiologic center, and also of referring the positives from the standard high risk screening tests for otoaudiologic evaluation. The information from these lists should be reported to the local public health agency.

Provision should be made to report to the managing physicians the names of the infants who have been placed in the "at risk for deafness" category. Follow-up of these infants can be made by the hospital screening program personnel or by the public health agency, whichever is appropriate. In any case, the managing physicians of the well-baby clinic to which the child will be taken must be aware of their responsibility in screening the child further for hearing loss or referring to an agency that can do the screening, and then reporting this follow-up to the proper agency.

The recommended screening procedures for office or well-baby clinic visits are outlined in the following section:

For the Older Infant in Office and Well-Baby Clinic

I. Hearing Concern?

Mother should be asked the simple question: Has she had any concern over whether her child hears normally or not? Of 300 children in our Congenital Deafness Clinic, the average age at which the mother suspected a hearing loss was 11 months; but the average age at which the losses were diagnosed was almost 2½ years.

The lesson here is self-evident: *Listen to Mother!* Her concern may be a valid one, and it is worth asking her this simple question to determine whether she has observed any abnormal behavior.

II. Ear Tests Normal?

The test of choice for the infant from 2 months to 2 years is production of an orienting response using noisemakers. Before the age of 4 months the response is largely reflexive in nature, and may be difficult to see outside of a sound-treated room. The same criteria should therefore be used for the birth to 4-month period that are used at birth.

In the presence of a lack of response, the tester should repeat the use of a particular stimulus at his discretion until the observer is satisfied that the failure to respond is genuine. Two repetitions should be adequate to establish this fact.

It must be kept in mind that failure of the child to locate the sound does not always indicate that the child did not hear it. The simple fact that he may not be interested in that particular sound can account for this lack of response. For this reason more than one stimulus in a particular range is available for use at the discretion of the tester.

Standards for criteria for failure may be set up by the individual programs. The failure to respond in any way to the sound stimuli is obviously a failed test. Depending on the type of stimuli used, the program may require that the infant respond at least once to one of the lower pitched sound and once to one of the higher range of sounds (see "Equipment and environment" below).

The failure to respond does not necessarily mean that the child has a hearing loss, but it does mean that his auditory behavior is not normal. The reason may be a physical or mental impairment. In any case, failure to respond satisfactorily for his age level should mark a child for referral to an audiology and speech center for more detailed testing.

A. Testing with one observer (a simplified procedure by Downs)

1. Equipment and environment

A quiet room is required, with little distraction from the outside. The suggested list of equipment is as follows:

a. Squeeze toy. A soft rubber squeeze toy should be selected that makes a breathy "whoosh" sound, not a throaty noise. When buying it, compare different ones and find the one that sounds the highest pitched and can be made to sound the softest.

b. Bell. A small gold East India import bell produces the highest pitch and also the softest ring. Compare the bells and select the one that is highest and softest. We have measured the output of such bells and found that they produce only frequencies around 4000 Hz when rung slightly, at levels as low as 30 dB SPL.

c. Rattle. The usual baby rattle is adequate, providing it can be handled to produce a soft rattling sound. One may often find a toy plastic block that has sand-like material in it, that produces a sudden rustling sound. (If you survive the scrutiny of the toy store clerk after making these selections, you are in business as an infant tester.)

One chair is needed, for the mother to sit in with the child on her lap. A colorful toy like a small doll should be available as a distraction, but it should not be too attractive or it will engage the whole attention of the child.

2. Procedure

The tester kneels at a 45° angle to the side of the child, with the distracting toy in one hand and the noisemaker well hidden in the other. When the baby's attention is engaged by the toy held in front of him, she makes the sound in the hand held close to the floor, out of the peripheral vision of the child. If an orientation response is seen after one or two presentations, the tester kneels on the other side and uses another noisemaker to test on that side. The tester will learn by experience that for the 0 to 4-month age level the noisemaker must be produced quite loudly; by 6 to 9 months, it can be produced more softly; and by 10 to 12 months it should be made as soft as possible.

The expected response is some sort of head turn toward the sound (see also Chap. 4). An exact description of the head turn and accompanying eye movement should be noted. The expected responses at each age level are as follows (Fig. 4.4):

0 to 4 months. Eye widening, eye blink (in a very quiet environment), or arousal from sleep as in newborn testing.

4 to 7 months. By 4 months, a "rudimentary" head turn is seen: a "wobble" of the head even slightly toward the sound.

This response gradually matures until at 6 months the head turn is definite, toward the side of the sound, but only on a plane level with the eyes. He does not fixate the sound source in the lower level where it comes from.

By 7 months there is an inclination to find the sound source on the lower level; the child will look first to the side and then down. He may even be mature enough to find the source directly.

7 to 9 months. At the beginning of this period he should soon find the sound source on the lower level directly, but if the sound is presented on a level above his head, he will only look toward the side. At the end of this period he may begin to look toward the side and then up, to fixate the higher sound source.

9 to 13 months. At 9 months, the beginning indirect localization on the higher level will be seen which soon turns to direct localization (Fig. 4.5). We thus see shortly after 1 year of age a direction localization of sounds in any plane.

13 to 24 months. The same type of orientation prevails for the older child as was seen for the 13-month-old. In other words, the full maturation of the auditory behavior of the child occurs at about 13 months and does not change significantly after that.

3. Interpreting test results

In making the observations described above, we are looking for more than a hearing loss. The hearing loss will be suspected if the child does not respond appropriately on either side, or if he orients to the wrong side. But there are other conclusions that can be drawn from the type of orientation he displays. The direction of the baby's orientation must be within the criterion levels described above if he is to be cleared. Take, for example, a 1-year-old child who is only able to turn his head on a lateral plane, level with his eyes, even though the sound source is below or above that level. Such a child should be referred for developmental evaluation, for he is certainly at risk for retardation or for central problems. He should be showing auditory behavior commensurate with the normative values for his age. Any deviation should be referred for in-depth testing of status of developmental communicative skills. With experience, the observer can derive additional information from the baby's behavior during the testing period. These include:

a. By 2 or 3 months the baby should give a smile response when you talk and smile at him. At later ages the young infant or child should make direct eye contact with you when you address him pleasantly.

b. By 3 months he should be able to follow visually a bright colored object as it is moved from side to side.

c. By 10 months he should be afraid of strangers holding him.

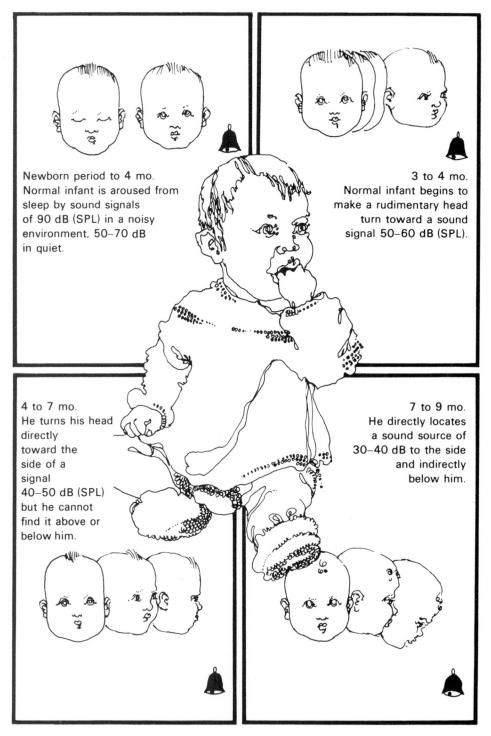

Newborn period to 4 mo. Normal infant is aroused from sleep by sound signals of 90 dB (SPL) in a noisy environment, 50–70 dB in quiet.

3 to 4 mo. Normal infant begins to make a rudimentary head turn toward a sound signal 50–60 dB (SPL).

4 to 7 mo. He turns his head directly toward the side of a signal 40–50 dB (SPL) but he cannot find it above or below him.

7 to 9 mo. He directly locates a sound source of 30–40 dB to the side and indirectly below him.

Fig. 4.4. Infant testing: newborn to 9 months.

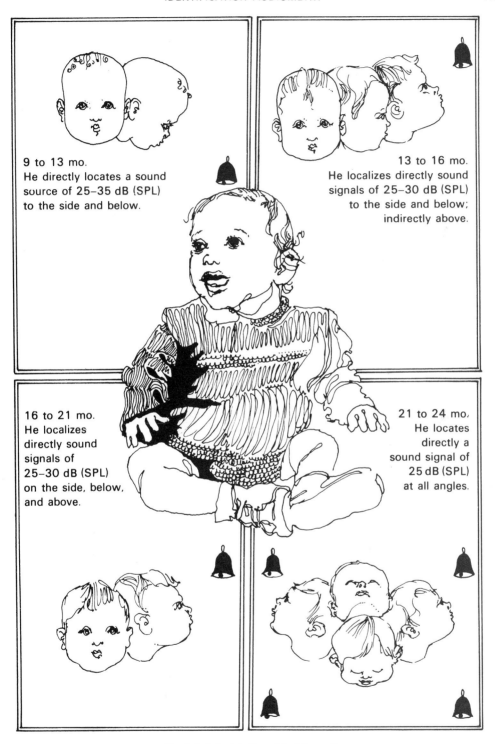

9 to 13 mo.
He directly locates a sound
source of 25–35 dB (SPL)
to the side and below.

13 to 16 mo.
He localizes directly sound
signals of 25–30 dB (SPL)
to the side and below;
indirectly above.

16 to 21 mo.
He localizes
directly sound
signals of
25–30 dB (SPL)
on the side, below,
and above.

21 to 24 mo.
He locates
directly a
sound signal of
25 dB (SPL)
at all angles.

Fig. 4.5. Infant testing: 9 to 24 months.

The child who deviates markedly in these behaviors should be referred for further developmental testing.

4. Follow-up

The ideal referral for children who do not pass the screening at office or clinic visit is to an otoaudiologic center—a center where an otolaryngologist can examine the child's ears and an audiologist can test the child's hearing in a standard sound room. The recommended tests in such a clinical situation are described in Chapter 5.

Even if the high risk children are passed at their office or clinic visit, they should continue to be screened at every succeeding visit, for the danger of developing a hearing loss in these children is never past.

5. Recommendations

Any child found to have an irreversible hearing loss of handicapping degree should be given the careful management described in Chapter 2.

More detailed explanation and demonstration of this procedure are found in the video tape "Auditory Screening of Infants" (1971b).

III. Arousal from Sleep?

A specific question that the mother should be asked is "When he is sleeping quietly in his room and you come in and talk or make noises, does he stir or awaken from his sleep?" He need not do this every time, but a few reliable reports are all that is necessary. The reason for this question is that it gives mother a specific, simple observation to make that is not concerned with slamming doors, stamping feet, or engine vibrations—all of which a deaf child will respond to.

IV. Responses to Developmental and Communication Scales Normal?

Here it is recommended that some screening scales be given which identify developmental and communication lags. The Denver Developmental Screening Test (Frankenburg and Dodds, 1967), Bayley Scale (Bayley, 1935), etc., are useful. In addition, a simplified questionnaire for various age levels should be given. The mother can be questioned either by written questionnaire or by oral query, depending upon which suits the needs of the population served. The questionnaire includes information on developmental status and communication abilities in addition to the questions concerning hearing status. It is recommended that this kind of questionnaire be used as a screening device to identify other problems which might benefit from treatment at an early age. The hearing questions are separated from the developmental questions because most of the commonly used developmental milestones are found to be present in otherwise normal deaf babies, and therefore would not identify a hearing loss.

Questions to Ask Mother at the
Well-Baby Examination

2 MONTHS

Hearing

1. Have you had any worry about your child's hearing?   YES   NO
2. When he's sleeping in a quiet room, does he move and begin to wake up when there's a loud sound?   YES   NO

Developmental and Communication

3. Does he lift up his head when he's lying on his stomach?   YES   NO
4. Does he smile at you when you smile at him?   YES   NO
5. Does he move both hands together in the same way?   YES   NO
6. Does he look at your face without your making gestures at him?   YES   NO

4 MONTHS

Hearing

1. Have you had any worry about your child's hearing?   YES   NO
2. When he's sleeping in a quiet room, does he move and begin to wake up when there's a loud sound?   YES   NO
3. Does he try to turn his head toward an interesting sound, or when his name is called?   YES   NO

Developmental and Communication

4. Does he lift his head up to 90° and look straight ahead?   YES   NO
5. Does he touch his hands together and play with them?   YES   NO
6. Does he laugh and giggle without being tickled or touched?   YES   NO
7. Does he coo to himself and make noises when he's alone?   YES   NO

6 MONTHS

Hearing

1. Have you had any worry about your child's hearing? YES NO
2. When he's sleeping in a quiet room, does he move and begin to wake up when there's a loud sound? YES NO
3. Does he turn his head toward an interesting sound or when his name is called? YES NO

Developmental and Communication

4. Does he lift up his head and chest with his arms? YES NO
5. Does he keep his head steady when sitting? YES NO
6. Does he roll over in his crib? YES NO
7. Does he reach for objects within his reach and hold them? YES NO
8. Does he see small objects like peas or raisins? YES NO

8 MONTHS

Hearing

1. Have you had any worry about your child's hearing? YES NO
2. When he's sleeping in a quiet room, does he move and begin to wake up when there's a loud sound? YES NO
3. Does he turn his head directly toward an interesting sound or when his name is called? YES NO
4. Does he enjoy ringing a bell or shaking a rattle? YES NO

Developmental and Communication

5. Does he support most of his weight on his legs? YES NO
6. Can he sit alone unaided for 5 minutes? YES NO
7. Can he sit and look for objects that have fallen out of sight? YES NO
8. Can he pick up two objects, one in each hand? YES NO
9. Can he transfer an object from one hand to the other? YES NO
10. Can he feed himself a cracker? YES NO
11. Does he make a number of different sounds and change their pitch? YES NO
12. Does he clap his hands in imitation and make noises at the same time? YES NO

10 MONTHS

Hearing

1. Have you had any worry about your child's hearing? YES NO
2. When he's sleeping in a quiet room, does he move and begin to wake up when there's a loud sound? YES NO
3. Does he turn his head directly toward an interesting sound or when his name is called? YES NO
4. Does he try to imitate you if you make his own sounds? YES NO

Developmental and Communication

5. Does he play peek-a-boo with you? YES NO
6. Can he stand for at least 5 seconds, holding onto crib or chair? YES NO
7. Does he try to hold onto a toy when it's pulled away? YES NO
8. Is he shy or afraid of strangers? YES NO
9. Can he pull himself to standing position alone? YES NO

12 MONTHS

Hearing

1. Have you had any worry about your child's hearing? YES NO
2. When he's sleeping in a quiet room, does he move and begin to wake up when there's a loud sound? YES NO
3. Does he turn his head directly toward an interesting sound or when his name is called? YES NO
4. Is he beginning to repeat some of the sounds that you make? YES NO

Developmental and Communication

5. Can he pick up a raisin or a pea? YES NO
6. Can he get to a sitting position without help? YES NO
7. Does he wave bye-bye or pat-a-cake when you tell him to? YES NO
8. Can he say "mama" or "dada"? YES NO

Some knowledge of the attributes of the deaf is necessary in order for the questioner to understand why the questions are worded as they are. For example, a deaf child will look around or will wake up when a door slams, when someone stamps a foot on the floor, when a large truck rolls by on the street, or when a very loud airplane flies low overhead. Therefore, if the mother states that the child awakens to a loud sound, she must be asked to specify the type of sound that he awakens to.

Another characteristic of the deaf infant is that he is unusually visually alert, and attends to movement in his peripheral vision. Therefore, if the mother reports that he turns around to an interesting sound or when his name is called, the question must be asked if she is sure that the sound is out of his peripheral visual field.

One of the erroneous assumptions that have been made in the past is that a deaf infant does not babble or make sounds like a normal hearing infant. Nothing could be further from the truth. Until the age of 6 months, the deaf infant sounds exactly like the normal infant; he babbles just as much; he increases his vocalizations when the parent appears and coos at him, just as the normal child; and only an expert phonetician could identify the subtle qualitative differences in the babbling sounds that the deaf child makes. Therefore, great care has been taken in the questionnaire not to assume that the baby's vocalizations are any index of his ability to hear.

A very misleading indication is a mother's report that her baby says "mama" at around the age of 1 year, and that therefore the baby must be hearing at that point. Oddly enough, the mothers of most deaf children have made just such a report, and it is universally true that a profoundly deaf infant will appear to be saying "mama" at around 1 year of age. Actually what he is saying is "amah," which is the most primitive sound that can be made, involving as it does the almost animal-like "ah" vocalization plus the coming together of the lips. It has been postulated that one of the reasons for its development is that in infancy the baby is carried close to the mother, and feels the vibrations or hears low frequencies of his mother's voice, and is thus stimulated to perpetuate the sounds. At any rate, the sounds soon drop off, and nothing remains but the "ah" vocalization in a strident voice.

With this background, the physician or nurse can use the questionnaire to determine whether the child should be more carefully examined at another time.

A. Acoustic impedance measurement

Interested readers are referred to Northern (1974) for clinical measurement procedures.

1. Tympanometry—measure compliance of tympanic membrane as a function of air pressure from +200 mm H_2O to −200 mm H_2O.

2. Acoustic reflex—stimulate test ear with sound and observe possible compliance change

of tympanic membrane (see Chapter 6).

3. Criteria for referral

A child should be designated as a failure under the following conditions:

a. If his tympanogram falls outside of the normal limits

b. If there is no acoustic reflex at 100 dB HL at 500, 1000, or 2000 Hz

Recommended Syllabus for Training Course

1 hour   Orientation and rationale for screening
            Movies: "Not Cleared for Hearing"
            (Downs, 1965) and "Auditory Screening
            of Infants" (Downs, 1971b)

I hour   Demonstration of techniques
            Test for sleep state
            Responses: Movie—"Auditory
            Responses of Newborns"
            (Downs, 1971)
            Instruments
            Specification of arousal response

2 hours   Practicum in nursery
            Measuring sound level in quiet room
            Demonstration of 90 dB sound level
            signal and responses of infants

2 hours   Logistics and mechanics
            Standard forms to be used
            Recording of light or deep state
            of sleep
            Checking batteries and calibration
            Ground rules of this nursery:
            orientation of how to behave,
            scrub, etc.
            Becoming familiar with the charts
            and how to read them
            High risk identification
            Questionnaire: written and oral
            Visually observed high risk
            categories: cleft lip or palate,
            and malformed ears
            Other high risk categories from chart

2 hours   Screening in office and well-baby clinic
            Films: State of Maryland
            ("Auditory Screening for Infants,"
            1959) and State of Nebraska
            ("Auditory Screening of Infants)
            (Downs, 1971b)
            Questionnaire: written and oral
            Demonstrations

8 hours   Practicum
            4 hours in newborn nursery

4 hours in well-baby clinic
Two weeks of supervised practice in newborn nursery and well-baby clinic.

Screening the Preschool Child, 2 to 5 years

Background

Ingenious efforts have been made to develop effective screening methods for the preschool child. The problems arise from the definition of screening as "rapid, simple measurements applied to large numbers of children." Any test that requires a voluntary response from a 2- to 5-year-old will be neither rapid nor simple. The 2- to 3-year-olds are particularly difficult to test. They can be negativistic, apprehensive, or "eager-beavers"—all attitudes which hardly make for easy testing.

Several solutions have been proposed to implement the screening of preschoolers, but none seem to have solved the 2- to 3-year-old problems. Among them are the following:

Speech Audiometry. Following the procedure utilized initially with the Western Electric 4-A speech audiometer, Newhart and Reger (1956), Watson and Tolan (1949), and Bennett (1951) reported presenting monosyllabic words to children who would then identify the corresponding picture. This procedure had the same inherent disadvantage as the Western Electric: it could fail to identify children with mild to severe high tone hearing losses, or even those with mild low tone losses. Meyerson (1956) attempted to eliminate this disadvantage by filtering spondee words through a high pass filter, a test which should identify children with high tone losses. Downs (1954) applied the filtering technique to familiar sounds: a cat meeow, a dog bark (250 to 750 Hz); a car horn, a cow moo (750 to 1500 Hz); and a bird song and a telephone bell (1500 to 3000 Hz). In the devoted hands of an experienced group of Junior League volunteers, the technique yielded satisfactory results on preschoolers for 12 years in the Denver public school preschool program. But even the expertise of this group was eventually defeated by the lack of proper instrumentation.

The VASC test culminated efforts to use non-pure tone signals for screening preschoolers. In this test, the child is told to point to the picture, on a stand in front of him, that represents the word that is spoken. The stimulus words consist of four randomized lists of the same 125 spondee words, beginning at a hearing level of 51 dB (re: normal threshold). Each subsequent word is presented at a 4-dB attenuation rate. The last three words reach a level of 15 dB.

The original study reported by Griffing et al. (1967) tested 175 preschool children with the VASC. All the failures were given pure tone tests, as well as every third child who passed. Five of the nine positives were found to have reduced hearing levels; four were normal. Because only one-third of the children were given the criterion pure tone threshold test, one cannot apply a sensitivity-selectivity formula to this report.

Mencher and McCulloch (1970) studied the VASC test by applying the VASC and also a pure tone screening test at 20 dB (ANSI), to all of 53 kindergarten children in an economically depressed area. The criteria for failure in the pure tone screening were any two frequencies between 500 and 4000 Hz above 25 dB or any hearing loss above 25 dB at 6000 Hz. The criterion for failing the VASC test was failure to correctly identify two of the last three words presented at 15 dB. The results can be charted as in Table 4.11. When looked at in this way, the co-positivity of 10% for the VASC approaches randomness, even though the co-negativity is perfect. Mencher concludes that the VASC does not identify hearing losses in the 30- to 40-dB range—losses which are critical to a child's learning.

Table 4.11. Pure Tone and VASC Comparison*

VASC	PURE TONE		
	Diseased	Nondiseased	Total
Positive	1	0	1
Negative	9	43	52
Total	10	43	53

* Co-positivity: $1 \div 10 = 10\%$; co-negativity: $43 \div 43 = 100\%$.

It is possible that modifications of the VASC test will overcome the problems pointed up by Mencher's study. For example, the use of filtered speech signals or familiar sounds might change the numbers of false-negatives. Certainly the instrumentation by the Zenith Corporation for the VASC is well designed and accurate. One of the questions, however, is whether it can be used for the 2- to 4-year-old group, particularly those in sub-marginal language areas. Four- and five-year-olds are screened routinely in public school programs using pure tone techniques so there seems to be no need for a new test for this age group. It remains to be seen whether this test can be made to be useful for younger children, 2 to 3 years old.

In view of the still unresolved status of preschool screening, it is well to review the goals that have been stated for screening this group and to formulate new principles of screening from them. The primary goal is to identify medically remediable ear disease; the secondary goal, to identify handicapping hearing loss of any degree. The purist will object to placing hearing loss as a secondary rather than a primary goal at this age, but he should reflect for a minute on what has happened by age 2 or 3.

The child with the severely handicapping hearing loss has been identified by now even if not covered by a screening program. His failure to develop speech or to respond to sound will have resulted in referral for testing. Most of the milder sensorineural losses should have been found in follow-up testing of high risk children by this time. But the child is now at the most vulnerable age for middle ear disease which, if left untreated, can ultimately cause permanent hearing loss. The hearing loss can be either conductive or eventually sensorineural, as Paparella and Brady (1970) and English et al. (1973) have demonstrated.

What are the best tools for screening for middle ear disease? First, of course, is the pneumatic otoscope examination. Properly performed, this test is the most perfect instrument for detecting middle ear disease.

Jordan and Eagles (1961) most effectively proved the case for otoscopic examination. They found that such evaluation identified 50% more ear diseases than did audiometric hearing screening tests. It is therefore time that a great leap be taken into the future: the consideration of large scale training of nonmedical people for the pneumatic otoscopic examination of the ears of preschool children.

Otoscopy has long been the province of the otolaryngologist, of whom there are not enough to go around; therefore it has not been considered as a screening tool. However, contemporary otolaryngologists and pediatricians are leading the way in proposing that nonmedical people can be taught to use this examination as effectively as medical personnel. Dr. Raymond Wood (1972) has successfully trained otolaryngology assistants currently being utilized in field health facilities on the Navajo Indian Reservation in the southwestern region of the United States.

Silver and Ott (1973) have demonstrated that nurses and trained "Child Health Associates" can effectively examine ears with a pneumatic otoscope. Supervision of the Associates by physicians is built into such programs.

The second most appropriate tool for detecting middle ear disease is the acoustic impedance test. It has been found effective for this purpose in any aged child, from birth on (Brooks, 1973, 1974; Renvall et al., 1973).

Guidelines for Hearing Screening for the Preschool Child

WHO Should Conduct Preschool Screening Tests? Any agency that attracts preschoolers in large numbers to its doors should undertake a hearing screening program. These agencies include (1) doctors' offices, (2) public well-baby clinics, (3) neighborhood health centers, (4) Head Start programs, and (5) public school preschool programs.

In each case the program should be planned and supervised by the medical staff of the agency, with the testing being done by personnel trained and supervised by certified audiologists, i.e., audiometric technicians, nurses, or well trained nonprofessional personnel.

WHY Should Preschool Hearing Programs Be Conducted? It is vital to the child's cognitive development that he hear well during these early years of life. Mild to moderate hearing loss may not have been identified during the first 2 years of life, and now is the time to look for it.

Studies have shown that even mild hearing losses can cause learning problems (Bond, 1935; Scottish Council, 1956; Ling, 1959; Holm and Kunze, 1969; Luke, 1965). These losses are of a kind that is due to otitis media. Of the hearing losses in children who reach school age, 90% are caused by otitis media, and can be remedied medically or surgically. Long before school age is reached these problems should be identified.

A small number of sensorineural losses will not have been discovered during the first 2 years of life. These may only number about 10% of all the hearing problems in children, but they are important to identify because of the severity of the handicaps they cause.

Even the slightest hearing loss may be significant to a child's development. The earlier it is found, the less the handicap.

HOW Should Preschool Hearing Programs Be Conducted? Three types of preschool screening tests are recommended and are listed in order of their ease of application. The ideal program would utilize all three evaluations; if this cannot be done, the first two can be used with satisfactory results; and in case only one test can be administered, the acoustic bridge gives the most adequate screening. Various studies have shown that acoustic bridge tests will identify from 90% to 95% of all the significant ear pathologies in children. The pure tone screening test may identify 50% of the ear pathologies (Melnick et al., 1964); the otoscopic examination will identify most of the middle ear pathologies, but has no way of finding the sensorineural loss.

1. Acoustic Bridge Test

Same as described in the section on infant screening above.

2. Pure Tone Screening Tests
   a. Play-conditioning procedure for testing the 3- and 4-year-old child (one child with three or four observing)
      1. Have available a peg board, a ring tower, plain blocks, or other simple toys that are motivating to young children
      2. With headphones on your ears, take a block (or peg, etc.) and hold it up to

one ear as if listening. Make believe you hear a sound, say "I hear it," and put the block on the table.
      3. Put the phones on the child's ear and hold his hand with the block up to his ear.
      4. Sound a 50-dB tone at 1000 Hz and guide his hand to build the block tower. Repeat once or twice and then see if he can do it alone. If he can, go on. . . .
      5. Set the hearing level to 25 dB and repeat the test. If he responds, go on to the other frequencies (2000, 4000, and 6000 Hz) and repeat the procedure. Praise him for each correct response. After each presentation, place another block in his hand.
      6. Switch to the opposite ear and repeat the test starting at 4000 Hz and descending to 2000 and 1000 Hz.
   b. Procedure for testing and referrals for the mature 4-year-old and the 5-year-old child are identical to that described in the next section, "School Screening Testing."
   Criterion for referral: Failure to respond to 25 dB (ANSI) at any frequency.
3. Pneumatic Otoscopic Examination
   a. It has been demonstrated that nonmedical people who have been well trained by otolaryngologists can perform pneumatic otoscopic examinations (Wood, 1972). It is necessary for an otolaryngologist to train the lay personnel who will conduct the examinations, and to make sure that they are able to identify ear disease. The instruction period should include an in-training experience that will allow the otolaryngologist to check on each trainee's ability to use the otoscope successfully.
   b. The personnel to be trained should be carefully selected for their ability to observe and to build rapport with children. Nurses, audiologists, audiometric technicians, and selected nonprofessionals are all eligible to learn the techniques.
   Criterion for referral: Examiner's judgment that either drum is abnormal.

Physicians can decide whether to include evidence of past disease, such as scarring, monomeric membrane, etc., in the criteria, or just evidence of active disease.

School Screening Testing

Background

School hearing screening has a long and honorable history. As early as 1924 a group of dedicated otolaryngologists utilized and reported a new instrument for testing the hearing of school children (McFarlan, 1927; Goldstein, 1933). The instrument was developed by Fowler and Fletcher (1926) for the Western Electric Company. The Western Electric 4-A audiometer was a phonograph connected to an assembly of 30 earphones which would simultaneously present well calibrated speech signals to the earphones. Numbers were spoken by both a man's and a woman's voice, starting at 33 dB and ending at 9 dB (re: normal threshold). Newhart and Reger (1956) and McFarlan (1927) were the physicians and audiologist most responsible for promoting the use of this instrument. It was used for school screening until the late 1940's, when the pure tone audiometer eventually supplanted it (Newhart, 1938).

The reason for the change to pure tone testing was that the gross speech signals used in the Western Electric test did not identify children with high frequency losses. West (1940), Johnston (1952), and Gardner (1947) were among those who evaluated the speech screening test and found it wanting.

For its time, the 4-A test was productive, identifying many otherwise ignored hearing losses. It established hearing screening as an effective part of the growing preventive health efforts. For example, the Denver Public School System reports a continuous, on-going hearing conservation program since 1927, initially with the Western Electric 4-A and subsequently with pure tone screening audiometry. Few screening procedures can boast such long term lineage.

Individual Pure Tone Sweep Test. In 1961 the Committee on Identification Audiometry of the American Speech and Hearing Association issued a monograph providing guidelines for school screening (Darley, 1961). It recommended individual pure tone screening as the most accurate procedure, but stated that group screening tests were less costly and could be used where cost is a factor. In Michigan it was reported that individual screening tests ran between 25 and 35 cents per capita, whereas group pure tone screening involved 15 to 17 cents per child.

The Committee on Identification Audiometry recommended that four frequencies be tested: 1000, 2000, 4000, and 6000 Hz; 500 Hz was to be omitted because testing environments often produce too high ambient noise levels. The intensity level recommended for screening was 10 dB (ASA) for 1000, 2000, and 6000 Hz and 20 dB (ASA) for 4000 Hz. The criteria for referral were failure to hear the 10 dB level at either 1000, 2000, or 6000 Hz, or failure to hear the 4000 Hz tone at 20 dB, in either ear.

The conversion to ANSI calibration would shift the hearing levels for screening to 20 dB for the frequencies 1000, 2000, and 6000 Hz and to 30 dB for 4000 Hz. However, the practicability of changing the hearing level dial twice during the testing of each ear, from 20 dB to 30 dB (ANSI), is questionable. The time consumed in making these shifts greatly decreases the efficiency of a screening program, and we see no urgent reason for it. A 25-dB screening level for the four frequencies of 1000, 2000, 4000, and 6000 seems to be an effective compromise. The criteria for failure can then be failure to respond to 25 dB at either 1000 or 2000 Hz, or failure to respond to both 4000 and 6000 Hz at 25 dB. In this way over-referral of the common 4000 Hz dip will be reduced.

Guidelines for Hearing Screening the School-Aged Child

WHO Should Institute a School Hearing Program? The Health Department or medical directors of all school systems, whether public, private, or parochial, should provide on-going screening programs. The organizational lines are as follows:

Supervisory
1. *The medical director* plans the program with the consultation of a Board-certified otolaryngologist and a clinically certified audiologist.

2. *The audiologist,* who should hold the certificate of competence in audiology of the American Speech and Hearing Association, supervises the organization of the program, the training of technicians, and the calibration and maintenance of equipment.

3. *The school nurses* may act as organizers, supervisors, or technicians, depending on the size of the school.

4. *Technicians* may be salaried such as 2-year college-trained Child Health Associates, or drawn from mother's groups, PTA's, or community service organizations (thus releasing professional workers for follow-up, diagnosis, and therapy). Short, intensive training courses by audiologists can prepare the technician for screening. Guidelines for courses in audiometric techniques are available (Northern, 1971b).

WHY Should a School System Institute a Hearing Screening Program? Because good hearing is essential to the child's socioeducational development. The following benefits accrue from a well planned screening program.

1. The prevention of handicapping hearing losses, through medical treatment which can be instituted when a child's ear problem is identified at an early age.

2. The maintenance of adequate hearing for the child in the classroom. Many hearing impairments that affect the child's class work may go unnoticed unless a testing program detects them. Medical treatment may be effective in 90% of the children found to have hearing problems.

3. Habilitation for those children with permanent hearing losses which are identified by the screening program. Audiologic, educational, and therapeutic approaches will help these children to function better in the classroom. Such children should be followed with monitoring audiometry and regular otologic examinations.

HOW Should a School Screening Program be Initiated? The following steps should be followed in instituting a program:

I. Organization

A. Preliminary arrangements should be made with the school principal to conduct the screening at certain times. The school nurse may be the contact person to arrange the schedule.

B. Selection of a quiet room for the testing should be made carefully, keeping in mind the class schedules and the traffic that occurs on any given day. (Ideal screening conditions call for commercial sound-treated booths, but realistically most schools cannot afford this purchase.)

C. Coordination of the class schedule with teachers, nurses, and technicians must be clearly understood by all. The teachers will instrust the children where to go and when.

II. Frequency of testing. Testing should be conducted annually in grades kindergarten, 1, 3, 5, and 7. Annual tests should also be conducted on all transfers into the school system (including high school students), and on all students with a history of previous hearing problems until, following treatment, no decline in hearing is shown for 3 successive years.

III. Procedure

A. The individual pure tone sweep check test. This is the standard screening technique which should always be employed, even if other tests are to be used as supplements.

1. Set the hearing level of screening audiometer at 25 dB (ANSI).

2. Screen one student at a time, at 1000, 2000, 3000, and/or 4000, and 6000 Hz. Sweep check each student, using hand- or finger-raising techniques.

3. At the completion of testing the group, rescreen any who fail to respond to the tone at the level of 25 dB at 1000 or 2000 Hz, or who fail to respond to two out of the three frequencies of 3000, 4000, and 6000 Hz.

B. Optional supplementary tests: air-bone gap screening. The yield of significant ear conditions from screening programs may be increased by screening for "air-bone gap" in addition to the pure tone screening. Many children who have ear disease may fall within the normal hearing range for air conduction (Jordan and Eagles, 1961). It has also been shown that many children with ear pathologies have markedly better hearing by bone conduction than by air conduction. For these reasons, consultants to screening programs may feel it worthwhile to add one of the following procedures for air-bone gap screening.

1. Audiometric air-bone gap screening (Lounsbury et al., 1965)
   a. An audiometer with a bone conduction unit should be altered by inserting an impedance matching T-pad within the bone conduction circuit to provide additional attenuation.
   b. Set the hearing level dial at a point 10 dB below the threshold of the normal ear.
   c. Using the techniques described above, screen bone conduction at the recommended frequencies.
   d. If the child responds at this low level, he "fails" the screening test, and is selected for the follow-up testing. (The rationale is that in the fairly noisy screening environment, a child with normal air and bone conduction will not hear the tones because of the masking effect. However, the child who has an air-bone gap will not be masked by the environmental noise, and will probably have increased bone-conduction hearing.) For further information, see Lounsbury et al., 1965.
2. Tuning fork testing for air-bone gap (Hildyard et al., 1963). The two classic tuning fork tests are used for this screening test.
   a. The Weber test. Strike a tuning fork and press the end of the handle against the midline of the child's forehead. Ask him where he thinks he hears the sound. His report as to where it is heard can be interpreted as follows:

"In the middle" indicates that both ears are most probably normal in hearing. Rarely, it can also mean the presence of equal sensorineural or conductive hearing losses in both ears.

"On the right (or left) side" indicates that the ear in which the sound is heard has an air-bone gap or that it is the better ear of a sensorineural loss. If both ears have an air-bone gap, the sound will usually be heard in the one with the greater gap.

   b. The Rinne test. Strike the tuning fork and place the tip against the mastoid bone behind the ear and then hold the tines at a point 1 inch from the ear canal. Ask the child where it is louder, in front or in back. Repeat the test to make sure he understands. His report as to where the sound is louder can be interpreted as follows:

"Louder in front than in back" indicates that he most probably has normal hearing, with no air-bone gap. It can also mean that the ear has a sensorineural hearing loss. "Louder in back than in front" suggests the presence of a significant air-bone gap. "Equal in loudness" indicates a smaller but significant air-bone gap.

Designate for otologic examination and threshold audiograms those children who either hear the sound on one side or the other in the Weber test; or hear the sound louder in back, or equal in loudness, on the Rinne test.

Because of the variability of tuning forks and tuning fork techniques, an otolaryngologist should be consulted for specific directions and training of the testers.

   c. Acoustic impedance test (As

previously described).

IV. Follow-Up of Failures: All children who fail the screening test are processed as follows:

A. Threshold audiometric tests are given for both air and bone conduction. These tests must be done in special sound chambers, by qualified audiologists.

B. Otologic examination is scheduled for those children whose audiometric test results show:

1. A hearing level of 25 dB (ANSI) or worse at any one frequency in the range 250 to 2000 Hz.

2. A hearing level of 35 dB (ANSI) or worse at any one frequency in the range 4000 to 8000 Hz.

3. An air-bone gap of 15 dB or more in the 250 to 500 Hz range; 10 dB or more at 1000 Hz.

Discussions of referral criteria may be found in the literature (Darley, 1961; Glorig, 1965; Newby, 1964; A Comprehensive Plan for Hearing-Impaired Children in Illinois, 1968; Berlin and Catlin, 1965). Variations in referral criteria may occur because of environmental testing conditions, otologist time, equipment used, and type of personnel doing screening and testing. Certainly, efforts should be made to avoid referring for otologic examinations large numbers of children who prove to be otologically and audiologically normal.

Those experienced in hearing conservation programs agree that some over-referral to otologic phases of the program is better than under-referral. How much over-referral can be tolerated may depend upon the availability of otologist's time, and upon the degree of understanding by all concerned of the objectives and limitations of hearing screening programs. Where there is a period of time between threshold testing and otologic examination, experience has shown that about 12% of the children referred for otologic examination will be found to be otologically normal. This percentage probably represents the spontaneous recovery of temporary ear conditions as well as some testing errors. However, a 21% figure may be used for a rough evaluation of the conditions under which testing is done, and the criteria which is used for referral for otologic examination. If all children at otologic examination show abnormalities, the program is probably missing some significant ear conditions that it is capable of identifying. If there are large numbers of otologically normal children referred, then valuable professional time is being used nonproductively.

C. Further consultant services are given those children who are found to have irremediable hearing losses even after medical treatment has been concluded. These services include further audiologic studies which may lead to recommendations for hearing aid use, special seating in classrooms, classes for lip reading and auditory training, or referral to special schools or classes.

V. Equipment and environment: At the present time, from the standpoint of their relative versatility, cost, and maintenance, the use of portable audiometers is recommended for school screening purposes.

Concurrent with the purchase of any audiometric equipment must be a plan to provide proper and periodic calibration and maintenance for the equipment. The reliability of an audiometer depends upon the accuracy of its setting, and no audiometer will indefinitely maintain the accuracy of its calibration. As a minimum, each audiometer should be calibrated at least yearly, and a 6 months schedule is better. Even new audiometers should be checked for calibration accuracy before they are put into use.

Arrangements for periodic calibration and repair service should be made with a laboratory which is equipped to provide calibration to the standards of the American National Standards Institute (ANSI). The firm manufacturing the audiometer may provide or suggest calibration services; larger universities or acoustic laboratories may have such facilities. Some laboratories and companies now provide calibration and maintenance services on a contract basis.

In addition to periodic calibration, daily monitoring by audiometric technicians is recommended to detect gross changes or breakdowns in audiometer performance. Monitoring procedures and audiometer performance are discussed in the literature (Eagles et al., 1967; Glorig, 1965; Newby, 1964; Eagles and Doerfler, 1961).

The yield of significant ear conditions and hearing losses is influenced greatly by the audiometric testing conditions. Ideal screening conditions call for commercial prefabricated, sound-treated booths. Although schools having continuing hearing conservation programs have been urged to provide such booths in school buildings (Darley, 1961), at the present time most school buildings do not have ideal conditions for audiometric screening.

The use of "ear muffs" with audiometers has been suggested by some as a means of cutting down ambient noise during screening. However, hearing conservation programs have been unable to demonstrate that the use of such muffs increases the yield of significant conditions in hearing screening programs. The use of "muffs" on an audiometer may frighten some small children, and may interfere with the proper calibration of the audiometer.

Mobile testing units consisting of sound-treated booths mounted on a truck, bus, or trailer have been found valuable in providing good acoustic testing conditions in large areas with small schools or sparse populations.

Where booths or mobile units are not available, the quietest room in the school building should be selected for audiometric screening. The room should be as far as possible from heating and other mechanical equipment, shops, music and typing rooms, and other sections where student traffic or scheduled activities create noise. The worst noises are steady or continuous such as those created by heating and ventilating equipment, traffic, and so forth.

The audiometric technician may check the masking effects of noise in a rough way by comparing her known hearing level with the screening intensities to be used. When the hearing levels obtained in the screening procedure will be greatly affected by excessive ambient noise, it may be necessary to transport children to a more suitable location or to schedule the screening at a quieter time.

Auditory Screening of the Mentally Retarded

Standards for institutions serving the mentally retarded as set forth by the Accreditation Council for Facilities for the Mentally Retarded (1971) provide operational guidelines for audiology services. In reference to audiometric screening, the standards state that all new residents, children under 10 at annual intervals, other residents at regular intervals, and any resident referred shall be screened. In addition, many facilities provide outpatient evaluation and services which include audiometric screening. As a result audiologists in such facilities are finding themselves faced with great numbers of retarded, of all ages and functioning levels, for audiometric screening.

Comprehensive audiologic assessment implies pure tone thresholds, speech audiometry, and any other significant diagnostic information obtainable. However, when large numbers of mentally retarded are involved, the need for a more efficient method of screening becomes evident. A variety of conditioning techniques, evoked response audiometry, special diagnostic procedures, as well as other auditory assessment techniques, have been suggested; although these may be reliable clinical tools, the technical problems of applying them to rapid mass screening have not been resolved. Subjective approaches which employ behavioral observation alone give limited information and no indication of cause of hearing loss.

We have developed a screening procedure for the retarded based on behavioral observation as a function of mental age (Downs, 1970) and acoustic impedance audiometry (Lloyd and Norris, 1970; Northern, 1971a). This project was carried out under the direction of Connie H. Knight, M.A., Audiologist at the Georgia Retardation Center in Atlanta. Our screening technique is designed for use with the severely and profoundly retarded and other patients who would be classified as difficult to test. It is not proposed as a substitute for pure tone screening when pure tone results are obtainable within the limitations of a screening program. Rather, it is designed for use when traditional clinical assessment techniques are not applicable.

The subject is seated or held in the sound suite facing one speaker. Initially the stimulus is presented through the opposite speaker so that if the subject localizes he must make an overt lateralization, which is very obvious, to seek the sound from the speaker furtherest away from him. If he localizes, as soon as his head is turned toward the speaker, the examiner quickly switches the signal to the other speaker in an attempt to get him to localize to the other side. Speech is primarily used as the sound stimulus, but a variety of other stimuli can be employed. It is sometimes necessary to change the stimuli during testing to pure tones, warble tones, white noise, or complex noise.

Observations are made by an audiologist and, if possible, trained observers. Response categories include (1) responses which indicate awareness such as eye opening, quieting, assuming a listening attitude, smiling, laughing, cessation of activity; (2) localization responses which are the overt learned responses which take the place of generalized body movements as the child matures; (3) startle responses which are the involuntary reflexive responses which are expected 65 to 85 dB above threshold and include eyeblink, orientation reflex, tonic neck reflex, Moro reflex; and (4) no response.

Step 1

An ascending approach should be employed in an attempt to obtain responses from the subject at levels of 45 dB HL or better.

Awareness, or preferably localization by 45 dB HL constitutes passing the observational portion of the screening.

Step 2

If no response is obtained by 45 dB, ascend in 10-dB steps in an attempt to elicit a response. It is necessary to vary the time between presentations in an attempt to catch the subject off guard. If the subject shows awareness or localizes by 65 dB HL and a startle can be elicited, it may be concluded that he either has grossly normal hearing or a mild-to-moderate hearing loss.

Step 3

Even when a subject shows awareness and/or localization at levels below 45 dB, an attempt is made to elicit a startle. If no startle is obtainable the subject fails screening and probably has a hearing loss. Even as the examiner attempts to elicit a startle at high intensity levels, it is important to continue to watch for awareness and/or localization responses. Responses at these levels will provide further inferences about auditory sensitivity.

Step 4

The final step in the screening procedure is impedance audiometry. Tympanograms are obtainable bilaterally; in addition, if the subject is cooperative with the bridge technique and especially if there are questions concerning observations, it has proven worthwhile to establish acoustic reflex levels at one or two frequencies. The objective measurements obtained with the impedance audiometer not only rule out or establish conductive problems but serve as an objective means of examining the more difficult-to-test students.

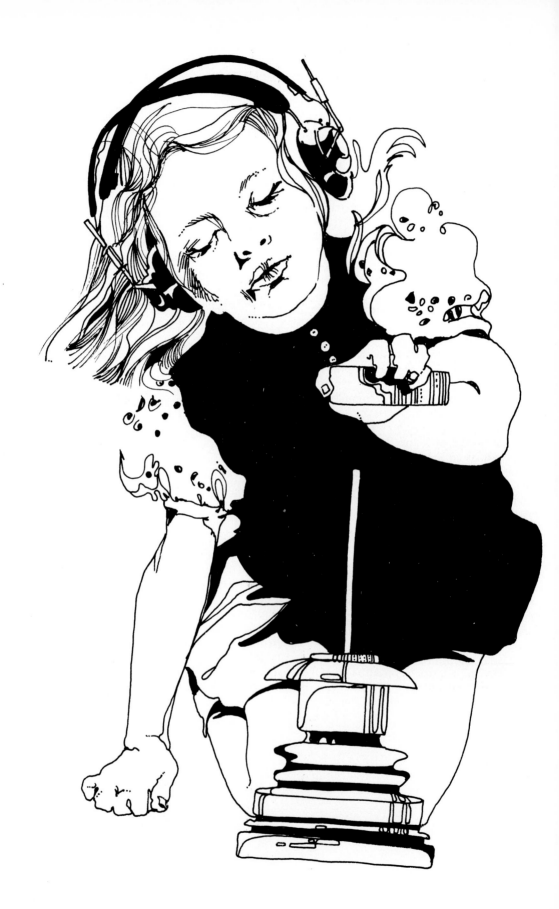

5 CLINICAL AUDIOLOGIC TESTING OF CHILDREN

Once the development of the auditory function is fully understood, it should hardly be necessary to describe the clinical testing procedures for evaluating hearing in young children. Given a keen observer with sharp clinical insight, all the procedures follow upon the developmental phenomena. However, most observers are made, not born; and clinical insight to some of us is a matter of seeing so many thousands of handicapped children that it is impossible to ignore the obvious after many repetitive exposures.

We will try to describe the techniques that have seemed most useful to us. Hopefully the born clinician will learn how to test children merely from reading; others will have to learn laboriously by repeated application of the observations suggested.

The testing procedures we will describe for children up to age 4 or 5 will include chiefly subjective kinds of clinical observations. Subjective techniques seem to be the most efficient ones in the large audiology clinic processing a large number of clients per day. Objective tests are described in Chapter 6; some of these are utilized when indicated. The acoustic impedance test is the only objective test used in the routine clinical evaluation. For hospital clinical needs, we have found that subjective tests supplemented by acoustic impedance testing are sufficiently accurate to meet the immediate needs of the medical examiner and of the habilitation clinician.

Questioning the Parents. In this chapter there will be no description of taking the case history. There are valid reasons for this omission. In the first place, we feel that the taking of a case history prior to the testing session gives the audiologist an adverse bias that may affect his observations. The audiologic evaluation should stand alone, uncomplicated by knowledge of historical facts which could be misleading. The audiologist should record only what he himself sees, not what he expects should be seen from his prior knowledge of the

case. After the testing has been completed, the physical and historical facts can be related to the auditory findings. If the two do not agree, further evaluation can be made at that time to resolve the discrepancy.

Another reason for omitting the case history is that the diagnosis of a hearing impairment should be a team approach. This approach is detailed in Chapter 2, which describes the physical and historical examinations that are made by various specialists. For the audiologist to take a detailed case history is an unnecessary duplication of effort and an unprofitable one. He cannot track down a family pedigree of associated disorders the way an experienced pediatric geneticist can. He cannot take a medical history covering all the pertinent health factors the way an otolaryngologist or a pediatrician can. Nor can he put together the picture of the family and psychologic environment the way a social worker or psychologist can.

What the audiologist can contribute, in addition to the actual hearing test, is his insight into the auditory and oral behavior of the child. No one understands better than he the effect of a certain degree of loss on the child's behavior, nor how the history of auditory development relates to the onset and degree of the loss. The audiologist's time will be most valuable spent in analyzing these aspects of the child's history. Therefore, the sequence of the audiologic session can be as follows:

1. Question the parent as to the chief concern which brought him here? Who referred him? (This is all the information that is necessary before the audiologic testing, and no details should be pressed.)

2. Give the audiologic test.

3. If a hearing loss appears evident, query the parent as to the child's auditory and oral development.

At 0 to 4 Months. When he was sleeping quietly, did sudden noises awaken him momentarily? Did he cry at very loud noises? Did he ever jump to sudden loud noises?

At 4 to 7 Months. Did he begin at 4 months to turn toward sounds that were out of his sight? Did he keep on making babbling noises of a large variety at 5 and 6 months? By 7 months did he turn directly to sounds or voices that were out of his sight? What kinds of babbling sounds did he make at 6 and 7 months? Could he sit alone at 6 months?

At 7 to 9 Months. Did he turn to find the source of sounds out of his vision? Did he gurgle or coo to voices or sounds that he could not see? Did he make sounds with rising and falling inflections?

At 9 to 13 Months. Did he turn and find a sound anywhere behind him? Did he begin to imitate some sounds? Did he have a large variety of different sounds, in different pitches? Were some of them consonant sounds (buh, guh, duh)? Did he say "ma-ma-ma-ma," or just "mama"? What specific sounds did he say?

At 13 to 24 Months. Did he hear you when you called from another room? Did he make a noise in response, or come to you? Did he have any other words or sounds than "mama"? Did his voice sound normal?

From this questioning, and from listening to the child's present voice quality and speech, the audiologist can derive clues as to the onset of the hearing loss and its degree. If the voice quality at the present time is strident, and only vowel sounds are made, an early severe hearing loss would be suspected. If the voice quality is good, in the presence of an evidently severe loss, a later onset would be suspected. Particularly if the child has some words or even sounds in normal intonation, a later onset is suggested. Such clues are helpful in determining the etiology of the loss. They can only be detected by the intuitive art of the insightful audiologist.

It is this kind of information that the audiologist should contribute to the team's diagnostic efforts. When put together with all the information the other specialties bring to the case review, a meaningful diagnosis can be made. All of the items of such an evaluation are discussed in Chapter 2.

You and the Child. A word about how the clinician relates to the child. Too often we have heard audiologists say "I don't like to work with younger children—I can't depend on their responses and they are too inconsistent to be relied upon." Nothing could be less true. Babies do just what they are supposed to do; the clinician often doesn't. The clinician has to give the right stimulus in the right structured situation in order to get the right response. There are no poorly responding babies—only inadequately prepared clinicians.

What are the general rules about working with children of all ages?

For Infants and All Children. Establish quickly an easy relationship with mother. Speak pleasantly and relaxedly to her; you will find the child looking back and forth between you two, and finally becoming content that all is well, he too will relax. In other words, the child absorbs the cathexis between you and mother and becomes at ease. Many people prefer to work with a child alone, and banish the mother from the room. This is fine if you have enough time to establish an easy relationship with the child. It may be quicker and easier to use mother in the testing situation; there is less apprehension in the child and he stays relaxed during the session. Mothers are usually quite cooperative and entirely rational. There are rumors around that most mothers are tense, over-protective, guilt-ridden, or rejecting; but it is amazing how much like you and me they are. In this chapter we describe the utilization of mother in the hearing test.

For Play-Conditioning Testing of the Older Child. Tell him what he is going to do—don't ask him. In this respect, the very young and the very old are alike, and one handles them both not by asking whether they would like to do something (they never do), but by telling them firmly and pleasantly that this is what they are going to do. Children do just what you expect of them, and if you firmly expect them to do what you want them to, they usually oblige. Of course, occasionally, one balks and yells like a banshee anyway—you can't win them all. But, give it a try—children are a great deal easier to handle than you think.

Believe in the Child's Responses. Develop a staunch and fervid belief that when children hear a sound, they will react in a stereotyped way that is consistent with their level of mental functioning. This holds true for the near-deaf child as well as for the normal child. The child with a threshold of 80 dB for a given sound will respond at 85 dB like the normal-hearing child who hears the same sound at 5 dB. A 2-year-old mentally retarded child with a mental age of 1 year will respond near his threshold in the way a normal-hearing child of 1 year responds near his threshold. There is no mystique about observing the hearing-impaired child's responses; other than having a hearing loss, he is a normal-behaving child or a "normal" mentally retarded child or even a "normal" aphasoid child, so far as peripheral hearing is concerned.

The trick, if there is any, is to become confidently familiar with the auditory behavior of normal-hearing children regardless of the integrity of their mental processing or central nervous system functioning. Once one knows the hearing level at which these children should respond, as well as the kind of response they will give, the deviation of the deaf child will become patently evident. The student who asks "How do you tell a deaf 3-month-old baby?" should be told "Go and test 100 normal-hearing 3-month-old babies, and then the deafness in any other child will become marvelously apparent to you."

We would add another principle, at the risk of becoming maudlin—and that is to love every child as a human being. The clinician is often hard-put to develop any charitable feelings toward the wall-climber, the temper tantrum expert, the withdrawn "Great Stone Face," or in some cases the misshapen, contorted face and limbs of the syndrome-ridden child. On one of my (M.D.) first contacts with Crouzon's syndrome, I was aghast at the little 2-year-old with the great bulging eyes, high head, and malformed nose and I wondered what resources of objectivity I could draw upon to relate to this blob for whom nature dealt a wicked blow. Suddenly, as I was hesitating the blob smiled at me—a smile so deeply compassionate for me that I hugged him in the joy of recognition of mutual humanity. The same humanity underlies the kicker, the screamer, the silent one—all of them humanly acting out their protests at a world that has given them less than it has to others. They too can be loved.

Clinical Testing of the Infant, Birth to 2 Years

The intensity levels and the observed responses that will be described for the birth to 2-year-old child are taken from an Auditory Behavior Index used in our clinic since 1966. The Index (Table 5.1) attempts to classify the type of response and the level of the adequate stimulus that will elicit a response at various ages of normal development. The Index was prepared in an effort to replicate an auditory behavior index reported by Dr. Kevin Murphy of Reading, England (1962). This remarkable observer of infants and children has diagrammed the quality of the behavioral responses of children to sounds, chiefly to noisemakers. Our study attempted not only to replicate his findings, but to add to it the level of the adequate signal that would first elicit a response. A comparison of our study with that of Murphy's showed less mature response levels than his, and we were forced to use general groupings that indicated an age period at the end of which the response should have developed. It may be that English babies are more precocious than American babies, or that the selection of our babies from a welfare hospital's pediatric clinic proved to be a significant variable. At any rate, we found too large a deviation in responses at any specific month of age to make as fine an analysis as Murphy's. Defining the upper limits of the ages at which certain responses can be expected has proved sufficiently useful for clinical judgments.

The value of such an Index lies in its consistency of reproduction in the clinical situation. Particularly reliable are the responses to a speech signal, as shown by the small standard deviations in the speech response column. Less reliable are the responses to pure tone signals as shown by the larger standard deviations in the pure tone column. This difference was to be expected after Eisenberg's (1969) description of the greater sensitivity of the infant to speech dimensional sounds. The requirement of speech dimensionality also explains our clinical findings that infants and children with high frequency losses do not respond to speech at normal levels for their

Table 5.1. Auditory Behavior Index for Infants: Stimulus and Level of Response†

Age	Noisemakers (Approx. SPL)	Warbled Pure Tones (Re: Audiometric Zero)	Speech (Re: Audiometric Zero)	Expected Response	Startle to Speech (Re: Audiometric Zero)
0–6 wk.	50–70 dB	78 dB (SD = 6 dB)	40–60 dB	Eye-widening, eye-blink, stirring or arousal from sleep, startle	65 dB
6 wk.–4 mo.	50–60 dB	70 dB (SD = 10 dB)	47 dB (SD = 2 dB)	Eye-widening, eye-shift, eye-blink, quieting; beginning rudimentary head turn by 4 mo.	65 dB
4–7 mo.	40–50 dB	51 dB (SD = 9 dB)	21 dB (SD = 8 dB)	Head-turn on lateral plane toward sound; listening attitude	65 dB
7–9 mo.	30–40 dB	45 dB (SD = 15 dB)	15 dB (SD = 7 dB)	Direct localization of sounds to side, indirectly below ear level	65 dB
9–13 mo.	25–35 dB	38 dB (SD = 8 dB)	8 dB (SD = 7 dB)	Direct localization of sounds to side, directly below, ear level, indirectly above ear level	65 dB
13–16 mo.	25–30 dB	32 dB (SD = 10 dB)	5 dB (SD = 5 dB)	Direct localization of sound on side, above and below	65 dB
16–21 mo.	25 dB	25 dB (SD = 10 dB)	5 dB (SD = 1 dB)	Direct localization of sound on side, above and below	65 dB
21–24 mo.	25 dB	26 dB (SD = 10 dB)	3 dB (SD = 2 dB)	Direct localization of sound on side, above and below	65 dB

* Testing done in a sound room.

† Modified from Deafness in Childhood, edited by F. McConnell and P. Ward, Ch. 2, pp. 25–33. Nashville, Vanderbilt University Press, 1967.

ages, despite the fact that the lower frequencies may be heard fairly normally.

This Index is used for testing peripheral hearing levels present in all auditory disorders. Where perceptual involvements exist, it is far easier to identify normal hearing in the first year of life than it will be later on. Most normal-hearing, centrally damaged children show excellent reflexive responses to sounds at the expected normal levels. The type of awareness responses they give at a later age may not be consistent, but their startle responses will be normal when they are infants.

A spin-off of the use of the Index has been its unexpected value in identifying mental retardation. As indicated in the Index, not only the level the infant responds to, but also the way he responds, show a maturational sequence

(Fig. 5.1). For example, the first localization of the young infant is a rudimentary head turn that may not reach a 90° angle. Later there follows a direct head turn to the side, but only in a lateral plane with the eyes. Direct fixation of a sound source in another plane follows, first on the lower level and then above the eye level; the final maturation is fixation of the source at a higher plane. Although individual differences exist in the rate of maturation, these are indeed guidelines for the kinds of behavioral activity that can be expected at any age.

Thus, if a 6-month-old baby gives only reflexive reactions to sound such as arousal and eye widening, but does not turn his head even rudimentarily, his auditory behavior age is lower than 4 months. If an 18-month-old child gives only a lateral head turn and cannot fixate a sound source below or above his eye level, he is behaving on a 6- to 9-month level.

Where developmental scales have been applied, the auditory behavior level usually corresponds fairly closely with the estimated mental age of the retardate. In several cases of infants, the mental retardation was first identified through the auditory behavior and referral was made for diagnostic work-up. In each case, developmental studies showed retardation commensurate with the estimate of auditory behavior level.

Conversely, the Index serves to confirm normal development in infants and children with mild to moderate hearing losses who have been suspected of being mentally retarded. If a child gives the type of response expected for his age level, but only at louder sound levels, he can be considered a hearing-impaired child who is fairly intact intellectually.

It is logical that one could correlate auditory behavior with mental age, in view of the fact that the mentally retarded child behaves consistently in all areas in the normal pattern for his mental age.

One cannot expect a 6-year-old with a 60 IQ to respond to finger-raising techniques in audiometry. If, however, we expect him to behave like a 3-year-old, the application of play audiometry will be as successful as it is with a normal 3-year-old. It is almost always true in mental retardation that behavior remains consistent with the mental age level.

We urge clinicians not to accept our norms for infant auditory behavior, but to generate their own index based on their instrumentation and their clinical style. Such an index should only be used by clinicians who have made the indicated observations on hundreds of normal infants in a structured, repeatable situation. Only then can they feel confident in separating the normal from the abnormal.

Clinical Testing of the Newborn Infant

There are three essentials to the clinical testing of newborns: an adequate sound room, measured noises, and a sleeping baby. With these given, even the least experienced observer can identify hearing levels as low as 35 dB in an infant.

The Sound Room. Newborns will respond only to very loud sounds when they are in their natural habitat, the noisy nursery. Noise levels of 70, 80, 90, and 100 dB SPL have been measured in the usual busy nursery. The newborn has been listening to sounds of 72 dB in utero, so he is accustomed to a background level of noise. We want to place him in the almost total isolation of a good sound booth in order to prepare him to respond to softer signals. It is best to leave him in the nursery crib, which can be wheeled into the sound room. Absolute quiet must be observed once the baby is in the booth. No more than two people should be in the room with him.

The best sound treatment available is necessary for the testing room. We prefer a double-walled sound booth, large enough for the crib and two people. We recommend that two observers be present when an infant is tested in a sound room, in order to increase the reliability of the observations.

The Acoustic Signals. For the kinds of responses we want to observe, toy noisemakers are the most useful signals, largely because of their sudden, rapid onset. They are also more complex than pure tones and include high frequency components that have the best arousal value.

Premeasurement of the noises on a sound level meter is requisite. Note that we do not use the term calibration of the noises; these toys cannot be calibrated like an electronic instrument. They can be measured so their output is known.

The noisemakers that we have found useful, in order of our preference are listed.

A Small Bell. We prefer the kind of Hindu bells found in import stores. With careful selection of the highest frequency-sounding bell, we have found some that when rung gently produce frequencies only around 4000 Hz at 25 to 35 dB SPL at 3 inches. When rung moderately, no more than 45 or 50 dB SPL should be produced with high peaks at 4000 Hz.

A Plastic Block or Rattle with Sand Inside That Can Be Shaken Suddenly. The sound made should peak at 1000 Hz or above, and with a quick, gentle shake should measure no more than 45 to 55 dB SPL at 3 inches.

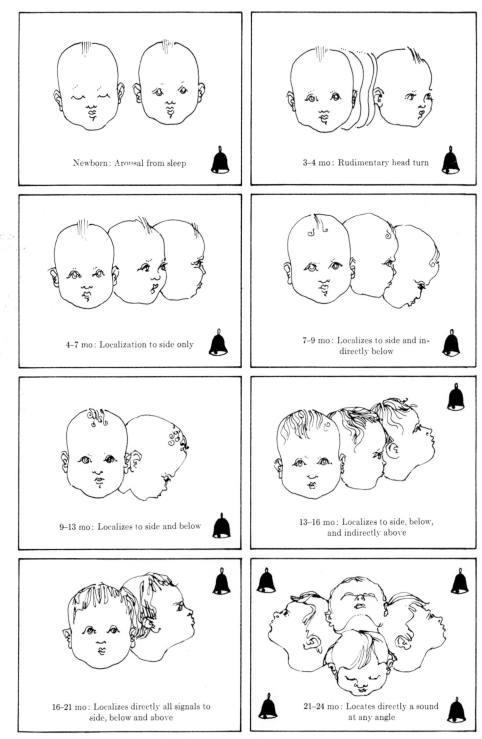

Fig. 5.1. Maturation of the auditory response.

A Rubber Squeeze Toy. This too should be carefully selected to produce the highest pitched and the softest sound that can be found. This sound should peak at 1000 or 2000, at no more than 45 dB SPL.

Tissue Paper (or Celophane from a Cigarette Package). When crushed, this produces 40 to 50 dB at around 1000 Hz and higher.

One Loud Squeeze Toy. One is needed which can produce at 50 to 85 dB SPL (all frequencies).

Other noisemakers may be found to be equally successful at producing responses. The above sound levels and frequencies give the tester some consistent measured levels that can be replicated.

The toy noisemakers should be held motionless within 3 inches of the baby's ear for at least 10 seconds before making the sound. The waiting period is necessary to obviate any response due to the hand's location in respect to the light source, or to any air movement. The short distance from the ear is deemed important by Sheridan (1957), who applies sound signals at distances commensurate with age. The distances used in her tests vary from within 30 inches at 6 months to 39 inches at 9 months, etc. She explains these differences in "distance hearing" as due to the incomplete experience of the infant with sounds and to his inability to discriminate foreground from background noises. Whatever the explanation, we have found it more effective to place the sound source close to the ear in the newborn period. The output of a loudspeaker 3 or 4 feet from the infant's ear has not proved effective for us at this age.

Speech, pure tone, and noise audiometry through loudspeakers should be available, but we have found that they fail to produce quite the rapid onset required in the testing of the newborn, and also change the structure of the situation unfavorably.

Sleeping State. It is quite possible to observe reactions to sounds in an awake baby. However, as Ling et al. (1970) pointed out, in this condition the chance is too high of observing random responses and judging them to be valid responses to sound. On the other hand, Mencher (1972) reports that the chance of recording a random response in a sleeping baby

is 1%. For this reason and in order to recommend the most foolproof method for testing infants, we prefer the sleeping state.

When necessary, a very experienced observer may validly note in an awake baby the kinds of responses described by Eisenberg (1969). A startle response should always be obtained to higher levels of intensity, as will be described later, in order to confirm that the responses to softer sounds are valid.

Two states of sleep can be operationally defined: a light state that is demonstrated by an eye or body movement to the flicking of the eyelid; and a deep state demonstrated by the absence of any movement when the eyelid is flicked (Mencher, 1972). Mencher found that the light sleep state is more productive of responses than the deep state. However, because this state of arousal may change from moment to moment, the baby should be tested regardless of which state is present.

Responses and Response Levels. The only response that should be accepted as valid is an arousal from the sleep state. By arousal we mean even a brief, transitory movement that indicates a marked change from the quiet, motionless sleep state. In the clinical situation, where repeated presentations of different stimuli can be made, we can accept the following responses as valid:

1. A definite eye-blink immediately following the presentation of the sound.

2. A slight shudder of the whole body.

3. An opening of the eyes, even briefly.

4. A slight head turn toward the sound.

5. A marked movement of arms, legs, or body.

6. Any combination of these.

The response must be seen within 2 seconds of the stimulus presentation in order to be considered valid.

It is always prudent to present a loud stimulus at the end of the testing period, in order to evoke a large startle response which will reconfirm the observations of movements that have been made.

Procedures. Maintaining complete quiet for at least a minute or two, the observers watch the baby carefully for on-going activity. If there is none, a flick of the eyelid should be made to determine the state of sleep. The fact of a deep sleep will change the judgment that is made of the subsequent responses, for the baby is less apt to give good responses when in a deep state of sleep. If a light state prevails, greater confidence can be placed in the responses or lack of responses that are seen.

A typical testing sequence with stimulus presentations and their intensity levels would be as follows:

1. Small bell rung at 35 to 45 dB SPL. Wait 30 seconds before the next presentation or until baby resumes the sleeping state, if he has moved. Usual response: arousal (body movement, head turn).

2. Soft rattle sound at 45 to 50 dB SPL. Wait 30 seconds. Usual response: eye-blink.

3. Soft rubber squeeze toy sounded at 35 to 45 dB SPL. Wait 30 seconds. Usual response: arousal (body movement, head turn, eye opening).

4. Loud, "squawking" squeeze toy at 85 dB SPL. Usual response: large startle (a sudden rapid movement of arms and other parts of the body; almost a small "jump").

Responses to each of these sounds should be seen in the normal baby. If in doubt, a sound can be repeated after a quiet interval. In a brief testing period, the baby's responses usually do not extinguish when a variety of sounds are presented at different time intervals. The state may change from time to time, however, and one must use clinical acuity as well as the eyelash test to estimate whether he has fallen into too deep a state to test. Shaking of the crib may arouse him sufficiently to test.

If responses are not seen to the softer noisemakers, other sounds should be employed. The crushed tissue paper, voice at 45 dB, white noise and narrow band noise at 45 dB (these last through the loudspeakers), and finally, sudden voice burst at 65 to 70 dB (re: audiometric 0). We have found that a "buh-buh-buh" at 65 dB usually produces a large startle response at any age.

If no responses are seen to the softer sounds, yet the baby responds to the louder ones, repeat tests should be made at another time. No greater than 5% false-positive (normal-hearing babies who do not respond at a given time) should be found with this technique. There has been a great deal of speculation as to why babies with normal hearing do not respond at a given time, yet will respond at another time. Some people have inferred the possibility of central disorders when a response is absent at any time, even when later testing shows normal hearing (Mencher, 1972). It seems to us that the demonstrated relationship between the state of sleep (state of arousal) and the occurrence of responses shows clearly that lack of response cannot be ascribed to central disorder. Also, the demonstration of the lack of inhibition of responses to continued stimulus presentations, shown in the brain-damaged and high risk child (Eisenberg, 1969; Downs, 1971a), mitigates against the theory of lack of response being related to central problems. We prefer to say that when a response does not occur it is due to the low state of arousal of the infant, resulting from a state of deep sleep that is unproductive of responses.

The kinds of responses we see in the infant's arousal from sleep are not high level, integrated reactions. They are rather varying degrees of reflexive responses which can be mediated in the brain stem or even the spinal cord. As such they relate only to the peripheral hearing mechanism, not to central auditory processing. We must look elsewhere to identify an aberrant auditory response that will lead to suspicion of central disorders. Our feeling is that we must look to the qualitative and quantitative nature of the response to find central aberrance. The two phenomena that are immediately open for further investigation are the response decrement and the latency of response.

It has been our experience that at least 95% of the normal-hearing infants—even those AT RISK—can be identified as normal on the first test by the kind of procedure described above. Most of the remainder will be identified in a repeat testing sequence, and only one-half of 1% will require a third visit to the sound room.

So far as warbled pure tones are concerned, the newborn infant requires around 70 dB (re: audiometric 0) before a response can be seen. The esoteric nature of the pure tones does not seem to arouse the infant to the degree that sudden complex sounds do. Therefore, the clinical usefulness of pure tones for newborns is reduced. When such high levels of sound must be used, there is always the possibility of a hearing loss with recruitment, giving the infant a loudness sensation equal to a normal ear. It is this possibility that reduces the effectiveness of a 90-dB screening level in identifying the more moderate hearing loss. Mencher (1972) has estimated that no hearing loss less than 75 dB can be identified by screening because the 90-dB signal will usually be responded to by the infant with 75-dB sensorineural loss.

Testing the Infant, Birth to 4 Months

During the first 4 months of life the infant's gross auditory behavior does not change markedly. In fact, by 3 months of age it may be more difficult to see a baby's response than it was at birth. This is probably because he is apt to be awake during the testing situation, and because he has been exposed at home to a great variety of acoustic stimuli from which he is still learning to select what is meaningful. He obviously has normal hearing, but neither his integrative processes nor his auditory-motor coordination have been well enough established to give the clear-cut responses we want to see. By 4 months he will make a great leap to responding overtly to softer signals than before. Until that time, both parents and clinicians are hard-put to see responses.

The requirements for testing the 0 to 4-month-old infant are almost the same as those outlined for the newborn baby: the adequate sound room, a quiet state, and measured noises. If the baby is sleeping, the protocol can be the same as described for the newborn. In addition we will add some speech audiometry to the protocol. The steps are as follows:

1. If the baby is awake, seat the mother with the baby in her lap, half reclining in her arm if under 3 months, and sitting leaning against her chest if over 3 months.

2. With a toy in one hand, engage the baby's attention straight ahead. Place your head as close to the toy as possible, so that the baby can look back and forth between you and the toy without much movement of his eyes.

3. With the other hand, hold the noisemaker 3 to 4 inches from one ear, and behind it enough so that it is out of the baby's peripheral vision. Hold it still for at least 10 seconds to be sure he is not aware of the positioning. Extreme quiet is essential.

4. Sound the noisemaker briefly—no more than 2 seconds.

5. Watch for immediate responses, which include (a) eye widening—the eyelids raise, and the eyes may turn toward you; (b) quieting; (c) a rapid eye-blink; and (d) by 4 months, a rudimentary head-turn that may not go farther than looking at you. It may go past you slightly, but until 5 to 7 months will not be a 90° turn.

Repeat the test with other noisemakers on the other side, as with the newborn protocol, ending with the loud noisemaker to produce a startle.

By 3 months of age it is possible to identify a monaural loss, when the baby may shift his eyes to the opposite side.

6. While observing from the instrument room, with the baby still on the mother's lap positioned between two loudspeakers located at 70° angles on both sides and slightly in front, repeat "buh-buh" into the microphone, in a slowly ascending presentation from zero. Keep the instrument room dark so the child will not see the tester. The observations will be made through the window of the suite. Present the speech signals at 20- to 30-second intervals for each ascending 5-dB step. Observe the first awareness response (eyes widening, quieting, eye-shift, or beginning head-turn), and record the level. Awareness should occur at an average of 47 dB in this age range. Use only ascending 5-dB steps. When a response is seen, do not repeat the test. The speech test is the most consistent of all, but should be repeated only at the end of the testing.

7. Present at 65 dB a sudden speech signal (buh-buh-buh) to produce a startle response. Warn mother not to startle. The child should give a typical Moro's response, almost jumping up at the signal. A startle confirms your previous observations if the infant has given normal responses; if he has a severe hearing loss he will not attend in any way to 65 dB; if he has a moderate loss he may only be mildly aware.

8. Repeat steps 5 through 7 using the bone conduction receiver pressed firmly by the mother on the midline of the top of the head. The bone conduction receiver should be calibrated for speech biologically, which usually

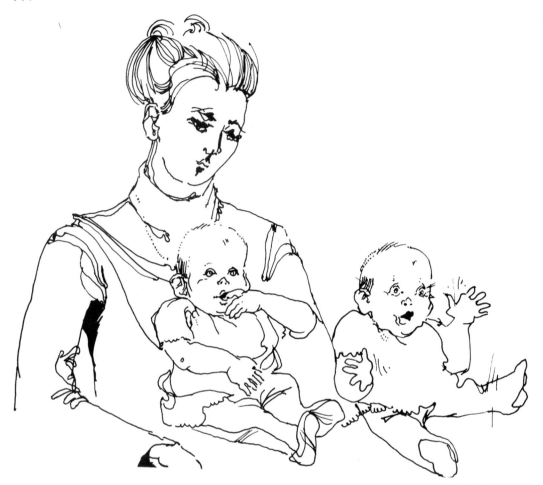

Fig. 5.2. Quiet baby shows startle response to sound presentation heard at 65-dB sensation level.

places 0 dB threshold at 35 to 40 dB on the dial. Make the same observations of awareness levels to speech as above, but keep in mind that the normal child or one with bilaterally symmetrical sensorineural loss will look to the front for the sound. If there is a conductive loss in one ear or a lesser sensorineural loss, he will lateralize to that side, thus providing a diagnostic clue to the type of loss.

A consistent difference of 10 dB or more between the air and bone conduction responses to speech is considered significant, and may represent a true air-bone gap. The standard deviation for the first response to a speech signal at this age does not exceed 8 dB. Therefore, even small differences are considered significant.

The degree of startle reaction to 65-dB speech is also significant diagnostically. An infant who gives only a mild startle to air-conducted speech at 65 dB, but shows a large jump to bone-conducted speech at that level should be suspected of having an air-bone gap. Infants, even newborns, with middle ear anomalies demonstrate a dramatic difference between their responses to air- and to bone-conducted speech signals. The fact that their conductive losses muffle their usual reception of air-bone sound makes the contrast between air and bone conduction literally startling.

9. Verify audiometric impressions with impedance audiometry (see Chapter 6).

Using the entire battery of tests in the Index, mild to moderate sensorineural losses become evident even in the first 4 months of life. The speech awareness level usually is consistent with the hearing loss around 500 Hz in cases of severe losses. In milder losses, it is closer to the 1000-Hz level. Care should be taken, however, in estimating the pure tone thresholds from the awareness level for tones. In these cases, an absolute correction cannot be made from the levels shown in the Index, because the presence of recruitment may permit responses closer to threshold than those shown. With sensorineural losses, the child's response to pure tones may be within 10 dB of the true threshold. In such cases, the degree of correspondence is close enough to allow us to recommend with confidence an appropriate hearing aid fitting after only a few testing sessions.

In the 0 to 4 months period, the infant's eye and motor coordination begins to develop. At 1 month he can raise his head from the surface while in prone position. At 2 months he smiles and coos; at 3 months he can follow a moving object with his eyes and hold his head erect. These abilities are important to remember because they should coincide with the same chronologic stage of auditory development. The infant who at 6 months of age is not able to follow a moving object or hold his head erect can be expected to fall into the 0 to 4 months' category for auditory responses. In this way, the Auditory Behavior Index can be used as a correlative of developmental landmarks.

The chart in Table 5.2 shows the rapid development check list that is approved by the American Academy of Pediatrics. Care should be taken in interpreting some of the landmarks as indicative of normal hearing. A deaf infant coos and chuckles quite normally at 2 to 3 months. He laughs aloud at 4 months; he can babble in two sounds before 6 months; he says something like "ma-ma" at 9 months; and by 12 months he may have a vocalization that sounds like "da-da." This can be misleading. The parents of one deaf child in our clinic insisted that their boy had normal hearing at 1 year of age because, they reported, he said "mama" and "dada." Yet polytomograms of the child's ears showed congenital gross bony abnormalities of the inner ears that were present at birth and precluded the possibility of any hearing at birth. It is well to view such

reports of early speaking with healthy skepticism.

Watch particularly for a baby who does not give a smile response by 2 months of age. The lack of this milestone of psychic development has been noted by Spitz (1959) to be an indicator of future problems. It is not only an index of development, but it also is a "psychic organizer," prerequisite to later milestones.

Testing the Infant, 4 to 7 Months

Around 4 months of age, the infant takes a giant step toward auditory maturity. Not only does he begin to turn his head toward a sound source, but he shows this response to a much softer level of sound than in the first 4 months. From a 47-dB average level of an adequate speech stimulus, he now becomes aware at 21 dB. During this period his muscle strength and his eye and motor coordination also show great improvement; he is out of the newborn period and on the way to becoming an active responder. He laughs aloud, he holds a rattle, reaches for objects and holds them, turns himself over, and sits by 6 months with a little support. By 7 months he can transfer an object from hand to hand and sit without support momentarily.

At this age the clinician should observe the visual acuity of the child: Can he track a bright object visually from one side to the other? Does he have good eye contact with you even for a brief period when he is 4 months and for longer periods of interest at 7 months? Smile and nod your head and say "Hi, Johnny." Is there integrity in the way he looks at you? Observations of many normal children of this age will give the necessary insight into an abnormal child's behavior.

The improved muscular coordination allows the child at 4 months to begin to turn his head toward a sound, but only on a lateral plane. He is not able to find a sound source below his head level or above it. The head turn at 4 months is a wobbly one which never gets around to a 90° angle. By 6 months the head should come around 90° toward the sound, but the eyes will not fixate the source when it is below or above him on that side.

Procedure. Present the same sequence of

Table 5.2. Rapid Developmental Screening Check List*†

NAME: .... D.O.B.: .... 1st Visit: ....

AGE				DATE
1 mo.:	Can he raise his head from the surface in the prone position?..	....YES	.....NO	
	Does he regard your face while you are in his direct line of vision?	....YES	.....NO	
2 mo.:	Does he smile and coo?	....YES	.....NO	
3 mo.:	Does he follow a moving object?	....YES	.....NO	
	Does he hold his head erect?	....YES	.....NO	
4 mo.:	Will he hold a rattle?	....YES	.....NO	
	Does he laugh aloud?	....YES	.....NO	
5 mo.:	Can he reach for and hold objects?	....YES	.....NO	
6 mo.:	Can he turn over?	....YES	.....NO	
	Does he turn toward sounds?	....YES	.....NO	
	Will he sit with a little support (with one hand)?	....YES	.....NO	
7 mo.:	Can he transfer an object from one hand to another?	....YES	.....NO	
	Can he sit momentarily without support?	....YES	.....NO	
8 mo.:	Can he sit steadily for about 5 minutes?	....YES	.....NO	
9 mo.:	Can he say "ma-ma" or "da-da"?	....YES	.....NO	
10 mo.:	Can he pull himself up at the side of his crib or playpen?	....YES	.....NO	
11 mo.:	Can he cruise around his playpen or crib, or walk holding onto furniture?	....YES	.....NO	
12 mo.:	Can he wave bye-bye?	....YES	.....NO	
	Can he walk with one hand held?	....YES	.....NO	
	Does he have a two-word vocabulary?	....YES	.....NO	
15 mo.:	Can he walk by himself?	....YES	.....NO	
	Can he indicate his wants by pointing and grunting?	....YES	.....NO	
18 mo.:	Can he build a tower of three blocks?	....YES	.....NO	
	Does he say six words?	....YES	.....NO	
24 mo.:	Can he run?	....YES	.....NO	
	Can he walk up and down stairs holding rail?	....YES	.....NO	
	Can he express himself (occasionally) in a two-word sentence? .	....YES	.....NO	
2½ yr.:	Can he jump lifting both feet off the ground?	....YES	.....NO	
	Can he build a tower of six blocks?	....YES	.....NO	
	Can he point to parts of his body on command?	....YES	.....NO	
3 yr.;	Can he follow two commands involving "on," "under," or "behind" (without gestures)?	....YES	.....NO	
	Can he build a tower of nine blocks?	....YES	.....NO	
	Does he know his first name?	....YES	.....NO	
	Can he copy a circle?	....YES	.....NO	
4 yr.:	Can he stand on one foot?	....YES	.....NO	
	Can he copy a cross?	....YES	.....NO	
	Does he use the past tense, properly?	....YES	.....NO	
5 yr.:	Can he follow three commands?	....YES	.....NO	
	Can he copy a square?	....YES	.....NO	
	Can he skip?	....YES	.....NO	

* Developed by the Committee on Children with Handicaps, American Academy of Pediatrics, New York Chapter 3, District II.

† This check list is a compilation of developmental landmarks matched against the age of the child. These are in easily scored question form and may be checked YES or NO by a physician or his aide, by direct observation.

"NO" responses at the appropriate age may constitute a signal indicating a possible developmental lag. If there is a substantial deviation from these values, then the child should be evaluated more carefully, taking into consideration the wide variability of developmental landmarks. (Adjust for prematurity, prior to 2 years, by subtracting the time of prematurity from the age of the child. E.G., a 2-month-old infant who was 1 month premature should be evaluated as a month-old infant).

It is our hope that the early recognition of such lags would lead to early diagnosis and treatment, the results of which can be very helpful to many of these children.

sounds as described for the 0- to 4-month olds, steps 1 through 9. For the noisemaker tests, the clinician can either kneel at a 45° angle to the child and hold the noisemaker unobtrusively down beside the chair, or kneel behind the baby and present the sound on the side at the lower level. The head-turn will be evident in this case, but the eye-widening and "aha" effect will not be seen.

For speech audiometry the baby should be held seated in his mother's lap, facing forward toward the window.

A small, not-too-attractive toy can be given the mother to hold in front of the baby on his lap. She should be instructed not to talk to him or to make any undue noise. Both loudspeakers are used. Present the speech first on one side until a head-turn is noted. Then quickly switch to the other loudspeaker and note whether the head turns back. The average level of the lowest speech which is responded to at this age is 21 dB.

At this age the speech testing should include saying the baby's name: "Hi, Johnny"; "hello, Johnny." Always find out which name the parents are using for the baby at home. It does not help to say "Hi, Johnny" to John Edwin who is called "Eddie" by his family.

As he approaches 7 months the infant may become responsive to "bye-bye" and that sound should be included in the speech reception battery with his name.

The entire battery of tests should always be used. One test confirms the other. Particularly, the startle to 65 dB should always be included at the end of each test period. If reduced hearing has been suspected, the lack of a startle or the reduced quality of the startle will confirm the previous findings.

Testing the Infant, 7 to 9 Months

In the 7- to 9-month period, the improvement in motor coordination allows the infant to sit steadily by himself and to change his position without falling. He manipulates two objects simultaneously, and transfers objects hand-to-hand and hand-to-mouth. This is the "explore-everything-in-the-mouth stage"—a good way to supplement information about the environment. We often see this stage represented in older mentally retarded children who are functioning at this mental age level.

He is able to play peek-a-boo, and may begin to learn pat-a-cake. He begins to be initially shy with strangers. He may be able to respond to bye-bye with a wave of his arm and a cupped hand. "Dada" and "mama" may be heard, but not with specific referents. He should imitate gross speech sounds nicely by 9 months.

Auditorally, the infant is now able to find a sound source below his eye level and to the side, but only by looking first to the side and then down. This is what is referred to as the "indirect fixation" of a sound source at a lower level. The transitional stage of his fixation ability becomes evident here. He is not yet ready to find the sound when it is above his eye level.

The level of an adequate speech signal now drops to a 15-dB average, showing the gradual maturation of the auditory response.

Procedure. 1. With the child seated on his mother's lap, let her hold a toy in front of him to play with—a small doll or a fuzzy animal. Usually he will be content to sit in his mother's lap and be mildly amused.

2. Present the same sequence of tests as before (steps 1 through 8). The noisemaker test again can be done by kneeling in front of the child at a 45° angle, being very careful not to let him see the noisemaker in your hand. Observe carefully the direction of his head-turn. At 7 months it may only be to the side but by 9 months, he should turn to the side and then look down.

3. For the speech awareness level, begin by saying "bye-bye Johnny." As in all the tests, you should develop a feeling for the moment when the child will be the most responsive. If he is still exploring his environment, wait until he settles down. If he is too engrossed in the toy in front of him, wait until his enthusiasm dies a bit.

Present the speech through one loudspeaker; if his head is turned toward one side, choose the loudspeaker on the opposite side. Once a head-turn is noted, switch to the other loudspeaker and repeat the signal. At this age, you can begin to manipulate the head-turn like that of people watching a tennis match, if you want. Not for long, however. It is not an interesting enough activity to sustain his interest.

At this age also, there may be a vocalization response to the speech signal. After listening to the voice, he may gurgle or respond with a questioning "eh" in a rising inflection. He may even imitate an "oh-oh" with inflection. He is a usually happy, out-going baby, not fearful of anything. He will submit to the impedance meter probe tip without complaint. Only at a later age does fear arise.

Testing the Infant 9 to 13 Months

It is normal by 9 months for the baby to be afraid of strangers if they come too close or attempt to hold him. "Strangeness" is one of the psychic organizers described by Spitz (1959). The child who will come to the arms of a complete stranger at this age may suffer a lack of psychic development. One should observe carefully the eye contact the child gives at this age. He should relate to you with interest, even if it becomes negative interest. Let mother handle him exclusively for the test. The advantage of testing from a dark sound room is evident at this point. It takes you out of the picture and allows the baby to relax and feel secure with mother. Normal babies do not mind the silence and confinement of the sound room. Occasionally an older child with cerebral dysfunction will object violently to the sound room, but even they usually settle down and enjoy the quiet.

By 11 months the baby is on his feet, cruising around his playpen or walking holding on to furniture. He is expected to say "mama" and another speech-like sound, but don't count on it. It may not be meaningful to him if he does make the sound. And remember that deaf children have been reported to say "mama" and "dada" by their hopeful parents.

The baby knows his own name now, and by 12 months can wave bye-bye. So we will now use "bye-bye Johnny" as our speech signal. It is an added premium if, as you present the phrase on an ascending threshold, he waves bye-bye to the loudspeaker at 5 dB. It is the best speech reception threshold obtainable.

The auditory behavior in this period progresses from the indirect to the direct localization of the sound source on the lower level. At the end of this period the baby should be localizing indirectly on the upper level; i.e., he will first look laterally and then shift his gaze upward. He is very interested in strange sounds in his environment, and will orient rapidly to the sound.

Procedure. 1. Go through the entire sequence as before. Include in the noisemaker test the presentation of a sound above and behind the baby's head, out of his eyesight.

2. In the speech sequence, the use of "bye-bye" will very often produce a hand wave in the direction of the sound. Another useful signal is "no-no," for by a year of age the child will stop what he is doing when he hears this signal, however faint. "Oh-oh" may produce an accurate imitation. The average threshold of response to speech at this age is 8 dB.

Testing the Infant, 13 to 24 Months

Once the child has reached 13 months, his orientation response is fully mature. After 2 years he may begin to inhibit his responses because of the strange social situation, but up to that time his reactions are still pure and untouched. In this period (by 15 months) he learns to walk—a skill that occupies him intensely for a while. He should be combining two words and be able to say three words other than mama and dada, but by 2 years it is not too alarming if he does not. He should, however, be using his voice meaningfully and in many variations. Up and down intonations, phonetic "grunts" of all sorts, and speech-like pauses in his vocalizations should be part of his repertoire if his hearing is normal. At this age in the deaf child the strident voice and the limitation of vocalization to the back vowels becomes evident. Once heard, the raucous "a-ah" of the deaf child can never be forgotten.

By 18 months he may know a few simple objects well enough to look for them. This ability can be used in testing. "Where's the meeow?" may elicit a quick look at the toy cat, or even a hit at it. By 2 years it is often possible to have him pick up toys on command during the testing session. So some simple speech audiometry can be added to the protocol. However, it is always well first to go through the testing sequence as for the younger infant, in order to have some information on his hearing level in the event he doesn't choose to cooperate.

Procedure. 1. Go through the test sequence as before, and record the results. The average level of response at this age is very close to 0 dB.

2. After the observations have been made of his orientation levels, try for some identification of speech in an ascending presentation: "Bye-bye." "Where's your nose?" "Where's mama?" "Where's the bow-wow?" "Want to go bye-bye?" As he becomes older he can pick up a few toys on command and give them to mama: "Give mama the airplane"—or the baseball, or the baby, or the kitty. Find out from mother which are his favorite toys, and use them in the presentation. In order to keep his attention on what you are saying at soft levels, you may have to set the carrier phrase ("Give mama the . . .") at 20-dB level and quickly shift down to the level you want to test, for the key word. Don't be alarmed if suddenly he stops responding. After a certain time you lose him to the game. Know when to give up—when you have exceeded the limits of his interest in what you are doing. This is even true of the 3-year-old during play audiometry. Every child has a limit to his period of interest. You must either change the game or give up testing when the limit is reached.

Remember that the speech games are just as effective using bone conduction as they are in free field. Although the child may not tolerate the earphones, the differences between his free-field threshold and his bone conduction threshold are significant. He will usually tolerate the bone conduction receiver held at the midline or behind his ear.

The use of the darkened instrument room is still indicated up to 2 years of age. The purity of his behavior includes an unquestioning response to the voice signal. At a later age he will be confused by the voice without a visible speaker, and it may interfere with the actions one wants to stimulate.

Clinical Testing of the Child Aged 2 to 5 Years

In this period the child grows into the independence of early maturity. He begins to separate from mother without much fuss; to dress himself, first with supervision and then without; and to understand his own identity. He becomes a wanderer, so don't turn your back on him or you will lose him. He begins to understand some abstract words like "cold" or "hungry," and can give his full name when asked. He becomes an eager beaver, happy to please you, and as a result gives the clinician a hard time in testing. Once he knows his cooperation in the play-conditioning pleases you, he may forget what he is supposed to listen for, in his eagerness to be praised. (Strangely enough, this attitude is often found in older deaf children—even in teenagers—who will give false responses in order to please, or to give a "good" test.) Therefore, one must temper one's enthusiasm with judgment, when dealing with this age child.

The learning of play-conditioning techniques starts at 2 years. But don't be deceived by the bright, talkative 2-year-old who appears certain to be able to learn the procedure. Play safe, and first get all the information obtainable from the observations of his behavior described for the younger child. Then when you draw a blank you have some valuable information as a basis for future tests or for a medical examination.

He may protest, however, when it comes to the acoustic bridge test. All of the audiologist's skills are called on to complete this test. Chapter 6 provides some suggestions for dealing with children and impedance measurements.

Until the child is 4 or 5 years, all the ingenuity the audiologist has must be brought forth. Short of standing on one's head, anything goes. But know when to give up. Don't traumatize him so much that he will be frightened the next time. There's always another day.

Occasionally it may be extremely urgent, however, that all the tests be completed in one day. A physician should then be consulted as to the advisability of giving a sedative to the child. If he prescribes and orders a sedative, the test may be accomplished. Such an extremity is resorted to most often in the case of an older, cerebrally damaged child who will not tolerate any handling. In this case the kind of sedative will be carefully considered by the physician. It should always be viewed as a last resort.

The darkened instrument room should not be forgotten even for these older children. A shy, immature child of 2½ may learn play-conditioning techniques easily, but the odd situation of a stranger's face in the window is too much for him to handle. The bodyless voice over the speaker can be coped with. It takes the stranger out of the situation. All the necessary instructions can be given through the speech circuit without being seen. So occasionally it will be useful to keep the instrument room darkened. A little experience with Braille will help the clinician manipulate the dials.

The description that follows of testing this age group is primarily related to double sound room testing. When the audiometric test is done in the same room with the child, the procedure can be easily adapted. The choice of audiometric testing in a double sound room or in a single seems to rest on personal preference. Whatever suits the individual's style should be elected. The speech reception tests will always have to be done with the clinician outside of the testing room.

The armamentarium of the child tester should include a carefully selected array of toys the names of which approach spondaic principles as closely as possible. However, in order to present children with easily recognizable toys, some compromise may be necessary. It is more important that the child knows and enjoys the toy than that it confirms to equal-stress-on-each-syllable principle. Among the small-sized toys available to the dogged shopper are the following:

Spondaic Words
   Airplane
   Baseball
   Toothbrush
   Hot dog (from the pet department)
   Cowboy
   Playground (a doll-house set of swings)
   Arm chair (a doll-house chair)
   Birthday (a play cake with candles)
Nonspondaic Words
   Baby (a small baby doll)
   Kitty
   Doggie
   Horsie
   Car

Truck
Lion
Hamburger (pet shop)

No more than 4 to 6 of these need be selected for the 2- to 3-year-old, and 6 to 10 for the 4- and 5-year-olds.

Procedure for Behavioral Play Audiometry

1. Placement. Place the young child in his mother's lap, with a table of toys in front of him. The older 4- or 5-year-old may prefer to sit alone with his mother in another chair, but mother's closeness may be important even at the older age.

2. Initial Rapport. Sit down and talk to mother first, developing an easy rapport with her. "What seems to be Johnnie's problem?" Let her tell you briefly why she is here, but don't belabor the history. Johnnie is the chief target. Turn interestedly to him and ask him how old he is, or comment on something he is wearing or has brought along. Little girls like their hair to be noticed. Ask him if he would like to play with your toys. "What is this?" If he doesn't answer, say "It's a big airplane, isn't it?" Try with other toys, and eventually he may tell you the name. Proceed to find out whether he can identify the toys. Eliminate those he isn't familiar with, and select those he seems to know best and enjoy.

During this period many observations can be made. Listen to his voice quality and how he articulates the words. Does he substitute for the high frequency consonants? If he omits or substitutes for the unvoiced consonants, either a mild sensorineural or a conductive loss can be suspected. If he misses the voiced consonants and some of the vowel sounds in addition, a more severe sensorineural loss may be predicted. Is he able to repeat words readily, but not to identify the corresponding toy? This is common in two types of children: those with sensorineural loss who have been given too much formal speech therapy or speech stimulation without sufficient experiences in hearing the word in connection with the object; and those with an auditory receptive disorder which allows them parrot-like imitation but no higher integration of the auditory-visual relationship. It may be difficult to decide which factor is present until diagnostic therapy reveals the degree of learning potential.

3. Introduction of Speech Test Procedure. Tell him what he's going to do. (Never ask him if he will do it.) "Now we're going to play a telephone game. You are going to put on the telephone like this, and I'm going to telephone to you. I am going to tell you which toy to show me. Won't that be fun? Now we'll put the telephone on you, and you can say hello to me. Hello!" Put the earphones gently but firmly on his head, saying "Hello, how are you? Now wait and I'm going to telephone to you from the other room." Try to get out before he balks at the phones, but if he does, don't fight it. Take off one phone and have mother hold it to his ear "like a real telephone." With the very young and shy child it may be preferable not to start with earphones at all. Do a trial run in sound field first, allowing him to become familiar with the situation. Then the earphones placement may be attempted.

4. Speech Test Procedure. In the instrument room, set the speech level at 40 or 50 dB (or as indicated) and say "Hello, Johnnie. We're telephoning, aren't we? Can you show me the airplane?" If he does, praise him and clap your hands. Then descend in 10-dB steps, asking him to show you a toy at each level. When he no longer responds, ascend 5 dB, but set the carrier phrase "Show me . . ." at a 10- or 15-dB higher level and switch quickly to the lower level. Too long a silent period will lose him to the game, so when searching for threshold the louder carrier phrase should be given. Accept two valid responses on the ascending presentation, and switch quickly to the other ear. Listening at low levels is not a child's cup of tea, and one must sacrifice some accuracy for the sake of holding his attention. If any discrepancies appear later, a recheck can always be done. It need hardly be said that the tester's mouth should be covered while giving the words.

Note that the speech reception threshold is obtained first in order to obtain information that will guide the clinician in the audiometric test. Too often a clinician will begin by training a child in audiometric techniques, starting at 40 or 50 dB, when the child has a 60-dB loss at that frequency. A complete, normal audiogram will then be recorded because the child plays

along with the clinician's silly little game of responding when he thinks he is supposed to. *Never*, never presuppose a level of hearing in a child. It is better to obtain an awareness level as in the younger child and confirm it with a startle response at 65 dB, than to enter blindly into a test with a young child. The greatest number of misevaluations occur because of this failure. The rare case of sudden bilateral deafness in a child is particularly subject to misevaluation. The normal speech pattern of such a child misleads the clinician into the wrong audiometric technique. If there is any doubt, a startle test will resolve it. At any age the normal or near-normal hearing child will startle to 65-dB speech coming out of complete silence.

Often masking must be used if the SRT in one ear is 40 or 50 dB worse than the other. At this age masking is more productive of valid results in speech reception tests than it is in pure tone testing. The esoteric nature of pure tones may confuse the child when a masking noise is present. Always prepare the child for the noise. "Now we're going to be on an airplane, and you can hear the airplane noise. See if you can hear me over the noise and show me the toys." It is rare that masking will interfere with speech reception once the child has learned the technique.

By 4 or 5 years, simple speech discrimination tests can be given. The challenge is to select a test on the basis of the child's present receptive language level. Even if his language level has been identified on the basis of previous language tests, there are no children's discrimination tests which will fit the language shortcomings of every age and of every degree of hearing handicapping condition. A great need exists to standardize speech with degree of hearing loss. Until then, a variety of picture discrimination tests are available for the 4- and 5-year-old: (1) the Siegenthaler and Haspiel Picture Discrimination Test (1966); (2) the Myatt and Landes Picture Discrimination Test (1963); (3) the Goldman-Fristoe-Woodcock Test (Quiet Subtest) (1970) (available on tapes, and is best done with two persons—an operator and an observer of the child's responses in the sound room); and (4) the Haskins PB-K, or Kindergarten Word List (1949). This test can only be used with bright and verbal 4- and 5-year-olds, but requires constant motivational techniques. It most resembles the standard PB word lists, and half of each 50-word list can be used.

Reinforcement techniques have been reported to improve the discrimination scores of both normal and hard-of-hearing children, 4 to 8 years old (Smith, 1969). The same is true of pure tone audiometric techniques for difficult children. The test results are enhanced by operant conditioning (Lloyd et al., 1968; Lloyd, 1970). However, for routine clinical purposes the social reinforcement of the enthusiastic and animated clinician is sufficient to obtain an optimal result.

5. Introduction of Pure Tone Test. Now begin the instruction for the pure tone test. Take the earphones off the child (he is bored with them by this time) and put them on yourself. Have available a number of sets of motivational toys geared to different ages: plain blocks for building a tower; a graduated ring tower; beads to throw into a container; a peg board with colored pegs (Put a horse or a car in the center and build a fence or a garage. Girls prefer the horses; boys prefer the cars.); and a piggy bank with pennies to put in (always give a penny as reward).

Other motivational games can be devised by the ingenious audiologist. Usually one is sufficient to accomplish the task, but you must be ready to switch to another one at the first sign of boredom. It is largely the enthusiasm of the clinician that keeps the child attending, but occasionally novelty must be employed.

Show the child what the game is about. "We're going to hold this peg (or block, etc.) up to our ear and listen for a little bell. Oh! I hear it, so I can put the peg in the board. Now I'm going to listen for a little one. Oh! I hear it, so I put the peg in. Now you can do it, and build a fence for the horse." In the case of the 2- and 3-year-old, instruct mother to hold his hand with the peg up to his ear, and to guide his hand to the peg board when the sound is heard. Then practice it through sound field so the mother will hear it. Three or four trials should be sufficient for the child to learn.

6. Pure Tone Procedure. Now tell the child he is going to do it all alone and switch to the earphone. Present the tone at 40 to 50 dB above the expected threshold. Praise him for a correct action by switching to the speech circuit. Instruct the mother to have another peg ready to give him the moment he has responded accurately by placing the peg in the board. Descend as rapidly as possible from 40 or 50 dB in 10- or 15-dB steps, indicating that he is to listen for a "tiny little baby bell." Again, work quickly to obtain threshold, accepting two responses on the ascending presentation.

Select 2000 Hz as the first frequency to be presented. It is the most important one so far as a sensorineural loss is concerned. If the SRT has not been normal, be sure the initial practice tone is loud enough to cover a possible high frequency commensurate with the SRT or the awareness level. Sometimes a child will seem to be cooperative at first, but soon forgets what he is supposed to do. In this case, recondition him with the mother's help, at levels you are certain he can hear. Several reconditioning periods may have to be run during a test. *Don't give up* until it is quite apparent that he is not about to stay with the task.

The next frequency will be 500 Hz, significant in a conductive loss. Then switch to the other ear and obtain thresholds at 2000 and 500 Hz. If by this time you have lost the child, at least you have some valuable information. If he stays with the task nicely, fill in the 1000- and 250-Hz thresholds, and then 4000 Hz. Know when to stop, because the bone conduction test is coming, and there must be some reserve of attention to carry him through it. It should be noted that when the child persistently refuses to wear even one earphone, sound field audiometry should be resorted to. Warbled pure tones, precalibrated to the location where the child is sitting, should be presented utilizing the play-conditioning techniques. The thresholds will represent the hearing in the better ear only, but will give the most essential information about how the child is hearing.

7. Now repeat the above with the bone conduction receiver. "We're going to use another kind of telephone—one that goes behind the ear. But you can hear the sounds just like the other telephone. That's like airplane pilots (or astronauts) use!"

Repeat the test as above, doing the more important frequencies first, and filling in with the others where possible. If there is any doubt about the bone conduction thresholds, give an SRT through the bone conduction receiver just as for the air conduction. The result can give a clue as to the actual situation. It is assumed that the bone conduction SRT has been precalibrated on normal-hearing people. The average normal threshold is generally around 35 40 dB on the dial of most instruments. Merely switching to the "microphone" input and the "bone conduction" output puts the speech circuit into the bone conduction receiver on most audiometers. If SRT's are all that can be obtained on a child, the difference between air and bone-conducted speech threshold gives significant information. In addition the bone-conducted speech can be masked effectively in the opposite ear without affecting the validity of the child's responses. The bone-conducted speech test is one of the most useful of the audiologist's tools. At the end, praise him or reward him with some token. This is insurance for future cooperation. You may have to see this child many times, so lay the groundwork for a happy return visit.

8. Verify Audiometric Impressions with Impedance Audiometry.

If the child should have to be sedated, one advantage is that he can then be retested in the sound room, if he has been over-active or uncooperative in the first trials. Mild sedation allows him to give consistent arousal responses, and the differences between his air and bone conduction thresholds of arousal may be very informative. Also, the startle response is no less effective under mild sedation than without it. The requisite is that the child be kept absolutely quiet in the sound isolation of the booth for a few minutes prior to an awareness test or a startle test.

Testing the Child 5 to 16 Years

By 5 years the child of normal intelligence can cooperate in the standard adult pure tone techniques and can repeat simple words. He will attend for fairly long periods of time to the hand-raising technique, given sufficient praise and encouragement. Not too much encourage-

ment, though, as he may begin to give false responses in order to please. He will repeat the PB-K words willingly, but a few errors should be expected even in the normal-hearing child.

The pure tone audiometric technique that is chosen is a matter of preference, so long as it fulfills the requirements of the descending-ascending technique that is a modification of the method of constant limits. Newby (1964) and Carhart and Jerger (1959) have described the most commonly accepted techniques for obtaining thresholds. In addition, a method proposed by Berlin and Catlin (1965) has some real advantages over the traditional procedures. The initial tone presentation is given at 0 (or −10) and ascends in 10-dB steps until the level is reached where the subject responds. Another signal is given at 5 dB above that level to confirm its validity, and then another presentation is given at 10 dB below the last one. An ascent is then made. If a response is given, the next tone is presented at 10 dB below that level and the next tone ascends 5 dB. Three no-responses must be found at 5 dB below the level of "threshold" and three responses at 5 dB above. Two or three responses must be seen at "threshold." Advantages to this method: (1) it structures the bracketing of threshold; (2) it confirms the first response on the ascent by obtaining a response at a higher level; (3) it eliminates the taking of false responses as the threshold, by confirming the lowest response level through a 5-dB higher level; (4) it accustoms the subject immediately to listen for softer tones rather than louder tones; and (5) in the case of a functional hearing loss, it minimizes the "measuring stick" of the subject by the presentation of lower hearing levels at the start.

Whether this precise method is used, the experienced clinician will routinely employ the confirmatory procedure of presenting a 5-dB higher level than the presumed threshold. False responses can be rapidly spotted through this maneuver.

Modifications of Standard Testing Procedures for This Age Range

5 to 10 Years. The younger child in this age group requires motivation to keep his attention on the test. Usually this can be done by social approval: smiling, nodding the head, clapping the hands, etc. It is rarely necessary to resort to bribery (commonly known as reinforcement technique). However, when the clinician has not enough resources or energy for social motivation, reinforcement can be used in the form of money, candy, etc.

The speech reception tests should be kept fairly simple at this stage. Usually 10 or 12 spondee words are sufficient to obtain threshold. Always familiarize the child with the words before the test. This can be done while sitting and talking to the child in an initial get-acquainted period.

The time spent in gaining rapport with the child is worth the effort. Talk to him about his clothes, his interests, his toys. Display a real interest in him. During this time you will make many useful observations about his voice quality, his articulation, the extent of his vocabulary, and the degree of cooperation you can expect.

Explain to him exactly what is going to happen, telling him this is what he is going to do—not "will you do this for me?" Be sure particularly to explain that he is to raise his hand (or finger) even when the tone sounds very faint and far away. He will have to listen hard for these little tiny sounds, because they are a long way off. A thorough explanation of this aspect of the test will preclude the possibility of his being falsely labelled "psychogenic" because he didn't understand what to do.

Speech discrimination words must also be kept fairly simple. Usually the PB-K's will suffice, but if not, the techniques given for the younger child can be used.

Always make certain of the mental age of the child. If a 5-year-old has a known IQ of 70, he should be treated like a 3½-year-old, not like a 5-year-old. The methods described for that age should then be used. Many children over 5 are labelled "untestable" merely because the clinician failed to apply the test procedure appropriate for the mental age level represented.

10 to 16 Years of Age. Very few modifications of the standard audiometric procedures are ever required for this age group. The development of rapport, the complete explanation of the test procedure, and the use of mild motivational techniques are usually sufficient for a valid test. However, there are a few precautions to take at this age, given below.

If the clinician has been presented with an audiogram from elsewhere showing a 30- to 60-dB loss, yet the child responds perfectly well to soft speech levels, suspect that you are dealing with a possible false-responder. Or you may note the personality characteristics described later for the "psychogenic" child. In this case, always start with a slow, ascending presentation of both pure tones and speech. He may give you lower, or normal thresholds with this technique than he would if you gave him a louder tone to use as a "measuring stick." Time will be saved in arriving at an understanding of the child's problem.

The deaf or hard-of-hearing child of this age must be handled carefully. Often he will attempt to respond when he does not hear, in an attempt to appear to have more favorable hearing than he actually has. It is best never to let such children see you during the test presentation. Face them completely away from you, because they can catch even a raised eyebrow out of the corners of their eyes. During the test, give them long periods of silence occasionally, and if they respond falsely, reprove them for the false response. Perhaps the clinicians who have tested such a child have been over-eager to motivate him, and he is merely trying to please. Reprimands are sometimes necessary to counteract this behavior.

At this age, and also at younger ages, the child has a right to understand what it means if he has a hearing loss, providing he has any receptive language at all. Too often we tend to "talk over" the child to the mother, in words that he doesn't understand. In the meantime, he is sitting there, wondering what it is about and worrying over what is wrong with him. The clinician should take time to explain to him in words that he can understand, just what kind of a loss he has, how severe it is, and what is going to be done for him. Often the clinician's explanation of the problem will ease the way toward his accepting the amplification and habilitation that will follow. Parents may be unable to explain these things to him, or may try to gloss over the facts, leaving the child bewildered and sometimes antagonistic. The child may be worried over what the other children will think of him in school. Explain that he is going to be a little different from the others, but only in this one respect. Otherwise he is just like everyone else, a good baseball player, a good game player, or a pretty girl who can play with the other girls. But in addition he will now hear his friends and his teacher better, and they will like that. We often tell the true story, particularly for the younger child, of the 8-year-old girl who took her hearing aid to school for the first time. Her teacher showed the aid to the class, saying "Susie has a little radio all her own that will help her to hear us all better." All the children then came up and listened to the little radio so they knew what it was. The next day the teacher had many telephone calls from parents who said "What should I do?—My child insists that he wants a little radio like Susie has." So sometimes the other children in a class envy the hearing aid!

Other Techniques of Behavioral Testing

The testing of infants and young children described above rests on direct subjective observations of the infants' responses under structured conditions. The weakness of such observations is in the pure tone tests, which do not consistently produce responses as close to threshold as the speech awareness tests. Whenever there is doubt about the validity of the observations made in pure tone tests, other test procedures are available to search for those thresholds.

Visual Reinforcement Audiometry

Liden and Kankkonen (1969) first coined the term "visual reinforcement audiometry" (VRA), based on a technique described by Suzuki and Ogiba (1961) and termed by them "conditioned orientation reflex" (COR) audiometry. This procedure as currently used employs lighted transparent toys which are flashed on simultaneously with the presentation of the auditory signal during a conditioning period. During the testing phase the light is flashed immediately following a response (looking toward the light). Liden and Kankkonen used interesting pictures on a slide projector to reinforce any response from the child, whether

the responses were merely awareness, eye-blink, orientation, or smiling. Matkin (1973) reports success using any of these responses as indicative of the child's hearing of the tone. Matkin also found that the technique is useful with earphones, and that VRA is successful with 90% of both normal-hearing and hearing-impaired children between the ages of 12 and 30 months. Furthermore, he states that speech stimuli are as effective as the warble tones usually prescribed. The VRA technique can also be used to test the child's responses with hearing aids.

In sound field it is apparent that VRA audiometry will test only the better ear in some children, even when loudspeakers on each side of the child produce the signals and the lights for localization. Hodgson (1972) states that the child with a severe hearing loss will not have learned to localize sound. He suggests that where there is confusion in localization, it is best to use only one loudspeaker in testing. In order to distract the child from looking constantly at the loudspeaker, an animated toy can be activated in another direction.

Fisher and Freedman (1968) simulated unilateral losses in normal children by plugging one ear, and found that they gave accurate sound localization. Thus, even with unilateral loss and one normal ear, such a child may locate the sound source. We feel that the localization skills depend upon the age of the child and upon the stimulus used. Warble tones are difficult for many infants under 12 months to localize consistently, whether the children are normal or hard-of-hearing. Matkin's suggestion for using speech as the stimulus would seem to be more productive of results for infants before 12 months of age.

Haug et al. (1967) described a procedure to overcome the problem of testing only the better ear. Their "Puppet in the Window Illuminated Test" (PIWI) was successful in obtaining thresholds in children under 3 years of age. With two loudspeakers, localization responses were reinforced by the appearance of a puppet behind a lighted window. After a conditioning period, earphones were placed on the child and the puppet again was illuminated every time the child responded to the tone by looking toward the window.

Despite many reports of using VRA audiometry on children, Matkin's (1973) estimate of 12 to 30 months as the most successful age for using this technique is probably most realistic. From 12 months down to birth, the response decrement becomes more and more evident, and would obviate success in evoking continued responses. No matter how attractive the play, the young infant soon loses interest in the game. Even when VRA audiometry is to be used, we prefer first to make observations of behavioral responses on an ascending threshold as described previously. In this manner one takes out insurance against the possibility of failing to obtain consistent information with VRA techniques.

Tangible Reinforcement Operant Conditioning Audiometry (TROCA)

Lloyd et al. (1968) described a technique of systematic reinforcement audiometry for use with mentally retarded children. The technique has also found favor among clinicians for testing normal young children (Matkin, 1973). TROCA procedure uses positive reinforcement (candy, cereal, or a trinket) for appropriate responses and a mild punishment (time out) for false responses. The child's behavior is conditioned until he pushes a response button on a feeder box whenever he perceives a sound. Lloyd et al. employed continuous reinforcement in their initial study of the technique. Others have used a fixed ratio scheduling (Bricker and Bricker, 1969; Spradlin et al., 1969), but there have been no studies determining which technique best maintains conditioning. A descending audiometric technique appears to be the method of choice (Lloyd, 1968), although Spradlin et al. failed to find any differences between ascending and descending threshold presentation. A film demonstrating the step-by-step operant procedure outlined by Bricker and Bricker (1969) has been produced by the Parsons Research Center, Kansas (available from Elizabeth Lawson, 6 Bailey Hall, University of Kansas, Lawrence, Kansas 66044).

Another operant procedure was reported by Spradlin et al. (1969). Their project demonstrated the use of escape avoidance and conditioned suppression procedures in searching for threshold.

While the clinician may not often have to resort to these techniques with mentally normal children, the tests should be available as back-up for testing the young child on whom clinical information is difficult to secure.

Nonorganic Hearing Loss in Children

The child who presents with a nonorganic, or functional, hearing loss is a quite different problem from the adult with a nonorganic loss. He is a much less sophisticated feigner of poor hearing than the adult, and his underlying motives, whatever the impelling factor, are sometimes more obscure. The needs which drive him to give an inaccurate hearing test are probably more honest, more unrecognized by him, and certainly engender more sympathy than in the adult.

The differences between the dynamics of simulated hearing loss in adults and those in children are striking. Under the age of 16 the secondary gains are never monetary, and the children are rarely consciously dishonest; i.e., the child is not often aware of the fundamental "wrongness" of his actions. He is impelled by such great needs that acting them out becomes a necessity to him. However, it is our belief that as in the adult, the "hysterical" or purely unconscious presentation of a hearing loss does not exist.

Any child who presents with a functional hearing loss has a problem, whether it be a minor transient difficulty or a deep-seated permanent disorder. It is a symptom of something, just as a runny nose or a fever is a symptom of something. It should never be disregarded or passed off as a temporary foible. It may represent a cry for attention, an apology for poor performance, or a rebuff to a hostile world. The child is saying "Help me, please." He is a lucky child, because the symptom he has chosen is the only one out of a host of possible physical and personality symptoms that can be accurately measured and definitely identified as being nonorganic and emotionally based.

Children who have some basic need that is unfulfilled may choose from a variety of symptoms that are available to them, ranging from the conscious to the psychosomatic. They may complain of stomachaches, headaches, poor vision, poor hearing, or specific pains. They may act out their needs in aggressive behavior or in withdrawal. Their symptoms may enter the psychosomatic realm, with disorders like eczema or chronic stomach disorders. Even psychosis may be present. When their behavior becomes outwardly aggressive and approaches delinquency, their disturbance becomes a threat to their families and to society. If in this chain of symptoms just one symptom is found that can be measured and identified as being purely emotional in origin, the progression of the symptoms can be halted by proper management. Hearing loss is such a symptom. Although not always serious, the problem is the only one which can be recognized for what it is, and its specific treatment outlined.

The clinician can recognize a possible "nonorganic child" almost immediately by his exaggerated behavior—exaggerated either in being too withdrawn, uncommunicative and lacking in affect, or in being over-talkative, brash, and manipulative. Both types are already acting out the individual personality dynamics that will be evidenced in the audiometric test. Most often they will understand what is said to them even if it is spoken low and out of their vision. The brash one will think to say "what?" occasionally, but will forget to do it when sufficiently interested. Even if these behaviors are not dramatically obvious, the clinician will intuitively feel some hostility in the child. Often the clinician is hard-put to control his own hostility, and may not understand why he feels it. One must keep reminding oneself that the child's behavior is not malicious and requires sympathy, not a reflection of the hostility.

The symptom of nonorganicity in children can often be said to be man-made, in that the opportunity for it has been created by the presence of audiometric screening programs. The large majority of children who present with such problems are referred because of failure on the screening test in school. Johnny sees that Joe, who has failed the hearing test, is given special treatment: he is excused from school to

have further examinations, and he is given special seating and attention in school. It is like having headaches or stomachaches—it gives an excuse for poor performance and a chance to bid for sympathy. Thus there is added another symptom to the choices possible to an upset child, and this time it is a man-made choice.

It should be recognized that this discussion of nonorganic hearing loss does not include those children who did not understand the instructions given them during a previous test. It should be obvious when the child has been confused over the directions, and has responded only to the loudness level of the first tone he heard. However, this is also the strategy used by the child with true nonorganic hearing loss, so care should be taken to ensure the fact that the child has completely understood the directions.

The continuum of the severity of emotional causes of nonorganicity runs a gamut from mild, transient problems to severe psychosis. We will give examples of three types in the order of their severity, keeping in mind that there will always be an overlapping between the ratings that are made.

Type I: Transient

Case 1. Alice B. is a healthy, attractive, out-going Caucasian girl of 9 years who moved to Denver from a smaller town out-of-state. She had been an "A" student and headed her class both in grades and popularity. During her first month at school, the audiometric screening program was given, and she failed the test. In the clinic she at first gave thresholds of 30 to 50 dB bilaterally, with large inconsistencies between thresholds. Her speech reception thresholds were zero in both ears. After the speech tests, she was asked this time to listen harder for the tones, which would be "beep-beeps" coming from way off in the distance. Ascending pulsed tones were then given, starting at −10 and ascending very slowly. She then responded at 0 to 5 dB at all frequencies bilaterally.

Management. Alice was told "you're doing fine," and was asked to wait outside while we talked to her mother. It was explained that, although her hearing was normal, Alice had not at first responded accurately to the test, and that this kind of behavior is often found in children who are upset for some reason. Mother immediately volunteered the information that Alice had been apprehensive about moving and going to a new school. She had worried about continuing to get good grades and to be liked by the other students. Mother felt that Alice had always been a stable, happy child, and suggested that perhaps the family could make a special effort to be supportive and understanding. This was considered to be sufficient handling for the time being. It was recommended to Alice's mother that she say nothing about the feigning of the loss, but simply to reassure Alice that she would be all right. A report was requested in 6 months to see whether any other problems had arisen. At that time her mother stated that Alice was satisfied with her grades even though she was not at the top of the class, had made many friends, and that no physical or emotional problems had arisen.

This case represents the very least amount of action that need to be taken. It requires well adjusted and understanding parents. The clinician will have to make a judgment as to the ability of the parents to handle the problem. In any case, a report should be sent to the schools so that they too will understand the situation.

Type II: Mild

Case 1. Susie S. was a thin, undersized 12-year-old Caucasian girl who seemed docile but withdrawn. She had failed the school screening test. Her audiogram at first stayed remarkably close to 50 dB at all frequencies, air and bone conduction, but on speech reception tests she would give half-spondee responses at levels of from 0 to 20 dB. Her pure tone audiogram could be manipulated on the basis of whether the initial orienting tone was high or low. If an 80-dB orienting tone was given, a straight 70-dB audiogram resulted; on another test sequence, if an ascending presentation was given, a straight 40-dB audiogram would be obtained. This behavior shows the use of a mental "measuring stick" in deciding what loudness level to respond to. It is relative to any reference tone that is given, and can change with variations in reference tones. However, when Susie was directed to listen for "tiny tones, miles away," and a very slow and

deliberate ascending presentation was made from −10, the picture changed. For 30 seconds or more the tone was presented at −10, with the clinician looking questioningly at her. Then at −5 dB for another length of time, and Susie obviously was beginning to wonder if she really could hear. Finally at 5 dB when she did hear, she was so relieved that she responded readily. Ascending technique at all frequencies produced normal thresholds, as did speech testing. This technique of "waiting them out" is an effective one for both children and adults, as it hoists them on their own petard. After long waits, they begin to worry about really not being able to hear, and will usually respond eagerly when they finally detect the tone.

Management. Susie's mother was told about the false responses Susie had given, and that "such behavior is often found in children who have some emotional upset." This produced a welling up of emotion in the mother, who recounted a series of upsetting family problems which were ending in a divorce. "I just can't handle it anymore," she sobbed, "Susie is sassy and won't do anything I tell her to. I've got to have help." Mother was asked if she would like to have counselling in the psychiatric clinic, and she agreed, with relief. It seemed that Susie's problems were actually mother's problems, and that the family situation required professional guidance. Their difficulties were not solved overnight, but after a year of counselling, both mother and daughter were working out their problems. This kind of acceptance of professional help is a happy result. The sad one is when a parent refuses to accept the fact that a problem exists, and rejects completely the idea that any counselling is indicated.

Type III: Moderate

Case 1. George T., age 14, represents a classic case of symptomatology. His psychiatrist father brought him to the clinic because George had failed the school screening test and said he couldn't hear the teacher. He appeared to hear everything that was said to him, and seemed eager to be tested. Father observed all the testing. George showed the usual intra-test inconsistency in responses, with an average of 40- to 50-dB apparent thresholds. On speech reception he gave half-spondee responses at 0 to

20 dB but as usual, ultimately yielded to the slow ascending technique and gave normal pure tone thresholds. A free-field speech reception test was given to demonstrate George's normal hearing to his father.

Management. Father was told, "I'm sure you know the implications of why George isn't responding accurately to the test situation. Have you observed any other symptoms?" He expressed relief that the hearing loss had been identified as nonorganic, because George had presented with a list of symptoms about which father couldn't be certain. He had had headaches that kept him from going to school, then a series of stomach upsets, and then complained of a visual problem which kept him from reading well. Now that he knew the hearing symptom was nonorganic, father assured us that he would be able to handle the problem. We cautiously suggested that perhaps outside counselling be sought, either by the school psychologist or someone of father's choice. This idea was rejected as being unnecessary. It was, however, suggested that George not be told that it was known he was feigning a loss, so that the symptom would not be taken away from him before his problems could be resolved. Father did not agree, but was confident all would be well.

A year later father very graciously called to report that finally he had realized that outside help was indicated. After the hearing symptom had been removed, George had developed severe eczema, and that was followed by behavior problems leading to delinquency. A fellow psychiatrist was counselling George and the family.

George's case represents a classic chain of events of which hearing loss is one. It is not always so easy to see the progression of symptoms, nor indeed are they always present. The possibilities should be kept in mind, however, and some follow-up assured if only by the schools.

Type IV: Severe

Case 1. Felicia R. was a 9-year-old Chicano child who did not answer to any greetings or questions. She did not smile or respond with any affect to anything that was said or done.

She had been referred by the school for having failed the screening test and for not attending to the teacher in class. Even on ascending threshold she would give no response until 70 or 80 dB. Speech tests under earphones gave sporadic results from 20 to 50 dB, but free-field speech was heard and responded to at 5 dB. At that level, such statements as "button up your dress," "all right, you can come out now," produced the indicated action.

Management. Felicia's mother, although sympathetic and devoted to her, had no explanation for Felicia's behavior. Five older children and one younger one were "all right," but Felicia "had never been like the others." She agreed readily to the offer for counselling, and was referred to the psychiatric clinic. There Felicia was diagnosed as having childhood schizophrenia, and was put under intensive psychiatric treatment. Her case represents the extreme disorder in which nonorganic hearing loss can be the identifying symptom of psychosis.

The above case histories represent the continuum of nonorganic symptomatology ranging from transient problems all the way to psychoses. It should be re-emphasized that the school screening programs identified the disorder in almost every instance. Although we have placed on the screening programs the onus of providing the opportunity for the symptom, yet in each case the programs have served a much needed function in detecting an emotional problem of some degree.

The prevalence of nonorganicity seems to rise and fall periodically over the years. In one year we estimated that 10% of all the children tested in the clinic had nonorganic hearing loss. In other years it has been as low as ½ of 1%. The lower figures coincided with the years when the school system employed an audiologist who rechecked the children in a sound room. Thus there was a recheck follow-up at which time the audiologist was able to identify most of the nonorganic losses.

Leshin (1960) reported a screening program which identified a number of cases of nonorganicity in children. He investigated the social dynamics of each case, and instituted a remedial program which would fulfill the children's needs that impelled them to a symptom such as hearing loss. Such a program can be highly recommended.

It is extremely rare that any of the classic auditory tests for nonorganicity need to be used on children. Their naiveté in giving normal threshold responses to the ascending technique and to speech reception tests usually renders further testing unnecessary. Occasionally in the case of a monaural feigned loss, it is useful to give the Stenger test to verify the true threshold level.

Summary

From the above discussion, we can list briefly the presenting symptoms, the recommended test procedure, and the management suggested for each personality type.

Presenting Symptoms

1. Exaggerated behavior: withdrawal and lack of affect, or verbosity and brashness.

2. Exaggerated straining to hear the sound.

3. Inconsistent intratest results: thresholds varying 15 to 20 dB with presentations at a frequency.

4. Variable intertest results, depending on initial orienting tone level.

5. Speech reception thresholds normal or markedly better than pure tone responses.

6. Better thresholds, usually normal, given on retesting with slow ascending technique.

Recommended Test Procedure. Once the inconsistencies above have been noted, apply the following procedure:

1. Inform the child (in the sound room, not over earphones) that this time the test will be different. This time he will hear the tone coming from miles away, and it will be a tiny "beep-beep." He is to tell you as soon as he hears it from far away.

2. Start presenting the signal at -10 dB, and keep it pulsing for at least 30 seconds. Look questioningly at the child as if you expect him to hear.

3. Repeat the same at -5 dB, and then at 0.

4. If the speech reception has been normal, make a special effort at 5 dB: while the tone is being pulsed, point first to one ear and then the other questioningly, to see if he will identify the ear where the tone is present. Usually he will respond in some way.

5. Repeat if necessary at 10 dB, but if the

speech reception has been normal, stop at that level.

6. Proceed to another frequency and repeat the technique.

If the speech reception threshold has not been quite normal, the same steps as above can be taken with spoken spondees, again "waiting him out," and looking quizzical when he fails to respond even at below threshold levels.

Observers of this technique have voiced their concern over the child's worrying briefly about whether he really can hear. Such critics can be assured that the gains accruing to the child from the information obtained will far outweigh any temporary discomfiture he may have.

General Management Recommendations

Type I: Transient. If in the judgment of the audiologist and the managing physician the parents have sufficient insight to fill any needs represented by the non-organic symptom, and if there appear to be no obvious psychologic problems, the treatment should be entrusted to the parents. A report should be sent to the school indicating the estimate of the transient nature of the problem.

Type II: Mild. If the parents report other evident behavioral problems and recognize a justifiable familial or environmental situation, referral can be made to the school psychologist, with the parents' full knowledge and acceptance. Report should also be made to the managing physician.

Type III: Moderate. In the presence of other identifiable symptoms or deep-rooted familial problems, psychiatric counselling should be advised. If such referral is rejected, the parents should be told that a report will be sent to the referring school and the managing physician, as a routine procedure.

Type IV: Severe. Given truly bizarre behavior and parental bewilderment over the cause, psychiatric counsel should be urgently advised, with the agreement of the managing physician.

The cry for help that is inherent in the presentation of nonorganic hearing loss in a child should not be taken lightly by the audiologist. Listen to the sound of his need.

Testing the Difficult-to-Test Child

The judgments the clinician makes on children's hearing abilities often necessarily involve a differential evaluation. In the presence of other disorders the child's behavior or his level of functioning may be so erratic that standard techniques of audiometry cannot be used. In order to apply appropriate tests for hearing, the clinician must be able to recognize the dysfunction that is present and to adjust the tests to it. The classical disorders that are to be differentiated are mental retardation, cerebral dysfunction, and autism (Myklebust, 1954). More than one of these may be present in one child. If the clinician has been trained in evaluating any of these disorders, he may also test the child's functioning in that specific area, as well as in the hearing area. But at the very least he has the responsibility of recognizing the disorder that exists. He must be able to apply the proper tests for hearing and to make referral for diagnosis and treatment of the other disorder.

In discussing the entities which must be recognized, it is necessary to reiterate an important fact—that neither cerebral dysfunction nor central auditory disorders nor mental retardation nor autism result, in themselves, in a decrease of auditory acuity as represented by the audiogram. The responses which can be elicited certainly require more ingenuity to obtain. But when credible responses reveal reduced hearing for pure tones and speech, a peripheral hearing loss is present, in addition to any central disorder that may exist (Goldstein et al., 1972; Kleffner, 1973). The clinical audiologist's task is to choose the appropriate test procedures that will reveal the presence or absence of peripheral hearing loss. It is not always a simple task to make this distinction.

To guide the clinician in fulfilling his charge, we will attempt to describe the salient features of the various disorders and to suggest appropriate tests that may be chosen.

Mental Retardation

One principle should be kept in mind when dealing with the mentally retarded child. If generalized developmental retardation is his only disorder, he will behave in all areas at the level of his mental age. This principle will hold up in all cases except those in which autistic behavior or cerebral dysfunction is superimposed upon the general retardation. Then the testing problem is further compounded, but is not insoluble.

0 to 5 Years. Infancy is an ideal time to test the retarded child's hearing. He has not yet developed the social behaviorisms, the self-stimulating activities, or the inattention patterns of the older retardate. In the first few months of life he sleeps a great deal, giving an opportunity for good observations of his responses in a sound room. Until 4 months the quality of his auditory responses cannot be distinguished from those of the normal child. It must be remembered that until 4 months of age we still apply the same criteria of hearing responses that are used at birth. Only after 4 months can we depend on searching activity to be present. So the hearing testing for 0 to 4 months will follow the procedures described for the normal child at that age, and the audiologist may not be able even to recognize the retardation. He can, however, make the observations suggested of the infant's developmental landmarks. Any impression of a deviation from these norms should be recorded and followed-up with referral for developmental testing.

After 4 months we begin to identify the retardate through his auditory behavior as well as through the developmental landmarks present. If by 5 months he is not making even a partial head-turn toward the sounds, determine whether he can reach for and hold objects, and if he laughs aloud. He may not even be holding his head erect, or be able to follow a moving object—behavior which would place him below the 3 month level of functioning. In this case one can expect only the auditory responses that are listed for the child under 4 months. If he then responds to all acoustic stimuli like a child under 3 months, his hearing is judged to be normal.

The same observations of auditory behavior and developmental behavior should be made of the older child, referring to the developmental landmarks. If all behaviors are consistent for a certain age level, and the auditory indices are within the normal limits listed for that age level, the hearing level is judged to be normal. For example, if a 15-month-old child's behavioral landmarks are at the 8-month level, a speech awareness level of 15 to 20 dB and pure tone awareness of 45 to 55 dB are considered to be normal hearing.

If previous developmental scales or IQ test results are available, the clinician will have no difficulty in correcting the auditory test results for mental age. It is when the intellectual status is unknown that the clinician must apply his own observations of developmental landmarks. If these are not consistent at a certain age level, another disorder should be suspected. The 5-year-old who has normal motor coordination and good personal-social adjustment for his age, yet is unable to identify all of a group of familiar toys should be evaluated further, providing that his hearing test is normal.

The severely mentally retarded child with random motor movements is the most difficult to test. One must apply the kinds of behavioral observations that are made for young infants, yet the noises of his movements and the inattention prevent responses to soft sounds. Sometimes the only observations that can be made are of startle responses to 65 dB speech. A good startle response indicates normal range of hearing, or at the least rules out everything but a mild sensorineural loss. If behavior is too hyperactive even for this test, mild sedation can be ordered by a physician. Even a little reduction of the hyperactivity may permit both the observations of responses in the sound room and the use of the acoustic impedance meter.

However, the behavioral responses previously described for infants (response to 45-dB speech level, and startle to 65-dB speech) have been shown to yield a high percentage of successes in severely mentally retarded children. Knight (1973) studied 100 mentally retarded institutionalized students from 2 to 35 years of age, and applied to them this technique and the related criteria, as suggested by the authors. The functioning levels of the students were classified predominantly as severe to profound retardation levels. Of these, 25 were designated as untestable for mental age. Knight also applied tympanometry tests to this population. The average test time for the subjective observations was 3 minutes 10 seconds. Impedance testing was done in an average time of 2 minutes per ear.

Among the audiologic and otologic studies on the prevalence of hearing loss and ear disease in institutions for mental retardation, the percentages of loss range from about 10% to 45% or greater. Lloyd (1970) has presented a review of the literature on the audiologic aspects of mental retardation in which a summary of the various reported incidences is given. Each percentage is affected by the chronologic and mental age of the population tested, by the testing procedures used, and by the criteria for failure which are applied. Thus, it is difficult to estimate an average incidence of hearing loss in this group. Lloyd's excellent review article is recommended to all who seek to study these problems in detail.

The objection may be voiced that 45 dB is too high a screening level and that it may miss milder hearing loss. But if we estimate the intellectual functioning level of these severe retardates as equivalent to the first 4 months of infancy, then response to a 45-dB speech signal is the normal threshold level for this group. True, some with mild sensorineural loss and recruitment may respond at the 45-dB level but these would be very rare. We feel that at the present time the procedure of behavioral responses plus tympanometry offers the most practical means of testing this group.

5 to 16 Years. The very severely retarded in this age group can be tested only in the way described by Knight (1973). However, a large number of these children will have a level of functioning that permits other tests to be used. If their mental age is over 2 years, the tests described for children of that age can be applied. Play-conditioning techniques often are successful with the older retarded child when standard techniques fail.

A period of pretest observation will reveal what can be expected of the child. Present him with toys and see how familiar he is with them. Can he hand them to you on a command? If he recognizes most of the toys and can give them to you on command, he is probably able to give both a speech reception threshold and play-conditioned thresholds. If not, the routine observations of behavioral responses can be made.

When precise thresholds are desired in such a borderline functioning child, the techniques of visual reinforcement audiometry and tangible reinforcement operant conditioning audiometry described under "Other Techniques of Behavioral Testing" above can be employed.

The Centrally Disordered Child

The suggested techniques for testing the brain-damaged child rest on two basic assumptions.

1. That any reduction in auditory acuity for pure tones, speech, or other signals is caused by lesions in the peripheral auditory system, not in the midbrain or higher pathways (see our discussion in Chap. 3 on "Disorders in Auditory Learning"). No real evidence has ever been presented that lesions central to the cochlear nuclei result in reduction in auditory sensitivity.

2. That only in the extremely severe centrally damaged child with gross motoric involvement will we see the complete absence of all of the four basic auditory reflexes: head-turn, eye-blink, startle response, and arousal from sleep.

The first rule in testing such a child is to determine his level of behavior. Pretesting will show what he can and cannot do. Sit and talk quietly and play with him in the sound room. Can he attend for any length of time to anything that you say or do? Can he give his name, age, or other appropriate information? Can he hand you toys or repeat words on request? In the case of a very young child, as well as an older one, is his eye contact steady and does it have integrity? Can he sit still for any length of time? Is he hyperactive and does he throw things around?

The child who has auditory perceptual dysfunction may be able to sit quietly and attend to visual stimuli but not be able to repeat words or to pick up objects on command. Such a child may, however, be perfectly able to do play-conditioned audiometry with pure tones and speech signals. Don't give up on formal testing unless it is proved to be ineffective.

If it is evident that formal testing techniques will not be successful, it is best to start at the lowest level of testing procedure, as has been described for the infant from 4 months on. The entire battery of observations should be made, from localization procedures to startle reactions. Remember that this child may be inconsistent in his responses to various stimuli, and at various times. A clear-cut response to one stimulus at 5 to 10 dB can be relied upon, even when responses to other stimuli cannot be seen at that level. The startle or the eye-blink response will always confirm the observation of some reactions to soft levels.

We have stated that it is rare for all of the auditory reflexes to be absent in a child. The reflexes are mediated at the level of the brain stem and are usually intact in the presence of higher cortical dysfunction. Auditory reflexes only tell us about the integrity of the peripheral auditory system through the brain stem. They tell us nothing about the higher orders of perception and integration.

In order to demonstrate the relationships between the peripheral, midbrain, and cortical auditory functions, and the levels of the auditory reflexes, Table 5.3 has been prepared.

From this chart it can be seen that only in the presence of degeneration of the brain stem at the olivary complex can the absence of the head-turn and eye-blink reflexes be expected. Even then, the startle reflex, mediated at a low brain stem level, should be active, unless there is widespread motoric damage that prevents the muscular system from coordinating. Even in severe cases of mental retardation, these reflexes are evident, as shown by Knight (1973). Although the startle or eye-blink reflexes to a 65-dB (SL) signal do not eliminate the presence of a mild sensorineural loss, one may be sure that the loss is not of a degree that would produce the severe degree of symptoms found in a child whose only testable avenue is the reflex. Often the audiologist's task is to identify the primary disorder; a hearing loss may only be secondary to the major problem. The startle reflexes will enable him to do so. When reporting on such a case, the audiologist can say with confidence: "Hearing loss is not the primary problem in this child's communication dysfunction." Where the clinician is equipped to apply tests for central auditory dysfunction, he will be able to include the type and degree of the disorder.

The Autistic-Like Child

It is seldom that one sees the purely autistic-like child; but when one does, the

Table 5.3. Relationships between Reflexes and Auditory Responses

Reflexes and Other Auditory Responses	Level in CNS	Auditory Dysfunction at This Level	Tests which Identify the Dysfunction
Startle reflex	Pontomedullary junction and below	None	Lack of response to 65 dB speech or noise (85 dB SPL) in quiet sound room.
Acoustic reflex (stapedus)	Pontomedullary junction or below	Amplitude regulation (mild tolerance problem)	Intra-aural reflex test with impedance meter (Anderson, 1969)
Head-turn reflex (perinatal period) Orientation-localization (4 mo. or older)	Lower pons accessory Olivary nuclei but dependent on temporal auditory cortex in man	1. Binaural integration disorder 2. Inability to localize sound source 3. Time integration problems for speech	1. Frequency fusion test in dichotic mode (Matzker, 1959) 2. Localization tests (Deatherage and Hirsh, 1959; Matzker, 1959) 3. Interrupted speech test (Bocca and Calearo, 1963; Berlin and Lowe, 1972)
Eye-blink reflex (auro-palpebral)	Pons	Same as above	Same as above
Higher level functions: Discrimination of parameters of speech signal Auditory memory Auditory closure Auditory sequencing	Secondary auditory area of temporal lobe; association areas of temporal lobe (superior temporal gyrus)	1, 2, 3. Auditory disorders 4. Auditory sequencing disorders	1. Dichotic speech tests (Kimura, 1961; Berlin et al., 1972a) 2, 3, 4. Identification of order of presentation signals (Efron, 1963; Jerger et al., 1969)

bizarre behavior he displays can be recognized almost immediately: refusal to meet any person's eye gaze, disregard of all human speech stimuli, long term fixation on some object, and refusal of physical contact with humans. He will consistently fail to attend to any speech stimulus, yet he will attend to some other acoustic signals. One such child will look for pure tone signals at low intensities, another will search for a cat "meow" at soft levels, and another will localize a white or complex noise signal at normal levels. All will startle or eye-blink to 65-dB voice in a structured sound room situation if hearing is normal. All the stimuli described for testing from birth on should be tried. Something is guaranteed to produce a response if the hearing is normal, even if it is only a startle reaction.

The real testing problem arises when autistic behavior is superimposed on central dysfunction. Indeed, one wonders whether all brain damage is not accompanied by some degree of autistic behavior. The symptoms are often so similar that they defy separation. In addition to the behavior described above, there may be the heightened activity and lashing out at humans. If such a child is difficult for the neurologist and psychiatrist to understand, so he is for the audiologist.

The testing procedures described for mental retardation and for central disorders are applicable here. Keep in mind the fact that autistic symptoms are sometimes found in the deaf child, so do not let anything mislead you in the search for peripheral hearing loss. The audiologist's task in identifying the hearing level is unique, and no other discipline can lend guidance here. One must simply remember that the auditory reflexes cannot be suppressed even in an autistic child when the properly structured sound room condition prevails. If one is lucky, a stimulus may be found that will confirm perfectly normal hearing, aside from the reflexes. Acoustic impedance tests may provide valuable information.

Freedman and Kaplan (1967) list the four chief identifying features of autistic-like children.

1. They exhibit aloneness, and will occupy themselves for long periods of time without attention to anyone.

2. Some fail to use any language or communication; others may show precocious speech with scholarly words that have no real meaning to the child.

3. They show an obsessive desire for the maintenance of sameness. Fearing new patterns, they endlessly reiterate old patterns, almost as rituals.

4. They have a fascination for objects in place of interpersonal relationships, and will occupy themselves endlessly with a familiar object.

The autistic-like child is different from the mentally retarded or the brain-damaged child in that he usually has a high intellectual capacity, as indicated in I.Q. tests when they can be performed.

One form of autistic-like behavior is demonstrated by extreme anxiety at being separated from mother. Freedman and Kaplan label this behavior as a "symbiotic psychosis" indication. When such behavior is evident, the clinician can overcome it by keeping the child close to the mother, on her lap if he is small enough or sitting next to her during the test situation.

The Deaf-Blind Child

Except for the eye-ear syndromes described in Chapter 9, most of the etiologies for deafness-combined-with-blindness fall at the present time into the maternal rubella category. These cases are most often confounded by central nervous system damage which makes it difficult to structure the testing situation properly. The rare cases of meningitis resulting in deafness and blindness may also have associated neurologic and cognitive dysfunction. Not all are as intact centrally as Helen Keller, nor do they all have a full 2 years of

auditory language experience.

In severe cases of multiple involvements, we have found it most expedient to rely again on the auditory reflexes, on orientation responses, and on quieting responses. In the absence of speech and language, one must apply the tests as for the infant proceeding to the upper limits of the auditory abilities present. As in the infant, the absence of auditory reflexes is the confirmatory evidence of a peripheral hearing loss. Reliance on the absence (or presence) of this response will rarely lead one astray. If a doubt remains, diagnostic therapy with a trial hearing aid will reveal the true condition in a short time. One rule we have been adamant about: the deaf-blind child should always be fitted with true binaural amplification, even if the hearing loss appears asymmetrical. A careful frequency-gain balancing will compensate for the differences. The blind child needs every binaural clue he can get to function at his best level and to locomote adequately.

It is the audiologist's responsibility to make the decision about the blind child's hearing abilities. It must, perforce, be a bold decision, for any equivocation is not useful to the child. The conservative hearing aid trial with careful observations by all concerned during a diagnostic therapy period will not hurt the child. Hesitance may deprive him of critical time for learning auditory skills and thus do him a disservice.

Management of the Child with Unilateral Deafness

Unilateral deafness has always been common among children, and its prevalence does not appear to be lessening. Chiefly due to mumps, it develops with a suddenness that often baffles both the child and his parents. Audiologists and otolaryngologists are not usually concerned over such deafness, other than to identify its etiology and assure the parents that there will be no handicap. The child is often left bewildered at the mysterious onset and the loss of his "stereo" hearing. Seldom is he able to express his bewilderment, yet the occurrence is more traumatic to him than adults can appreciate. He is infinitely relieved if someone takes the time to explain to him what has happened, how it will affect him, and what he can do to compensate for it. In addition, the vestibular mechanism can occasionally be affected by mumps, as well as the cochlea being involved, and this poses another problem that needs to be understood.

The following points should be made in interpreting the problem to the child.

1. Assure him that he will be able to go through school and learn just like any other child.

2. Explain what has to be done to compensate for the monaural loss: special school seating, using the eyes to find the sound source, and placing oneself with the good ear toward the speaker.

3. If there is vestibular involvement, ask the doctor if some things like scuba diving or scaffold climbing should be done.

4. Give hearing conservation rules to protect the good ear: (a) stay away from loud noises; (b) get prompt medical care for any ear infection; (c) avoid putting anything into the ear; (d) avoid oxotoxic drugs unless absolutely necessary; (e) take special care of general health, especially during flu seasons; (f) have an otologic and audiologic check once a year; and (g) don't get advice on treatment from anyone but qualified otolaryngologists and audiologists.

5. Inform the patient that a CROS hearing aid is available if he ever is in a position where it may be needed.

Parent Management

Often it is the audiologist who must inform the parents that they have a deaf or hard-of-hearing child. It is always best to have the parents observe the child's responses in a free-field situation so that they can see for themselves that the child does not hear normally, and what he can and cannot hear. It will be an extremely traumatic situation for them. Whether they show grief openly or contain it within themselves, you may be sure that they will be deeply disturbed over the knowledge. The audiologist must find ways to help them over this initial shock.

It is the usual tendency of parents to want to find out immediately everything that concerns the future of the child and his functioning. One must resist the temptation to go into great detail about the prognosis for the child's development. Whatever is said will only be half-absorbed and largely distorted on the first visit. One should limit the amount of information to the relative degree of loss that seems to be present—mild, moderate, severe, or profound—and concentrate on the implications of the loss and what is going to be done for the child. If the parents press the question as to whether the child will speak, what kind of school he will go to, or whether he will ever communicate, assure them that you will be able to answer these questions, but only after a period of diagnostic therapy. No one can ever guarantee what a child will be able to do with training; only the results will demonstrate that.

There is perhaps no way to cushion the shock of finding out that a child is hearing-impaired. Any attempt to minimize the problem would be a disservice and would avoid the reality of the situation. But a sympathetic attitude and an understanding of the parent's feelings will help as much as possible; "You probably feel pretty upset about this news," or "It's perfectly natural for you to feel badly about this." Let them air their questions and fears. Allot sufficient time for them to express their feelings. Offer to be available for any questions that they might have and let them feel that you will work with them closely on finding out what their child can do with his loss. Emphasize that he is a child first, and has a hearing loss only secondarily. He is just as lovable as any other child.

Wherever possible, parents' groups under qualified psychologic counsellors should be organized, in order to provide on-going guidance. If further help seems indicated, psychiatric or psychologic counsel should be sought for the individual parents. The audiologist should be aware of his limitations in providing psychotherapy for parents who cannot handle their problems.

In his relationship with the parents, the audiologist's responsibility includes the following points.

1. A complete explanation of what the audiogram means, and what the child can and cannot hear.

2. A description of the type of loss, whether conductive or sensorineural, and what it means in terms of whether medical treatment may or

may not be possible.

3. A thorough explanation of the educational programs that are available for the child: auditory, oral, or total. The parents should be directed to visit each program so that they may participate in the decision as to which program will be chosen. With proper guidance, they should be able to make this decision themselves.

4. Psychologic support. This may take the form of a one-to-one relationship, or the parents may require group programs or even individual psychiatric counselling. The audiologist should remember that in this difficult role he can and should seek counselling for himself and for the parents if he feels unable to cope adequately with the situation.

The Audiologist's Understanding of Himself

In the audiologist's zeal to help the hearing-handicapped child and his parents, he often overlooks his own motivations and how they will affect his relations with the parents. These relations may be critical to the parents' acceptance of the problem. Quite without meaning to, he may leave the parents with fears and with pent-up emotions that can adversely affect the habilitation process. At some point the audiologist must look at himself introspectively to see what his own feelings are in relation to the way he gives information to the parents, and how he handles them. If he has gone into the audiologic profession with an emotional zeal for "do-gooding," he may see himself as the authoritarian figure who directs the lives of people. He will not permit the parents to express themselves because he is in charge of operations. If he has gone into the field through an objective interest in the scientific manifestations of hearing, he may shrink from becoming emotionally involved and committed to the parents' problems.

So the audiologist too may have problems in feeling comfortable in his role as protagonist in the drama of the parent-clinician interplay. This subject deserves extensive coverage because it is vital to the ultimate emotional health of the child. The most meaningful exposition of the subject has been written by two experts in parent management, Dr. Brian Hersch, a psy-

chiatrist, and Carol Amon, an instructor of deaf children, who have been studying parent-clinician dynamics in the Hearing Habilitation Program of the University of Denver. We are indebted to them for permission to use their analysis of the dynamics of the parent-clinician relationship (1973), which is presented below.

"To parents who are anxious to hear that their idealized child is perfect, the statement that 'Your child has a hearing impairment!' may be painful words. Those words can cause many emotions . . . shock, bewilderment, depression, anger, guilt, or anxiety. If these emotions are outwardly expressed by the parents, the audiologist, too, will experience feelings which may also be painful.

"In order to avoid this uncomfortable experience, many audiologists today choose a painless method of reporting the diagnosis—a way that, although it is painless for themselves, may have devastating effects on the parents and their child. After listening to many parents relate their experiences and frustrations, we began to realize that the act of reporting the diagnosis was not only of paramount importance, but also that it was the beginning of a process that would include the habilitation and education of the child as well as the crucial involvement of the parents. This process could be enhanced or interfered with, by the interpersonal relations of the initial contact.

"An approach toward lessening the trauma of the initial contact is proposed. It is an outgrowth of an idea that an interdisciplinary approach to understanding hearing impaired infants and their families (the disciplines being audiology, deaf education, and psychiatry) is far superior to an isolated fragmented approach of one profession (Schlesinger and Meadow, 1972a).

"Schlesinger and Meadow describe three ineffective professional stances which are often seen today in the reporting of the diagnosis:

"(1) The "hit-and-run" approach. The diagnosis is reported very quickly and matter-of-factly in passing. "Your child didn't respond too much today . . . his hearing loss is probably severe to profound. I'll see you in six months for another evaluation." The parents are left with their feelings of bewilderment as to what to do next. The reporting of the diagnosis appears to be a dead end with no source of help.

"(2) *Minimizing the problem.* The clinician infers that there is really nothing to worry about. "In this day and age, deaf children can be given hearing aids and go to regular school just like any other child." These words give false hope to the parents, but the audiologist says them in order to make the parents feel better.

"(3) *The objectivity approach.* Many audiologists are hidden behind objectivity, using the "big word" technique. In one hour's time, they report the diagnosis, explain the audiogram and the hearing mechanism, and how their child differs from normal, describe methods of habilitation, demonstrate the use and maintenance of a hearing aid, and schedule the child for the first habilitation session. The audiologist does most of the talking, often using professional jargon which leaves parents confused and feeling lost. The audiologist avoids listening.

"(4) *The action-oriented approach.* This fourth approach is also a popular one. The audiologist states the problem, and almost before he completes the reporting of the diagnosis he tells the parents what they are going to do to take care of the problem. The action part is essential, but only if there is adequate provision for exploring the feelings of the parents.

"Such approaches by the audiologist greatly interfere with the process of acceptance of the handicap. A lack of acceptance prohibits the parents from helping their child grow both emotionally and educationally. The parents may deny the information and shop around for a professional who will tell them that their child is normal. Beck (1959) and Meadow (1968) have pointed out that parents are more likely to listen and to integrate painful and unpleasant information from interested and "feeling" individuals.

"The ineffective approaches used by the audiologist stem from a number of complex variables. First, he may lack knowledge and understanding of the habilitative process, and of the effect of his initial report. Secondly, he may be uncomfortable with the range of emotions that these parents may feel. Often audiologists state that they simply do not have the time to devote to reporting. This reasoning, however, may actually be a way of avoiding a more significant factor . . . that is, the audiologist has not yet worked out in his own mind what it means to him to tell someone some painful news. It is natural for people to avoid pain. The audiologist and the parents in a way become secretly and jointly involved in an agreement to avoid dealing with feelings.

"There is no painless way to inform parents that they have a child with a hearing loss. However, pain does not have to be regarded negatively. It is part of a process that facilitates and encourages a family's involvement. Even though there is no way of softening the blow, there is a way to help parents accept the realities of the situation and to make use of the resources available to them. The goals of this important first discussion of the diagnosis are multifold.

"(1) *Statement of the facts.* Initially, it is important to state the facts as clearly and as emphatically as possible. These parents want up-to-date and accurate scientific information about their child's problem presented to them authoritatively, but in language they can understand. If an alliance is going to be created with these parents, it is most important that the audiologist admit any lack of information or knowledge about the problem that he has, doing so confidently and without strain. Throughout the giving of this information, the audiologist must convey a true interest in this family. The tone of voice and non-verbal behavior of an audiologist can convey callousness, or it can convey concern. It is essential to convey concern rather than the idea that you are just doing your job.

"(2) *Support through listening.* Perhaps the most important goal is to provide support through listening. By listening patiently and non-judgmentally, you may be able to bring some of the parents' feelings out into the open—feelings of which they may not have been aware. Many parents have indicated during the initial conference that they had been anxious about their child for a long period of time, but had never shared that anxiety with anyone, not even the spouse. This may be the first opportunity they have had to express what they have been feeling for months.

"In order that these feelings be expressed by both parents together, they should both be present to discuss the diagnosis unless it is physically impossible. During this discussion, we can begin to assess the parents' interactions and begin to decide whether they have the kind of relationship that will provide support to one another or whether they will require some help from outside. It is important that the audiologist note and report his initial impression of the parents, as these notes may be valuable to others involved with the family.

"(3) *Giving the parents a role.* Another important goal of this first contact is to convey to the parents that they have a great deal to offer, even though they may have little formal knowledge about hearing loss and child development. Focusing on the parents' interaction with their child during that initial contact can give them some confidence. "You seem to sense Joey's needs very well." "That's beautiful, you called Joey's attention to that sound." "That's one of the most important ideas you will learn and you already appear comfortable with it." You can provide initial reinforcement of attributes that the parents are already equipped with, that will help their child's development.

"During the initial discussion, the parents need to be made aware of the resources available to them—not only resources for habilitation and educational programming, but also resources available to help with emotional needs. Ideally, the audiologist will remain in contact with the family periodically, in order not only to give repeated evaluations, but also to act as a coordinator of professionals working with this family. It is vital that there be an interface between the person delivering emotional supportive services and those people primarily responsible for the habilitation program. This interaction will provide an opportunity to share and be aware of mutual concerns and will prevent the traditional approach of professionals working in isolation of each other.

"In order for these goals to be realized, four criteria need be present: First, the clinical audiologist must have some knowledge of the rehabilitative process; second, he must be comfortable dealing with feelings; third, adequate time must be provided for the reporting; and fourth, an atmosphere of mutual respect must be created.

"For many years the clinical audiologist has accumulated experience in diagnosing and fitting hearing aids, but has known little about the habilitation process. There is a trend today to provide audiologists with more information about habilitation, a trend which we see as positive. Perhaps as audiolo-gists become more familiar with rehabilitative methods, they can objectively direct parents toward programs suited to their child's needs and alleviate the emotional controversy so often found among the educators of the deaf.

"Many audiologists are sensitive and concerned about their role in helping these families, but this does not necessarily mean that they feel comfortable in dealing with feelings. Sensitivity in raw form can potentially be a valuable tool and an asset for the audiologist, but just because the potential is there does not mean that it will automatically be used in a facilitative way. To learn how to use one's sensitivity effectively is a delicate process and cannot be taught. This exemplifies the necessity for an interdisciplinary approach where the audiologist who is uncomfortable in this area may take advantage of the mental health professions that deal with feelings routinely.

"A seemingly minute detail in the criteria for effective reporting of the diagnosis is the allotment of time; however, this is probably an essential factor in reporting. One of the most consistent complaints of parents in their dealings with audiologists initially is that the situation was regarded lightly and not enough time was devoted to this important problem. It is our feeling that the audiologist must allocate a minimum of forty-five minutes to this initial reporting. Should this not be possible, or should both parents not be available during this initial session, it is critical that an appointment be scheduled within the next twenty-four hours to discuss the problem thoroughly. As was indicated earlier, parents may experience a number of feelings at the outset, the most frequent being shock. Then may come anger, guilt, or depression. It is very important not to tell parents what they may feel because people experience different emotions. It is important to provide an open-ended approach, however, such as, "Today I have told you about your son's hearing loss. Over the weeks and months to follow, you may or may not experience some uncomfortable feelings as many parents naturally do. We will be available to you to discuss whatever feelings you may be having. Let's plan to talk again in a month or anytime before that, should you desire."

"The approach to effective reporting of the diagnosis is not only dependent upon the audiologist's knowledge, his comfortable feelings and the allotment of adequate time but also upon the atmosphere created. It is the universal observation of those who have constructed programs for special groups of young disabled children that unless the parents' emotional needs are adequately dealt with, the programs themselves have limited benefit for the children (Mindel and Vernon, 1971). Thus, it is critically important that an atmosphere of mutual respect and honesty be created—an atmosphere which allows the expression of feelings in non-judgmental and accepting ways.

"Often the atmosphere of mutual respect is interrupted when the parents' depression explodes into external anger which sometimes is directed at the audiologist. If the audiologist does not understand that this expression of anger is only an indication of the parent's internal struggles, he may become defensive. The parents will be aware of his defensiveness even if it is only conveyed non-verbally, and thus the climate of mutual respect is destroyed."

The above insightful description by Hersch and Amon (1973) of the audiologist's dilemmas should be useful to him in his relationships with parents. Introspection will reveal in many of us the dynamics that have been detailed.

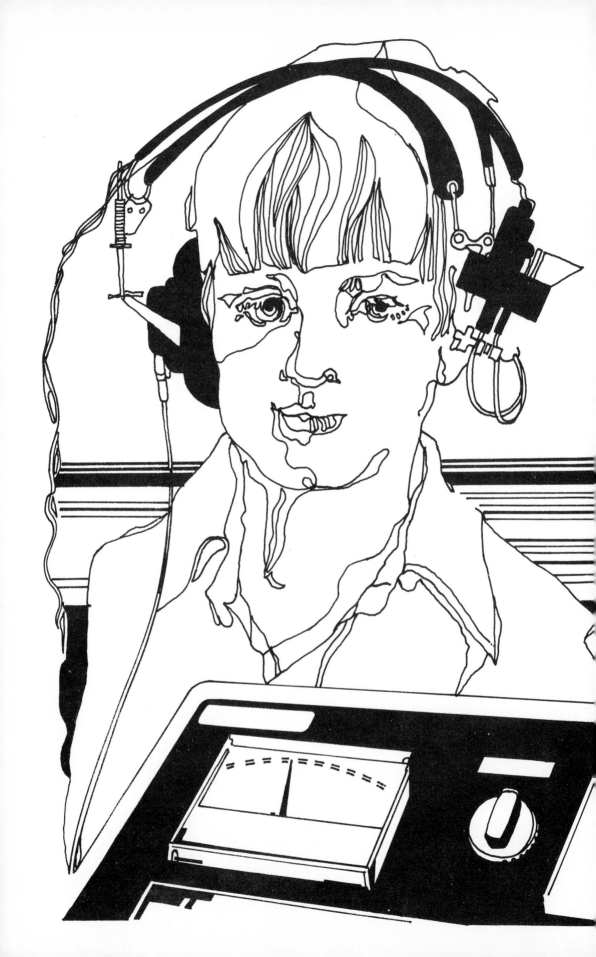

6 OBJECTIVE HEARING TESTS

Nothing can be more frustrating to an audiologist than to work with a 2-year-old child who needs to have his hearing evaluated, but who refuses to cooperate with any of the testing procedures. It seems impossible that a youngster who sat quietly and politely in the patient waiting area can suddenly turn into a crying, yelling, totally noncooperative subject as soon as he enters the sound-treated booth. And what causes a child who has been happily playing while waiting for his hearing test, to suddenly become an overly self-conscious, introverted, and unworkably shy patient? How does a clinician establish rapport with a youngster who is hidden in his mother's skirt or wrapped around his father's leg? Every clinician ultimately faces the child whom he just can't test. There are, indeed, means of handling such children, but the skills necessary to evaluate the hearing in uncooperative children are gained only through experience and insight.

One may expect the behavior of "normal" children to occasionally be obstinate. What about testing the hearing of a hyperactive, mentally retarded child? How does one elicit cooperation and establish play-conditioning techniques with an autistic or mentally disturbed youngster? Can you fit earphones on a child with hydrocephaly? Play-conditioning techniques are obviously not possible with a patient who won't even sit down! Just when the audiologist thinks that he has seen every conceivable situation, a child will show up who once again baffles every attempt to evaluate his hearing. Audiologists continue to seek a simple and accurate objective hearing test that can be used with any uncooperative child much like the early Spanish explorers continued to hunt for the Fountain of Youth! Almost no other aspect of audiology stimulates interest in the same manner as a new report describing a promising objective hearing test to solve problems associated with testing the hearing in difficult-to-deal-with children.

To deal with these difficult-to-test patients, the field of audiology has worked long and hard in the development of "objective" tests of hearing. An objective hearing test is one which defines a patient's hearing ability without the patient's active participation or cooperation. In the case of children, many factors may influence his ability to cooperate. He may not have the mental or physical capabilities to fully cooperate or to attend the hearing test task set before him by the clinician. The child's interest span may be too short. A clinician's skill in evaluating the hearing of these children often depends on his ability to establish rapport with the youngster, and at the same time, make an accurate evaluation of the child's capabilities in performing some task. A false start with these children may alienate them toward the testing situation, making additional test sessions necessary, and possibly more difficult.

Many "objective" hearing tests, usually related to an autonomic physiologic response, have been suggested and reported. Waldon (1973) proposes the term "Audio-reflex-ometry" as the method of measurement of hearing levels through the observation of involuntary responses resulting from presentation of acoustic stimuli. The Ewings of England in the early 1940's (Ewings and Ewings, 1944) observed eye-blinks, squinting, involuntary jumping, and sound localization with body or head movements while testing young children. Froeschels and Beebe (1946) evaluated the cochleopalpebral reflex (also known as the auropalpebral reflex)—defined as the involuntary closing of eyelids due to acoustic stimulation—in children and infants. The cochleopalpebral reflex has received the attention of a number of investigators including Galambos et al. (1953) and Albrite et al. (1956). Recently, Ames et al. (1970) report that they utilize the cochleopalpebral reflex as part of a test battery to differentiate normal children from children with central auditory imperception, peripheral hearing loss, and mental retardation.

Hardy et al. (1959) used informal tests with noisemakers and observed a wide variety of involuntary reflexes in young children including the Moro reflex, crying, eye-blinks, facial expression changes, immobilization to movement, eye-widening, head-turning, etc. Murphy (1962a) pointed out the value of the startle reflex in estimating hearing levels in children. Observation of such responses in infants and young children takes a trained eye and skilled clinician.

Unfortunately, new objective hearing tests are formulated with older children or cooperating adults, and these results are then generalized to young children. Another common means for new objective procedures is initiated with nonorganic hearing loss adults. Somehow, the generalization that such procedures which work well with adults, therefore should apply also to children, comes to a sudden lack of credibility when the clinician comes face to face with a screaming, wall-climbing, mentally retarded, 2-year-old patient!

Nonetheless, with the advent of each new "objective" hearing test, the inevitable flurry of excitement passes among audiologists, pediatricians, and otolaryngologists. We should pause to reflect that the presence of some physiologic response, seemingly related to the presence of an auditory signal, does not insure that the child does indeed "hear." Hearing, in this sense, implies meaningful interpretation of the sound so as to produce thought and language with verbal or nonverbal encoding and decoding. The toughest test for a new clinical procedure is to withstand clinician criticism by proving itself to be reliable, quick, easy to administer, inexpensive, and worthwhile over a long period of time.

The remainder of this chapter deals with five important "objective" hearing test procedures used to evaluate hearing in children—impedance audiometry, electrodermal or psychogalvanic response audiometry, cardiac audiometry, evoked response audiometry, and electrocochleography. Our selection of objective procedures reflects our own bias and interest. We have included testing techniques we feel are important, historically interesting, or that show future potential to the practicing clinician who deals with children daily.

Impedance Audiometry

The task of evaluating hearing in children has improved substantially in the last few years with developments in impedance audiometry. The testing techniques are especially well-suited for children since they are objective, accurate, quick, easy to administer, and create little discomfort to the patient. Often children who will not cooperate with conventional audiometric techniques will not object to the impedance test battery. Impedance audiometry results are of special benefit to the physician who is unable to perform adequate otoscopic examination on a youngster, as well as to the audiologist who has difficulty in establishing valid hearing thresholds on an uncooperative child.

Vast numbers of children have been tested with the impedance technique and a wide variety of normative impedance test values are available. Studies by Brooks (1968, 1971), Jerger (1970), and Robertson et al. (1968) have validated the tremendous benefits of impedance audiometry in children. Keith (1973) has shown that impedance audiometry can be conducted with neonates as young as a few hours of age.

The clinical impedance technique in the evaluation of the auditory mechanism was originally proposed by Metz in 1946 and has been used routinely in Scandanavia since that time. North Americans, however, were slow to accept the clinical utility of this testing procedure until Alberti and Kristensen (1970) and Jerger (1970) independently published articles exhalting impedance audiometry as a valuable routine procedure for assessing the nature of hearing loss in patients. Jerger succinctly stated the significance of impedance audiometry by commenting, "We frankly wonder how we ever got along without it." Impedance audiometry is now included as routine testing technique in many otologic and audiologic clinics, and we have found it to be particularly useful in the evaluation of hearing in children.

By definition, impedance audiometry is an objective means of assessing the integrity and function of the peripheral auditory mechanism. The electroacoustic impedance meter may help determine existing middle ear pressure, tympanic membrane mobility, eustachian tube function, continuity and mobility of the middle ear ossicles, acoustic reflex thresholds, and nonorganic hearing loss. The electroacoustic impedance bridge is equally practical for private office work and institutional clinics.

The electroacoustic impedance technique is based on the principle that sound pressure level (SPL) is a function of closed cavity volume. A diagram of the impedance meter is shown in Figure 6.1. An air-tight seal is obtained with a small probe which is inserted into the external auditory canal of the patient. The probe has three small holes. From one hole a 220-Hz probe tone is emitted; a second hole is an outlet for an air pressure system which is capable of creating positive, negative, or atmospheric air pressure in the cavity between the probe tip and the tympanic membrane; the third hole leads to a pick-up microphone which measures the sound pressure level of the 220-Hz probe tone in the canal cavity.

The sound pressure level of the 220-Hz tone in the external auditory canal cavity is determined by the compliance of the tympanic membrane and integrity of the middle ear system. The pick-up microphone quantifies the sound pressure level of acoustic energy that is reflected back into the external auditory canal. A high amount of reflected energy is measured when the middle ear system is stiff or heavy as in such pathologic conditions as ossicular fixation, otitis media, or cholesteatoma. In contrast, discontinuity of the middle ear system creates a flaccid tympanic membrane which absorbs most of the probe tone sound energy and reflects very little sound back into the external auditory meatus (Northern, 1971a).

The impedance audiometry test battery includes tympanometry, static compliance, and acoustic reflex threshold measurement. Although each of the test procedures can provide significant information, their diagnostic capabilities are strengthened when results from all three procedures are considered together (Table

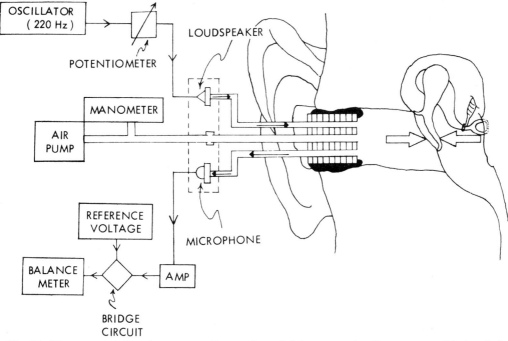

Fig. 6.1. Electroacoustic impedance meter. Note probe sealed into external auditory meatus with three holes for (a) 220-Hz probe tone from oscillator; (b) air pressure system from air pump and manometer; and (c) pick-up microphone to compare sound pressure level in the cavity between the eardrum and probe tip with the reference voltage of impedance bridge. (With permission from J. Jerger: Clinical experience with impedance audiometry. Arch. Otolaryngol. 92: 311-324, 1970.)

6.1) (Jerger, 1970). The entire battery of three tests can easily be administered by an experienced person in 60 to 90 seconds per ear.

Tympanometry

Tympanometry is an objective technique for measuring the compliance, or mobility, of the tympanic membrane as a function of mechanically varied air pressures in the external auditory canal. Lilly (1972) points out that the general term, tympanometry, refers to methods and techniques for measuring, recording, and evaluating changes in acoustic impedance (or resistance of the auditory mechanism) with systematic changes in air pressure. The compliance of the tympanic membrane at specific air pressures is plotted on a graph known as a tympanogram.

Tympanic membrane mobility is of particular interest since almost any pathology located on or medial to the eardrum will influence its movement. The otolaryngologist routinely creates air pressure against the eardrum with a pneumatic otoscope and makes subjective judgments regarding the mobility of the tympanic membrane. Tympanometry, however, is more objective than the otolaryngologist's eye, and the air pressures involved with the technique are very small compared with the air pressures created with a pneumatic otoscope. Often, eardrums noted to have normal mobility by pneumatic otoscopy examination, can be

Table 6.1. Summary of Impedance Audiometry Applications in Children

Tympanometry
  Objective measurement of tympanic membrane
    mobility
  Measures middle ear pressure
  Identifies perforations of tympanic membrane
  Confirms patency of ventilation tubes in
    tympanic membrane
  Estimates static compliance
Static Compliance
  Differentiates middle ear fixation from
    disarticulation
Acoustic Reflex Threshold
  Objective measure of loudness recruitment
  Validates nonorganic hearing loss
  Validates conductive hearing loss
  Differential diagnosis of conductive hearing loss
  Objective inference of hearing sensitivity

shown to have abnormal mobility with tympanometry.

The compliance of the tympanic membrane is at its maximum when air pressures on both sides of the eardrum are equal. That is, the eardrum achieves its best mobility when the air pressure in the external auditory canal is exactly the same as the existing air pressure in the middle ear (Fig. 6.2). The electroacoustic impedance meter permits the compliance of the eardrum to be evaluated under systematic variance of air pressure which is controlled by the clinician. Thus, when the clinician finds the air pressure value where the eardrum reaches its maximal compliance, he can then infer that the middle ear pressure is the same as the ear canal air pressure. The air pressure at the point of maximal compliance is also the middle ear air pressure. This fact has been shown experimentally by Eliachar and Northern (1974) and Eliachar et al. (1974). Jerger (1972) regards tympanometry as a "dynamic compliance" measure.

The knowledge of middle ear pressure is important clinical information. When the process of aeration in the middle ear is halted, as in closure of the eustachian tube, the now static air in the middle ear space is absorbed by the blood vessels in the mucosal lining (Ballenger, 1969). This situation produces negative air pressure in the middle ear space causing transudation of fluid and retraction of the tympanic membrane. If the aeration process of the middle ear cavity is blocked for an extended period of time, fluid may totally fill the middle ear space. Thus, the early identification of negative middle ear pressure may permit the physician to practice preventive medicine and avoid the condition of otitis media.

The presence of unequal pressures on either side of the tympanic membrane usually occurs when negative pressure exists in the middle ear space. This may be sufficient to cause a retraction of the eardrum accompanied by mild conductive hearing loss in spite of the fact that no fluid may be observed in the patient's middle ear. The most explicit example of this occurs when air pressures are changed in the passenger cabins of commercial aircraft. A normal-hearing passenger will first experience discomfort due to unequal air pressure in the

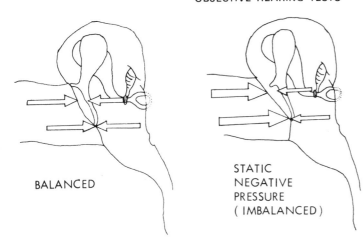

BALANCED

STATIC
NEGATIVE
PRESSURE
(IMBALANCED)

Fig. 6.2. Compliance of the tympanic membrane is at its maximum when air pressure is equal on both sides of tympanic membrane as shown on the left. When air pressure on either side of the eardrum is unequal, as shown on the right, the tympanic membrane does not move well and a conductive-type hearing loss can often be noted.

middle ear cavity and external ear canal. When the passenger forces open his eustachian tube in order to alleviate this discomfort, he will also notice that, when the air pressures are equalized and the eardrum is again in a most compliant condition, the environmental sounds in the aircraft become suddenly louder. This may be a practical explanation of the numbers of children seen by audiologists to have mild conductive hearing loss, and they are found by the examining physicians to have no evidence of otologic problem. Audiologists are quick to blame the patient or the audiometric test condition for this "unexplainable" conductive loss which may be due to the presence of negative middle ear pressure.

Jerger (1970) and Liden et al. (1970) have described basic tympanogram patterns and related them to conditions of the middle ear. Jerger's classification system of tympanometry curves, which he also calls "pressure-compliance functions," is summarized in Figure 6.3. For simplicity, Jerger ascribed alphabetical letters to each type of curve. This classification is convenient, but it may be more explicit to describe each tympanogram in terms of its dynamic compliance and the air pressure at which maximal compliance is noted.

Tympanogram Type A. Type A curves are found in patients with normal middle ear function. The curve shows adequate relative compliance and normal middle ear pressure at the point of maximal compliance. Some controversy exists concerning the limits of normal middle ear pressure values. Alberti and Kristen-

sen (1970) recommended the use of ± 50 mm H_2O as normative values, but we have noted many instances of negative middle ear pressure as great as -150 mm H_2O in patients who demonstrated normal audiograms and normal otoscopic examination. Brooks (1969) evaluated 1053 children in England and determined "normal" middle ear pressure from a statistical distribution to be from -170 mm H_2O to 0 mm H_2O. Decisions regarding "limits of normal" in terms of middle ear pressure will undoubtedly vary depending on the clinical situation and circumstances.

Tympanogram Type A_S. This pressure-compliance function is characterized by normal middle ear pressure and limited compliance relative to the mobility of the normal tympanic membrane. This type of curve may be seen in cases of otosclerosis, thickened or heavily scarred tympanic membranes, and some cases of tympanosclerosis. The $_S$ nomenclature is indicative of "stiffness," or "shallowness" of the tympanogram.

Tympanogram Type A_D. This curve is represented by large changes in relative compliance with small changes of air pressure. The A_D curve is noted in middle ears where discontinuity of the ossicular chain has occurred, or the eardrum demonstrates a large monomeric membrane. The significance of this curve is its representation of an extremely flaccid eardrum, with the $_D$ indicating "disarticulation" or a "deep" tympanogram curve.

Tympanogram Type B. The type B tympanogram is characterized by a function representing

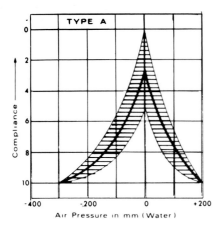

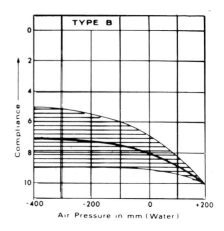

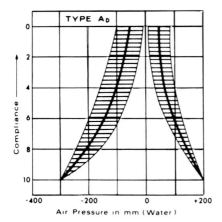

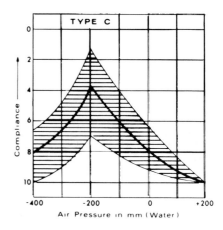

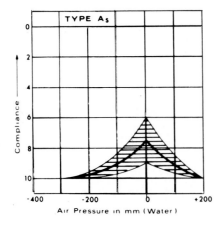

Fig. 6.3. Classification of tympanograms according to Jerger (1970). Lined areas of tympanograms represent range of results, while solid lines represent average tympanogram of each pattern. See text for clinical significance of each type of tympanogram.

little or no change in compliance of the middle ear as air pressure in the external ear canal is varied. Often no point of maximal compliance is observable with air pressure as low as −400 mm H_2O. This curve is seen in patients with serous and adhesive otitis media and some cases of congenital middle ear malformations (Northern and Bergstrom, 1974). This curve is also noted in patients who have perforations of the tympanic membrane, ear canals totally occluded with cerumen, or with a patent ventilating tube in the eardrum.

Tympanogram Type C. This tympanogram is represented by near normal compliance and middle ear pressure of −200 mm H_2O or worse. This curve may or may not be related to the presence of fluid in the middle ear, but one can conclude that the eardrum still has some mobility. Bluestone et al. (1973) report a very low incidence of middle ear effusion in children with type C tympanograms upon whom they performed myringotomies. Their results, however, differ markedly from our experience in which greater than 80% of children with type C tympanograms have fluid at myringotomy. Persistence of the type C tympanogram infers poor eustachian tube function in the presence of an intact tympanic membrane. Sometimes patients can be instructed to "pop their ears" or perform the Valsalva procedure (patient holds his nose and forces positive air pressure into the middle ear cavities). If the patient can open his eustachian tube, a repeat tympanogram may show that the type C curve has changed to the type A curve. Youngsters, however, with upper respiratory infections seldom can alleviate the type C tympanogram with the Valsalva maneuver.

A major drawback to the use of such categories to classify tympanograms is that the clinician inevitably comes across a tympanogram that does not clearly fit into one of the expectant categories. Such tympanograms may be few, but they do exist. In addition, various categorical systems do not always agree on the same nomenclature for the tympanogram patterns. The clinician should describe the mobility of the eardrum in terms of compliance and middle ear pressure, or draw a simple picture of the tympanogram if possible.

The technique for obtaining a tympanogram is quite simple. The eardrum is put into a position of known poor mobility with an air pressure of +200 mm H_2O pumped into the cavity created by the meter's probe tip and the patient's tympanic membrane. Then the clinician mechanically removes the positive air pressure and observes or records relative changes in the compliance of the eardrum. The compliance change is actually measured by the electroacoustic meter as a decrease in the sound pressure level of the enclosed cavity. When the compliance of the eardrum is permitted to increase, with the release of air pressure, more of the sound energy is transmitted through to the middle ear creating a decrease in the sound pressure level of the enclosed cavity.

As the air pressure variation approaches the point of maximal compliance, the mobility of the tympanic membrane increases. Maximal compliance is, of course, achieved when the air pressure in the external auditory canal equals the existing air pressure in the middle ear space. The clinician continues to reduce the air pressure in the enclosed cacity, which unbalances the equalized air pressure on either side of the tympanic membrane, and therefore creates a decrease in eardrum compliance again.

Clinical uses of tympanometry are many. The type B tympanogram quickly and easily identifies children with stiff middle ear systems even when the presence of the conductive problem is not sufficient to cause hearing loss. The diagnosis of otitis media, for example, does not pose a problem for the trained otolaryngologist as long as the eardrum can be clearly visualized. But less experienced examiners, or audiologists working outside the environment of an otolaryngology clinic, often benefit from the use of tympanometry to identify the nature of conductive hearing loss.

Tympanometry can be used to follow the entire progression and resolution of serous otitis media in children without the use of otoscopy or audiometry. Typical tympanograms obtained under such circumstances are shown in Figure 6.4. Imagine a 2-year-old youngster who demonstrates a type A tympanogram under healthy conditions. As the otologic disease process begins with a closed

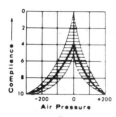

Time 500 1K 2K 4K

	500	1K	2K	4K
RE	85	90	90	95
LE				

Acoustic Reflex

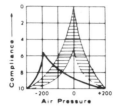

Time 500 1K 2K 4K

	500	1K	2K	4K
RE	110	110	a	a
LE				

Acoustic Reflex

ONSET OF OTITIS MEDIA

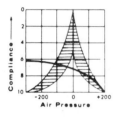

Time 500 1K 2K 4K

	500	1K	2K	4K
RE	a	a	a	a
LE				

Acoustic Reflex

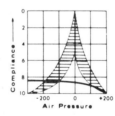

Time 500 1K 2K 4K

	500	1K	2K	4K
RE	a	a	a	a
LE				

Acoustic Reflex

OTITIS MEDIA

Fig. 6.4. Tympanometry and acoustic reflex thresholds may be utilized to follow otitis media through various stages of pathology. These hypothetical tympanograms are shown as a solid line against the tympanogram normative curve. Prior to the onset of otitis media, the tympanogram is type A with normal acoustic reflex levels. The onset of the disorder is noted with a type C tympanogram, elevated and absent reflexes on the involved ear; during otitis media type B tympanograms and absent acoustic reflexes prevail; as the pathology resolves the tympanogram and acoustic reflex return to normal.

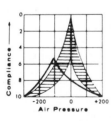

Time 500 1K 2K 4K

	500	1K	2K	4K
RE	110	105	100	105
LE				

Acoustic Reflex

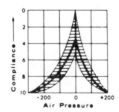

Time 500 1K 2K 4K

	500	1K	2K	4K
RE	85	90	90	95	.
LE				

Acoustic Reflex

RESOLUTION OF OTITIS MEDIA

eustachian tube, negative pressure is created in the middle ear space which produces a type C tympanogram. As fluid develops medial to the tympanic membrane, the compliance of the eardrum is decreased, and a type B tympanogram will be demonstrated by the child. If prescribed medications are effective and the fluid conditon of the ear begins to resolve, we would expect to once again see the type C tympanogram, and finally the type A tympanogram when the middle ear is back in its normal healthy condition.

Tympanometry is also useful in monitoring recovery of the middle ear following surgical precedures. Tympanoplasty grafts, for example, are thick and heavy immediately following surgery and produce a type B tympanogram. As the graft heals and becomes thinner with improved mobility, the tympanogram approaches the type A pattern. Resolution of Gelfoam in the middle ear can be followed with tympanometry. And, of course, this technique is valuable in evaluating post-surgical ears in which the air-bone threshold gap persists or reappears following the surgical procedure.

Static Compliance

Static compliance has traditionally been known as acoustic impedance, particularly in the United States. Compliance refers to the mobility, or springiness, of a system while impedance refers to the immobility or resistance of a system to movement. The choice of terminology between compliance and impedance is much like the old adage of describing a glass of water as either half full or half empty. We have chosen to orient our thinking in terms of mobility of the middle ear system; since this compliance measure is made during resting conditions of the system, we use Jerger's suggested nomenclature, "static compliance."

The concept of acoustical impedance, or static compliance, is a direct outgrowth of applications made by electrical engineers and physicists to describe the willingness of an electrical system to permit electron flow, and the ease with which a mechanical system moves. Impedance can be a technical topic, and readers interested in more exacting descriptions of this subject are referred to excellent materials prepared by Zwislocki (1963) and Lilly (1972, 1973).

The impedance of any mechanical system involves a complex relationship between three factors—the mass, friction, and stiffness of the system. In the middle ear mechanical system, mass is represented primarily by the weight of the three ossicles. The weight of the three ossicles, however, as is immediately obvious to one who has ever held the ossicles in his hand, constitutes very little mass. Friction in the middle ear is due primarily to the suspensory seven ligaments and two muscles which support the ossicular chain. This intricate suspension of the ossicles, however, lends to ease of mobility; thus friction as a factor in mechanical impedance constitutes meager influence in the impedance of the middle ear. The third element of impedance, stiffness, has a much more prominent role in the middle ear. The stiffness element has been identified as occurring at the footplate of the stapes, where a large resistant component must be overcome to move the fluids of the cochlear ducts. Thus, the impedance of the middle ear mechanical system is stiffness-dominated (Zwislocki, 1963).

Acoustic impedance is traditionally expressed in acoustic ohms; acoustic compliance is measured in equivalent cubic centimeters (cc) of volume. The measurement of compliance with the electroacoustic impedance meter is based on the fact that sound pressure level is a function of volume cavity size. That is, for a given probe tone of known intensity and frequency, the sound pressure level of the tone will increase as the cavity size is decreased, or the sound pressure level of the probe tone will decrease as cavity size is increased. Thus a specific relationship exists for a tone of known frequency and intensity (measured in dB sound pressure level) and cavity volume (measured in cubic centimeters). The electroacoustic impedance meter uses a pick-up microphone to measure the intensity of sound energy within the cavity created by the air-tight probe tip and the tympanic membrane. This intensity in dB is read in cubic centimeters of equivalent volume for ease and clarity of measurement.

Compliance is technically the inverse of impedance. A system with a great deal of mobility, or high compliance, has very little resistance to motion, or low impedance. Likewise, a poorly mobile system has low compliance and high resistance. This small equivalent volume in cubic centimeters of compliance is equal to a large impedance in acoustic ohms, and vice versa. In the middle ear pathologies, serous otitis media, for example, creates a middle ear system of very low compliance or very high impedance. On the other hand, a disarticulated ossicular chain in the middle ear creates a condition of high compliance or low impedance.

Static compliance is actually tested by making two equivalent volume measures with the tympanic membrane under specific conditions. The first volume measurement (C_1) is made with the eardrum clamped with +200 mm H_2O pressure. The second volume measurement (C_2), which is really an equivalent volume measure, is done with the eardrum in its most compliant air pressure condition. These two volume measures have little actual significance individually because they include the volume of the external ear canal. However, simple subtraction of the two volumes, $C_2 - C_1$, cancels out the contamination of the ear canal from both measures and gives an answer equal to the static compliance of the middle ear.

One of the major weaknesses of static compliance is its wide variance in values related to specific pathologies of the auditory mechanism. The central tendencies of small sample populations may reflect significant differences among various ear pathologies which make the measure look quite valuable. However, in clinical patient populations, the variation in static compliance values create considerable overlap among normal middle ears, otosclerotics, and ears with discontinuity shown clearly by Alberti and Kristensen (1970). Jerger (1970) has shown that differential diagnosis based only on static compliance measures may be difficult (Fig. 6.5).

Jerger (1972) has also shown normal static compliance to vary as a function of age and sex. Men show higher acoustic compliance than females at all ages, while both men and women show a general over-all decrease in compliance as they grow older. These facts caution against

attempts to construct norms for static compliance. As a guideline, however, the middle ear can be considered abnormally stiff when the static compliance is less than .28 cc of equivalent volume and abnormally flaccid when the static compliance is greater than 2.5 cc of equivalent volume. Serous otitis media often creates poor compliance of .1 cc of equivalent volume or less. Jerger et al. (1974b) found static compliance to be the least informative test of the impedance battery in children under 6 years of age.

Since the electroacoustic impedance bridge is able to measure volume in cubic centimeters, information about the absolute cavity size medial to the probe tip can be quite significant. In the presence of an intact eardrum, the typical enclosed cavity between the probe tip and the tympanic membrane should be approximately 1.5 cc or smaller. In young children this value may run closer to 1.0 cc and in infants the value may be as small as .5 cc. This value may vary depending on how far into the external auditory canal the probe tube and cuff are inserted. When the absolute volume size is greater than these suggested norms, the clinician may reasonably assume that the enclosed cavity includes the middle ear space and possibly even the mastoid air cells and entrance to the eustachian tube orifice. This procedure is particularly valuable in identifying perforated tympanic membranes or in the evaluation of patency of ventilating tubes which have been placed in the tympanic membrane as shown in Figure 6.6.

Acoustic Reflex Thresholds

The third test in the impedance audiometry battery is the determination of the signal threshold level at which the stapedial muscle contracts. Metz (1952) and Jepsen (1963) reported that in normal-hearing individuals, a bilateral stapedius muscle reflex can be elicited by stimulating the subject's test ear with pure tone signals between 70 and 100 dB HTL and approximately 65 dB HTL for white noise.

The function of the stapedial muscle is still open to question, but the classical interpretation offered by Wever and Lawrence (1954) is that the stapedial muscle reflex is responsible

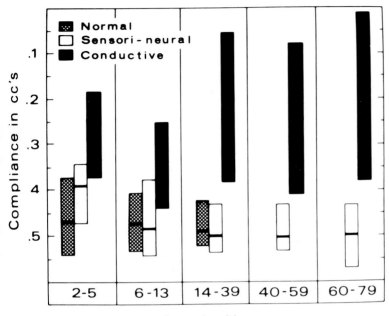

Fig. 6.5. Static compliance distribution from Jerger (1970) as a function of age and nature of hearing problem. Static compliance should separate conductive, or middle ear disorders, from normal and sensorineural loss ears. Considerable overlap may be noted especially in 2 to 5 and 6 to 13 age groups. Numbers of normal-hearing patients in the 40 to 59 and 60 to 79 age brackets were too small to be included. Each vertical box encompasses semi-interquartile range, and solid horizontal stripe is the median value for the group.

for protection of the inner ear from loud sounds. Anatomically, the stapedial muscle is attached from the neck of the stapes to the posterior wall of the middle ear cavity. When the stapedial muscle contracts, it pulls posteriorly on the ossicular chain, thereby decreasing the compliance of the middle ear system and attenuating the intensity of the sound which actually reaches the cochlea.

Much emphasis has been placed on the clinical value of the acoustic reflex measurement, particularly by the Scandinavians. Since the acoustic reflex is mediated by loudness, it is a sensitive indicator of cochlear pathology. The acoustic reflex threshold level in patients with cochlear pathology may often occur at sensation levels less than 60 dB above the auditory pure tone threshold. The patient with cochlear pathology hears the test signal as though it were much louder, due to abnormal appreciation of loudness. Thus, the acoustic reflex threshold provides an objective, simple technique for the measurement of loudness recruitment.

The ability to establish the presence of the loudness recruitment phenomenon permits the clinician to localize the site of auditory lesion to the cochlea. Anyone who has ever attempted

the traditional psychophysical loudness balance procedures on a youngster under 6 years of age to determine whether loudness recruitment is present, will immediately appreciate the simplicity and objectivity of this technique.

The presence of the acoustic reflex is quickly and easily obscured in the case of conductive hearing loss. In fact, Klockhoff (1961) states emphatically that a recordable stapedius reflex is proof of the absence of a conductive or middle ear component to a hearing disorder. Anderson and Barr (1967) obtained distinct acoustic reflex responses in 16 of 19 children with subsequent surgical intervention for ossicular malformations that exhibited conductive hearing losses. It may be that the acoustic reflex is indeed contracting in the presence of a conductive hearing loss, but generally the mechanism that is altering the conduction ability of the middle ear system is also inhibiting the tympanic membrane from showing a change in compliance as the muscle contracts.

An intriguing and valuable clue to the identification of unilateral conductive hearing loss lies in the fact that the acoustic reflex is often bilaterally absent. When the stimulating

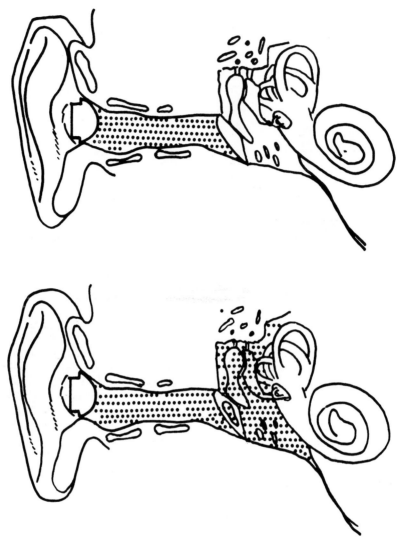

Fig. 6.6. Diagnostic representation of utilization of the electroacoustic impedance meter to measure absolute volume size. Top scheme shows volume between probe tip and intact eardrum; bottom view shows greater volume measurement when eardrum is perforated or has a patent ventilating tube in place. (With permission from J. L. Northern: Clinical measurement procedures. In J. Jerger (ed.), Handbook of Impedance Audiometry, American Electromedics Corp., New York, 1973.)

sound is presented to the conductive loss ear, the hearing loss may be sufficient to prevent the signal from being perceived loudly enough to elicit the acoustic reflex. When the head-set is reversed so that the earphone is placed on the good ear and the probe tip is in the conductive loss ear, the mechanism of the conductive loss prohibits the tympanic membrane from showing a change in compliance, and the reflex

appears to be absent. In a group of 154 patients with unilateral conductive loss, Jerger et al. (1974b) showed that the amount of air-bone gap necessary to abolish the stapedial reflex was approximately 25 dB with the earphone on the bad ear, and approximately 5 dB with the probe tip in the bad ear.

Other types of unilateral hearing loss do not obscure the stapedial reflex bilaterally. A unilateral sensorineural hearing loss with a contralateral normal-hearing ear will usually show bilateral acoustic reflexes as long as the unilateral hearing loss does not exceed 80 dB HTL (Jerger, 1970). A unilateral "dead" ear with a contralateral normal-hearing ear, however, will show absence of the acoustic reflex unilaterally when the stimulating earphone is on the "dead" side. Thus interpretation of acoustic reflexes in unilateral hearing losses can be diagnostically important, and of particular value when the patient is a youngster in whom audiometric masking for unilateral hearing loss is impractical or impossible.

Clinical Application of the Impedance Test Battery with Children

While tympanometry, static compliance, and the acoustic reflex threshold each provide some information about the function of the auditory system, their results become more meaningful when relationships between the three tests are considered. Diagnostic judgments and patient referral are made with greater authority and assurance when the over-all pattern is considered. Jerger (1970) indicates that tympanometry alone is useful to only a limited degree, static compliance norms are too variable for accurate diagnosis, and the absence of the acoustic reflex may occur from several factors. When considered together, however, the limitations of each test are reduced while their combined implications are enhanced.

Examples of the impedance test battery and its relation to clinical diagnosis are shown in Figures 6.7 and 6.8. Impedance test results from a case of negative middle ear pressure in a youngster's right ear are demonstrated in Figure 6.7. The audiogram shows a mild hearing loss with a 20-dB air-bone gap on the patient's right ear and normal hearing in the left ear. The audiogram gives no clue as to the etiology of this unilateral conductive hearing loss. The tympanogram for the left ear is superimposed on the normal tympanogram pattern, while the tympanogram for the right ear shows slightly reduced compliance and middle ear pressure of -200 mm H_2O. Static compliance is reduced in the right ear suggesting stiffness, thereby corroborating the reduced compliance noted in

the tympanogram. Static compliance in the left ear is within the normal range. The acoustic reflexes are present, but show elevated thresholds when the stimulating earphone is on the involved ear. The 20-dB air conduction hearing loss in the right ear is not severe enough to prohibit loudness from eliciting the acoustic reflex when the earphone is on this ear. When the earphone is placed over the normal-hearing left ear, the acoustic reflexes are absent. The probe tip is now in the involved conductive loss ear, and the conductive loss element prohibits compliance change in the right tympanic membrane. Knowledge of only the impedance audiometry test battery results, accompanied by experience in test interpretation, would permit a close estimation of this patient's audiogram if audiometry could not be successfully accomplished.

Figure 6.8 demonstrates findings in a patient with unilateral otitis media. The audiometric results show a stiffness-type air conduction curve with an approximate 30-dB air-bone gap in the right ear. Hearing in the left ear is normal. The tympanogram on the involved right ear shows a type B pattern, substantiated by a rather low static compliance measure. These results insure the presence of a stiffness component to the etiology of the right conductive hearing loss. The fact that the stapedius reflex is absent bilaterally, in view of a unilateral hearing loss, confirms that the loss must be conductive in nature. This over-all pattern could also represent cerumen packed in the right ear canal, a perforation of the right tympanic membrane or otitis media. Diagnosis is in the realm of the physician, but these impedance test findings, even without the audiogram, would suggest referral of this child to a physician.

Robertson et al. (1968) were among the earliest investigators to utilize impedance measurements in children. Although primarily interested in determining the youngest age at which the stapedius muscle reflex could be elicited with consistency, they suggested several other applications for impedance measures in children including validation of air-bone gaps in conductive hearing loss and demonstration of invalid air-bone gaps by observation of stapedius reflex measurements. They suggested

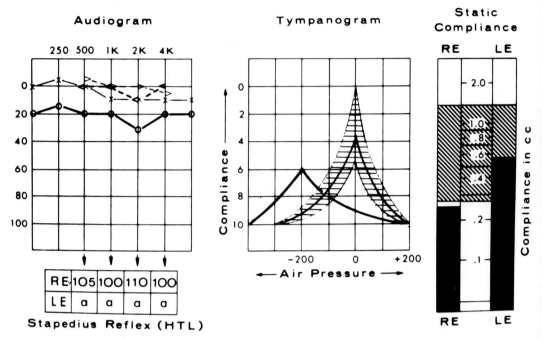

Fig. 6.7. Audiometrics and impedance audiometry results accompanying a right-sided conductive hearing loss caused by significant negative middle ear pressure. See text for full explanation.

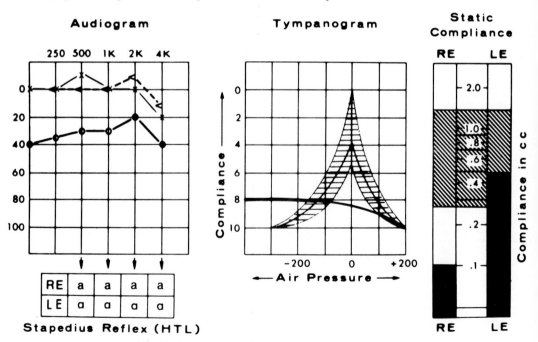

Fig. 6.8. Audiometrics and impedance audiometry results in a unilateral conductive hearing loss of otitis media etiology. See text for full explanation.

that children who have problems accepting amplification with hearing aids may have tolerance problems resulting from loudness recruitment which can be identified with the acoustic reflex. A further application suggested by these authors is consideration of the acoustic reflex as an index of residual hearing in children who offer no response to sound or speech in any form.

Keith (1973) performed impedance audiometry on 40 newborns ranging between 36 and 151 hours of age. He tested the babies following their feeding, and reported no difficulty in obtaining hermatic seal of the probe tip in the infant's ear canals. Most babies slept through the entire impedance audiometry test battery which included stapedial reflex measurement with stimulating pure tones of 500 and 2000 Hz. All three test components were completed on all babies except for reflex measures on one baby for both ears and two babies for one ear. In each of these instances, the babies became too fretful to complete the evaluation. The range of static compliance values found in infants was .54 to 1.75 cc with a median compliance value of 1.1 cc. The data showed little correlation between age and compliance during the first few hours of life. The test/retest reliability coefficient was approximately .85. The tympanograms were characterized by being quite compliant with a mean middle ear pressure from 80 ears of 4.5 mm H_2O with a range from -30 to $+60$ mm H_2O. Stapedial reflex testing yielded 23 of a possible 80 responses to the 500-Hz tone and 24 responses to the 2000-Hz tone. Keith concluded that impedance testing is indeed possible in infants, but he felt that the technique was not indicated for mass infant screening. These authors conclude strongly, and we agree wholeheartedly with them, that impedance audiometry is the single most powerful tool in pediatric hearing evaluations. They warn, however, that impedance test results can be interpreted only in combination with some independent assessment of hearing sensitivity level. Table 6.2 presents a paradigm developed by Jerger (1970) showing how results from impedance audiometry can be used to help confirm audiometric impressions in the evaluation of hearing in young children.

Bluestone et al. (1973) compared air conduction audiometry and tympanometry in 84 youngsters with concurrent or recent middle ear disease to determine which procedure could better predict the presence of middle ear effusion. They concluded that tympanometry is far more sensitive than air conduction audiometry for detecting common conduction defects in children. They caution, however, that tympanometry cannot detect sensorineural hearing loss and thus cannot be substituted for pure tone audiometry as a screening technique. They suggest that tympanometry in combina-

Table 6.2. *Use of Impedance Audiometry to Help Confirm Audiometric Impression in Evaluation of Young Children* *

Tympanometry	Static Compliance	Acoustic Reflex	Confirm Behavioral Audiometric Impression
Type A bilaterally	Within normal range, bilaterally	Normal bilaterally	Bilateral normal hearing or bilateral mild-moderate sensorineural hearing loss or unilateral mild-moderate sensorineural hearing loss
Type A in one ear; type B or C in other ear	Normal in A ear; low in B or C ear	Absent, bilaterally	Unilateral conductive loss
Type B or C bilaterally	Low bilaterally	Absent, bilaterally	Bilateral conductive loss

* With permission from J. Jerger: Clinical experience with impedance audiometry. Arch. Otolaryngol. 92: 311-324, 1970.

tion with air conduction audiometry appears to constitute the best method available for detecting middle ear disease and hearing impairment in large groups of children.

S. Jerger et al. (1974) reported an extensive evaluation of impedance audiometry in 398 children less than 6 years of age who were seen for routine clinical audiometric evaluation. Complete impedance results were obtained with 77% of the group, while satisfactory audiometry on the initial visit could only be obtained from 55% of the group. Impedance findings offered supplementary information not available from behavioral audiometric testing in 67% of these patients. They reported that the unsuccessful impedance results were generally found in children less than 3 years of age, who could also not be tested by standard audiometric techniques.

The main limitation in impedance testing of young children is that the test battery cannot be completed while the youngster is vocalizing—speaking, crying, moaning, yelling, or any combination of these factors. The reflex arc prior to each vocalization causes the stapedius muscle to contract spontaneously, thereby altering the compliance of the tympanic membrane at random and making impedance measurements impossible. The skilled clinician needs only a short time to complete the essentials of the impedance test battery, but his most difficult task is often to make the patient stop vocalizing.

Permitting the youngster to suck on candy or a bottle is no answer to the problem because the sucking motion also causes middle ear muscle activity. Each clinician must devise his own techniques to momentarily distract the child so the vocalizing will stop and testing can be completed. Figure 6.9 illustrates the manner we use to hold difficult patients for impedance audiometry testing.

Lamb and Norris (1969) point out that a certain amount of subject cooperation is needed to complete any audiologic test, although in impedance audiometry the cooperation is mostly passive. The patient must allow the probe to be put into his ear and manipulated until an air-tight seal is achieved. Because the mentally retarded child is often hyperactive, he may be held in his mother's lap

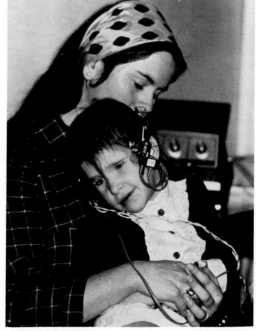

Fig. 6.9. Impedance testing can be accomplished with difficult-to-test patients as shown above with this mentally retarded rubella youngster.

or in a restraining harness. Simple toys or noisemakers may hold his attention long enough to complete the test. It may be necessary to hold the probe tip in place in one ear and the earphone over the other ear for children who refuse to accept the headset mechanism. Richards and Kartye (1973) have shown impedance audiometry results to be independent of the type of probe tip used. Sometimes even a tympanogram or acoustic reflex measure will be a valuable result since the clinician can then make assumptions regarding the presence or absence of middle ear problems and the need for medical referral. Impedance audiometry is also valuable in the evaluation of the severely mentally retarded, "mattress care" children, who are virtually impossible to test with any other testing procedure. These institutional youngsters are at high risk for developing chronic middle ear disease.

Impedance Audiometry with the Mentally Retarded

The evaluation of hearing in the mentally retarded patient presents a most difficult task.

The problems are so vast that an entire book devoted to audiometry for the retarded has recently been published (Fulton and Lloyd, 1969). Many retarded children do not condition well to pure tone play audiometry. They may not have sufficient maturation to perform auditory localization tasks or may lack consistent startle response. They may be too hyperactive to cooperate or too lethargic to be aware of changes in the environment. Difficult problems are commonly encountered with other physiologic tests in patients with questionable cortical function. Yet, in many of these patients, the determination of hearing function may be critical for their placement and treatment.

Even audiometric screening is very difficult with the retarded, and the majority of testing techniques recommended for use with the retarded do not fit the criteria of efficiency inherent in hearing screening. The purpose of any audiometric screening program is to identify those with hearing impairments or health problems as quickly and as economically as possible. Incidence studies have established that there is a higher incidence of hearing impairment among the retarded than among the nonretarded (Lloyd, 1970; Rittmanic, 1971). Yet the retarded are excluded from traditionally recommended screening techniques because of their limited capacity for responding.

Comprehensive audiologic assessment implies pure tone thresholds, speech audiometry, and any other significant diagnostic information obtainable. However, when large numbers of mentally retarded are involved, the need for a more efficient method of testing becomes evident. Of the variety of available techniques, evoked response audiometry, special diagnostic procedures, as well as other auditory assessment techniques that have been suggested, the impedance audiometry battery is in our opinion and experience, the most illuminative and efficient technique for evaluating the auditory mechanism of mentally retarded children.

Impedance Audiometry with the Congenitally Deaf Child

The work-up of patients with substantial sensorineural deafness will usually not identify superimposed middle ear anomalies. Impedance audiometry provides a useful means of evaluating the conductive hearing mechanism in patients with sensorineural hearing loss. Wilber et al. (1970) reported impedance data from 17 children with hearing loss associated with maternal rubella and found the group mean impedance to be 2700 ohms, somewhat higher than the range of impedance values for normal-hearing children which was 900 to 1800 ohms. None of the rubella cases in her series had a positive acoustic reflex. Our clinical experience with rubella deafness in youngsters supports Wilber's finding of resistant middle ear systems as identified with impedance audiometry. This stiffness may occur unilaterally, or bilaterally, or be within the normal limits. It is possible that the rubella group impedance mean values will be substantiated by other clinicians, but it seems unlikely that any individual rubella case can be diagnosed by this one particular result of increased middle ear stiffness.

Early identification of patients with congenital deafness is, of course, essential for successful habilitation. Decisions regarding educational placement and referral, possible exploratory tympanotomy, or selection of appropriate amplification devices may be made with increased authority when the specific condition of the middle ear is known. Audiometric evaluation of profoundly deaf children may be very difficult and often can only be successfully accomplished by experienced audiologists.

Older children in schools for the deaf are not routinely evaluated by otolaryngologists. These children seldom complain about their ears or of changes in their hearing levels. Yet, they no doubt suffer the same incidence of otitis media as found in normal-hearing children. Impedance audiometry has significant value in schools for the deaf as a means by which to identify middle ear pathology in these children with sensorineural hearing loss.

Impedance Audiometry with Diagnostic Problem Patients

Regardless of the skills of the audiologist and the otolaryngologist, a certain number of patients exist in whom diagnosis remains elusive. These patients seem to defy all attempts to detect or define their degree of hearing loss—which may be clouded by other abnormal manifestations. Peripheral responses to noisemakers, free-field speech, white noise, and warble tones may be equivocal, unreliable, or simply lacking. Speech and language development in these patients is often missing or untestable and questions also exist concerning the relationship of these communicative deficiencies.

Impedance audiometry can differentiate patients with a normal middle ear. Bilateral presence of the acoustic reflex, with normal tympanometry and impedance measures, can substantiate normal-hearing. Absence of the acoustic reflex, in light of normal tympanograms and acoustic impedance, suggest more severe sensorineural hearing loss. These findings may be critical for an abnormally developing child in whom fitting with a hearing aid might be needed.

Other Applications of Impedance Audiometry

Impedance audiometry is rapidly changing the routine of audiometric testing, and new uses of the technique are appearing in the literature at an amazing rate. One of the most revolutionary applications was reported by Niemeyer and Sesterhenn (1972) at a recent meeting of the International Society of Audiology in Budapest. These investigators have determined a means of calculating the air conduction hearing level threshold from stapedial reflex measurements. They verified their results on 50 normal-hearing subjects and 223 ears from 125 patients with sensorineural hearing loss. They conclude that this technique of calculating hearing thresholds from reflex threshold measurements can be accomplished bilaterally in 10 minutes or less, without great expenditure of additional equipment, and predicts hearing level with an accuracy that is at least sufficient for a rough rating of hearing loss.

The Niemeyer and Sesterhenn procedure involves several steps and easy mathematical manipulations. First, acoustic reflex thresholds are established for pure tone stimuli between 125 to 8000 Hz, and a mean stapedial reflex threshold is determined from these measures. Then a reflex threshold is established for a broad band white noise stimulus, which should occur at a lower intensity level than the pure

tone thresholds. The white noise threshold is subtracted from the mean pure tone threshold and this difference is multiplied by a constant factor of 2.5. The final step in the procedure is to subtract the derived difference value multiplied by 2.5 from the mean pure tone acoustic reflex value. This number represents the "calculated hearing threshold."

Jerger et al. (1974c) presented data from 1156 patients with normal hearing or sensorineural hearing loss as a follow-up study to the report of Niemeyer and Sesterhenn. The test procedure used was an attempt to predict the degree of sensorineural hearing loss from the relationship between acoustic reflex thresholds for pure tone and broad band noise stimuli. The underlying concept of this impedance procedure, known as the Differential Loudness Summation Test," is that the presence of sensorineural hearing loss predictably reduces the normal expected difference between acoustic reflex thresholds for pure tones and noise.

The Jerger procedure is a simplified version of the original German technique. The loudness summation differential test attempts to predict sensorineural hearing loss within four categories of impairment (normal hearing sensitivity, mild loss, severe loss, or profound loss). Jerger establishes pure tone acoustic reflexes at only 500, 1000, and 2000 Hz and a white noise acoustic reflex to predict the degree of hearing loss. In addition, the *slope* of the hearing loss is predicted by establishing reflex thresholds for a low pass band of noise and high pass noise band. Audiometric contour is predicted to be flat, rising, or steep configuration.

In the Jerger et al. series of over 1000 patients, the predictive error of the differential loudness summation test was insignificant in 63% of the group, moderate in 33%, and seriously erroneous in only 4% of the patients.

These findings have important implications for the auditory evaluation of babies and young children. The fact that this technique can be done with a child of virtually any age, with or without sedation, in minutes with a minimum of difficulty recommends the technique highly to those clinicians concerned with the accurate assessment of hearing in infants and children. Two limitations have affected the successful application of this new technique to all children. First, the technique is successful only if both middle ears are normal; and second, brain-injured children may fail to demonstrate an acoustic reflex in spite of apparently normal hearing. With these qualifications in mind, the technique promises to have a profound effect on the audiologic assessment of young children.

Electrodermal Response Audiometry

During the years of the late 1940's and early 1950's, many clinicians believed that electrodermal audiometry was the final solution to their problems in the evaluation of hearing in difficult-to-test patients. Electrodermal response audiometry (EDA or EDR) considered by many to be an objective hearing test, is also known as galvanic audiometry (GA) and psychogalvanic skin response audiometry (PGSR). Regardless of name, the testing technique utilizes a conditioning procedure of pairing a tone and electrical shock so as to elicit an autonomic change in sweat glands of the skin of the patient, which can be observed on most any type of recorder.

As one reviews the professional journals of some 20 to 25 years ago, it is easy to understand the optimism created about electrodermal audiometry as an objective type of hearing test. Later articles identified numerous problems associated with the EDA techniques, and the critical reviewer can sense a more cautionary and concerned viewpoint toward this testing procedure. More recently, many clinicians feel that the EDR audiometry should be reserved for adults, and that it currently has little clinical applicability for testing hearing of children. We share this latter view and do not include EDR in our testing with children, nor do we recommend this procedure as a children's hearing test.

Anyone who has ever attempted to entice a youngster into a sound-treated booth, when the child's previous exposure to having his hearing tested was with the EDR audiometric procedure, can appreciate our feelings toward this testing technique.

Background

The galvanic skin reflex was initially identified by Féré in 1888 and actually named by Veraguth in 1909. Goldstein (1963) states that the autonomic change in state of the sweat glands, which is the physiologic basis of the galvanic skin response, may be the most commonly used index of autonomic activity. This activity is measured as a change in resistance to a small electrical current flow or as a change in electrical potential between two points on the skin. When one evaluates the resistance of the skin to an applied current, the result is known as the Féré effect; but if the measurement is of the electrical potential which arises from currents within the skin, we speak of the Tarchanoff effect. Lindsley (1951) labels these two effects as "exosomatic" when applying an external current, or "endosomatic" relating to current from the skin. By either set of standards, the galvanic skin reflex is very small and often difficult to observe, especially with early physiologic equipment. Accordingly, clinical application for its use was not developed for many years.

Stimulation of the sympathetic nervous system increases activity of the skin's sweat glands which may secrete large quantities of sweat. The sweating reflex may have emotional or environmental thermal origins, although the actual neural mechanisms related to the emotional response activity is largely undefined. According to Hogan (1969) the emotional origins for sweat reflex activity are initiated in the cerebral cortex, and neural impulses are conducted by some central pathway such as the reticular tracts to sudomotor nerves which reach the sweat glands through cutaneous branches of the somatic nerves. Hogan attributes innervation of the sweat glands solely to the sympathetic division of the autonomic nervous system. Guyton (1971) states that the sweat glands are stimulated by nuclei in the hypothalmus that are usually considered to be parasympathetic with cholinergic innervation. However, the sweat glands also have adrenergic innervation, especially in the hands and feet, and so many emotional states that are alerting to the adrenergic portions of the sympathetic nervous system will cause sweating in the hands and feet. The sweat reflex increases saline on the skin, and lowers resistance to a small current flow between two electrodes on the body surface. With sweat on the skin, current flows more freely and the changes in resistance to passage of the current can be recorded in wave-like form and related to the time of a stimulus presentation.

Heart Rate Response Audiometry

Change in heart rate response to presentations of auditory signals is a well established feature of electrocardiac measurements. Zeaman and Wegner (1956) note that upon presentation of a brief, moderately loud tone, the human patient will display a temporary wave-like alteration of the electrocardiogram. This is an unconditioned response often used by psychophysiologists in cardiac conditioning experiments (Zeaman et al., 1954; Zeaman and Wegner, 1956).

The early evaluations of heart rate change due to auditory stimulation did not attempt to use the technique to establish auditory thresholds. The physiologic measurement is based on the fact that immediately prior to each cardiac contraction, an electrical impulse is initiated and travels through the heart. As this electrical impulse passes through the muscle of the heart, small electrical currents spread into the tissues surrounding the heart. Some of this current reaches the surface skin of the body and is measured with sensitive electrodes. If the electrodes are generally placed on either side of the heart, the potentials are recorded with an electrocardiograph. For complete description of this cardiac activity, the reader is referred to Guyton's *Textbook of Medical Physiology* (1971).

The unconditioned heart rate response noted by Zeaman and Wegner (1954) identified two types of subjects. One group showed a decelerative type of heart rate response, while the other group demonstrated an acceleration in the heart rate following presentation of an auditory signal. The investigators noted that the unconditioned cardiac response was greatly influenced by the subject's respiration, and in each subject the response accelerated during inspiration and decelerated during exhalation. Evaluation of the cardiac response rate over time was virtually impossible because the variable cardiac rate associated with respiration produced an average response rate that showed little change related to auditory signals. There-

fore, examination of the unconditioned cardiac response to auditory stimuli requires a beat-by-beat analysis, an extremely tedious and time-consuming task.

The Zeaman and Wegner study (1956) established that changes in the heart rate patterns of adults were specifically related to the intensity of the auditory signal. Bartoshuk (1962a, b; 1964) examined cardiac responses to acoustic signals in some 100 neonates. His cardiac recording technique (1964) utilized an electrode on the infant's left leg and the second electrode on the head in the frontal area. A cardiotachometer was used to determine stable heart rate, and ancillary recordings included electromyograms from the right forearm extensors, bipolar EEG electrodes on the left frontal and parietal area, respiration, and body movement measurements. The analysis of results was done by comparing the five or six cardiac beats immediately prior to stimulus onset with the initial five or six beats following termination of the stimulus. His results verified that cardiac acceleration to auditory signals was reliably observed in all neonates; that cardiac acceleration was greater in 4-day-old infants than 1-, 2-, or 3-day-old infants; and that repeated stimulus presentations created cardiac response decrement exhibited by a shortened period of acceleration. Keen et al. (1965) tested 40 infants and found consistent heart beat acceleration following auditory stimulation of moderate intensity which showed response decrement to long, 10-second stimulus presentations. No response decrement, or habituation, was evidenced to short, 2-second auditory signals.

In a clinical study of heart rate change in infants, Schulman and Wade (1970) tested 30 high risk babies between 6 weeks and 9 months of age. A computer program was used to present auditory signals and average responses over trials. Heart rate change was measured by sampling the cardiac record at each 2-second interval during a prestimulus period until 2 seconds before the onset of the next stimulus. Each trial period was composed of 10 sampling points which were averaged across trials to compare prestimulus and poststimulus heart rate. Since gross motor movement can influence test results, the infants were tested during quiet sleep or following feeding. According to these clinicians, it is not necessary to sedate babies for this test, but the infants must be observed closely so that stimulus presentations can be made during periods of minimal body movement. Under the conditions of their evaluation of the 30 infants, cardiac rate responses were obtained in 27 subjects at 34 dB SPL. The other three subjects appeared to have elevated auditory thresholds, even with repeat testing.

Stimuli used were band-limited noise signals centered at 500 and 3600 Hz. The intensity of the signal was controlled in increasing steps of 10 dB, ranging from 34 to 84 dB SPL. Initial stimulus presentations were at 34 dB SPL, and if no response was observed, the signal was raised 10 dB until a response was noted. Stimuli were presented in blocks of five and consisted of 3-second duration bursts separated by 30-second quiet intervals. The resulting heart rate change was averaged with a special purpose computer over the five stimulus presentations (see Fig. 6.10). Total testing time for obtaining heart rate responses to the screening stimulus of 34 dB SPL was approximately 20 minutes.

Schulman (1970a, b) tested a hypothesis proposed by Luria (1963) and Eisenberg et al. (1966) that infants with central nervous system damage fail to habituate to repeated stimulation. Schulman used 80-dB SPL stimuli presented for 3 seconds at 20-second intervals. Examination of heart rate change averaged across time for trials 1 to 5 and trials 26 to 30 showed significant habituation for both the experimental group of high probability CNS-damaged babies and a matched control group of normal full term infants. Butterfield (1962) was unable to obtain positive heart rate responses in three retarded patients, although normal patients were easily tested. He reported difficulty in finding mentally retarded patients who could cooperate with the testing procedure.

Schulman attempted to use the heart rate response in audiologic evaluation of children. In a study of 24 children, ranging in age from 3 weeks to 13 years, heart rate change, cortical evoked potentials, and conventional audiometry results were compared in the assessment of auditory response levels. Heart rate responses were obtained at approximately normal-hearing levels, and agreed closely with other test results in subjects with documented hearing loss. The authors concluded that heart rate change is a sensitive measure of auditory function, and is within clinical feasibility. In comparison to evoked cortical potential measurement, the heart rate technique had a number of advantages because it is technically simpler, electrode placement is not so critical, a superior signal to noise ratio exists, and fewer stimulus presentations were needed to obtain a response. The heart rate procedure was less time-consuming, more reliable, and less expensive to perform.

Electroencephalographic Evoked Response Audiometry

Some 30 years ago Davis (1939) noted that the electrical activity of the brain as indicated by electroencephalographic recordings showed a change when the subject heard a loud sound. This led numerous clinicians to attempt to use the standard EEG technique as a test for hearing acuity. Results, however, were disappointing. The electrical response in the cortex to auditory stimuli is so small that it is difficult to see in the normal on-going electrical activity of the brain; particularly when the stimuli are low level pure tones.

In the early 1960's a number of special purpose computers appeared on the commercial market. These computers, known generally as signal-averager computers, utilized a summation technique to cancel out random on-going background physiologic "noise," which created an improved signal-to-noise condition, which in turn enhanced specific, time-locked potentials of small magnitude. These computers store and average potentials which are related in time to the onset of a stimulus, while "random" noise which consists theoretically of an equal number of positive and negative electrical potentials, is averaged out to be of zero value. Thus, only the wanted potential activity summates in the computer and can be read out on any recording device. When this technique is used to study cortical response to auditory signals, it is known as evoked response audiometry (ERA), electroencephalographic audiometry (EEA), or cortical audiometry.

The cortical evoked response results from generalized electrical activity on the cortex due to the presentation of various sensory stimuli

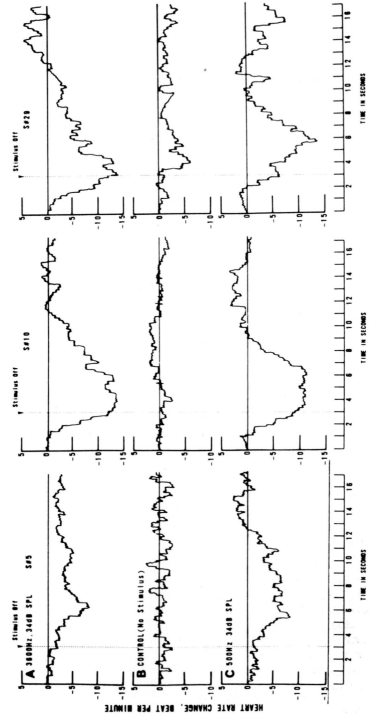

Fig. 6.10. Heart rate change averaged over five trials on a special-purpose computer. A, response to band-limited noise peaking at 3600 Hz, presented at an intensity of 34 dB SPL; B, random heart rate change during control trials; and C, response to band-limited noise at 500 Hz at 34 dB SPL. (With permission from C. A. Schulman, and G. Wade: The use of heart rate in the audiological evaluation of non-verbal children. II. Clinical trials on an infant population. Neuropaediatrie 2: 197-205, 1970.)

including light, vibrotactile stimuli, and sound. In fact, the presentation of any sensory stimulus of sufficient intensity, or the abrupt change of any stimulus, produces a widespread evoked potential from the human brain (McCandless and Rose, 1970). By the mid-1960's, evoked response audiometry was being hailed as "the answer" to audiometric testing problems and the inevitable difficult-to-test patient. Unfortunately, this did not prove to be the case; technical problems, equipment expense, and time-consuming clinical testing arrangements made routine use of evoked response audiometry impractical for most clinical facilities. Researchers found test results to be influenced by so many variables that work is still under way to sort out the primary parameters of cortical audiometry. Volumes of information have been written about this testing procedure, yet the technique is still beyond the "routine application" stage. Excellent chapters in other books provide extensive literature reviews of evoked response audiometry and interested readers are referred to the works of Goldstein (1963, 1973), McCandless (1971), and Skinner (1972). This already copiously covered topic will not be given extensive attention in this book, since its use as an adjunct to conventional testing procedures has been well acknowledged.

Procedure

Although as many clinical procedures exist for evoked response audiometry as clinicians who use it, a "typical" procedure has been described by McCandless (1967).

Infants are tested while held in their mother's arms or lying in a crib. Older children are seated in a chair. Younger children often doze or fall asleep naturally during the clinical procedure. Testing may be done in a sound room or other quiet environment. Recording electrodes are attached with electrode paste to the vertex of the skull on the interaural plane, and clipped to an earlobe. The ground electrode is clipped to the opposite ear. Standard pure tone test signals are used as stimuli, of 700-msec duration, once every 4 seconds, with

a rise-decay time of 20 msec. The stimulus programmer stimulates the averaging computer for a total scan time of 1 second following each stimulus presentation. The test tones may be presented through earphones, free-field speaker, or bone conduction oscillator. In the hands of an experienced clinician, the evoked response audiogram may be completed in 60 to 90 minutes.

A total of 50 stimuli are presented for each evoked response measure. The summed result of the 50 presentations is read out on an oscilloscope or X-Y plotter. The evoked response threshold is defined as the stimulus intensity which produces a visually detectable response when a 10-dB lower intensity does not produce a similar waveform. A high level initial test, 80 dB HL, is often made to serve as a reference pattern for subsequent runs. In order to obtain what is considered to be the most important audiometric information in the least amount of time, thresholds are obtained at 2000 and 500 Hz initially.

The average evoked response is not a unitary response, but rather a composite reflecting general cortical activity. An idealized response is characterized by a multiphasic wave having fairly consistent latencies. The negative and positive peaks and valleys in the classic waveform have been labeled P_1, N_1, P_2, N_2, and P_3 (Fig. 6.11). The characteristic latencies of the specific peaks for a 2000-Hz tone at a moderate intensity signal level are $P_1 = 50$ msec, $N_1 = 100$ msec, $P_2 = 175$ msec, and $N_2 = 300$ msec (Derbyshire and McCandless, 1964; Davis, et al., 1966; Price et al., 1966). Goldstein (1973) presents an idealized evoked response that separates the peak components into early (50 msec or earlier), late (50 to 400 msec), and contingent negative variations (later than 400 msec) (Fig. 6.12). The amplitude of the evoked response is generally related to the intensity of the stimulus; the more intense the stimulus, the larger the average evoked response to a certain point. The growth in amplitude of the wave is accompanied by a decrease in latency of the peak components. As the stimulus signal is decreased toward threshold levels, the presence or absence of the averaged evoked response becomes difficult to separate from the biological baseline activity (Fig. 6.13).

*Influencing Factors in Evoked
Response Audiometry*

The variables that are capable of influencing the average evoked response are so numerous that researchers have been busy for several years trying to delineate the influence of each factor.

Electrode placement has been studied exten-

sively. Electroencephalographic audiometry generally uses one active, one inactive, and one ground electrode. The placement of the active electrode has been the subject of some controversy among investigators. Geisler (1960) found the occipital area to provide the largest amplitude for click-type acoustic signals. Bickford et al. (1964) recommended the inion as the site for the active electrode and inactive electrode

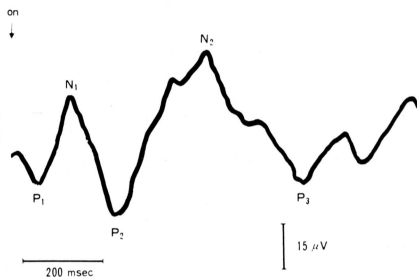

Fig. 6.11. Typical pattern of an averaged auditory-evoked response from a 3-year-old girl. Test tone was a 1000-Hz signal at 30-dB sensation level. (With permission from T. Suzuki and K. Origuchi: Averaged evoked response audiometry (ERA) in young children during sleep. Acta Otolaryngol. [Suppl.] (Stockh.) 252: 19-28, 1969.)

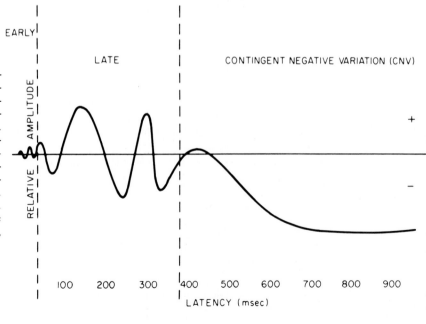

Fig. 6.12. Schematic averaged electroencephalic response. (With permission from R. Goldstein: Electroencephalic audiometry. In Modern Developments in Audiology, edited by J. Jerger, Ed. 2, pp. 407-435. Academic Press, New York, 1973.)

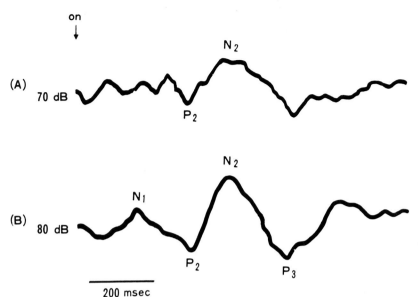

on

(A)
70 dB

N_2

P_2

(B)
80 dB

N_1

N_2

P_2 P_3

200 msec

Fig. 6.13. Averaged evoked response in a 15-month-old infant. A shows questionable response at 70 dB HL; B shows definite response at 80 dB HL. (With permission from T. Suzuki and K. Origuchi: Averaged evoked response audiometry (ERA) in young children during sleep. Acta Otolaryngol. [Suppl.] (Stockh.) 252: 19-28, 1969.)

on the earlobe. Davis and Yoshie (1963) favored the vertex as the place for the active electrode. The vertex response varies from the inion response in terms of response latency and myogenic influence from neck muscles. Most recent investigators have used vertex placement of the active electrode, while position of the inactive electrode seems to be nonsignificant (Davis and Zerlin, 1966). Accordingly, the evoked response is sometimes called the vertex or V potential.

The nature of the acoustic stimulus must also be considered. The important signal parameters include the rise and decay time, the signal duration, the intensity of presentation, and the number of stimuli presented to the subject for each trial period during which the raw EEG is summed or averaged. Lamb and Graham (1967) reported that clicks were more effective stimuli than pure tones with 10-msec rise-decay times. Pure tones with longer rise and decay times produced fewer evoked responses. Lamb and Graham also reported that rise and decay time of the signal affect the latency and amplitude of the response. The suggested number of signal presentations recommended by Liebman and Graham (1967a) and McCandless and Best (1966) is 50; Davis et al. (1967) recommend 64 presentations of approximately one per second. The McCandless and Best (1966) study indi-

cated that the frequency of the stimulus had no effect on the form of the response, but increases in signal intensity caused an increase in response amplitude.

In the evaluation of each evoked response, the clinician must be prepared to note latency amplitude and consistency of peaks within the waveform. These parameters are the result of subject variables including physiologic state and age. Most reports agree that sleep causes an increase in response latency (Williams et al., 1962; Ornitz et al., 1967; and Suzuki and Taguchi, 1965).

The influence of subject age on the evoked response has received considerable attention, and is especially pertinent to our theme of testing hearing in children. Price et al. (1966) found greater response amplitude in children over 10 than for adults; Suzuki and Taguchi (1968) found children under 14 to have consistently smaller amplitude responses than adults. The latency of the evoked response has been found to decrease with increases in age. Barnett and Goodwin (1965) as well as Davis et al., (1967) confirmed this latency change as a function of subject age. Actually, Davis and Zerlin (1966) and McCandless and Best (1966) concluded that the evoked response is highly variable at all ages, between subjects and test/retest reliability with the same subjects

(Fig. 6.14). McCandless (1967) reported good success with 90 of 102 hard-of-hearing children, and that his evoked response measurements indicated thresholds that were ultimately within 10 dB of behaviorally determined thresholds on children older than 2 years of age. In his study, 10 of the 12 children whose thresholds could not be determined by ERA were between 3 days of age and 2 years.

Response Criteria

The basis of the decision as to whether an evoked response is indeed present in the summed tracing is crucial to the clinical utilization of evoked response audiometry. Derbyshire and McCandless (1964) published a template of the "ideal" evoked response. They indicated that individual variation in response was considerable, and thus the template could really only serve as a guide. Rose and Ruhm (1966) made a significant contribution to clinical procedure with the evoked response by suggesting the use of a silent run, during which time the EEG activity is averaged but no acoustic stimulus is presented to the subject. Results from the silent run are then compared to results from a stimulus presentation run. Davis, et. al., (1967) suggested the use of a strong tactile stimulus in order to elicit a clear evoked response to serve as an individual template. The Davis technique of using an alternate stimulus such as vibration or light is informative to insure that the equipment is in good working condition during the testing procedure. The problem may be summarized by stating that the variability of the evoked response makes it impractical to employ rigid response criteria. Cohen et al. (1971) reported intraobserver agreement in scoring the presence

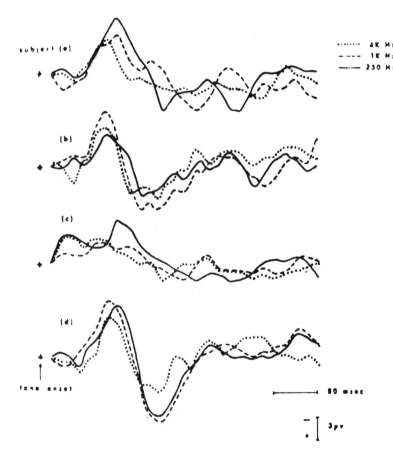

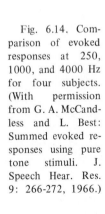

Fig. 6.14. Comparison of evoked responses at 250, 1000, and 4000 Hz for four subjects. (With permission from G. A. McCandless and L. Best: Summed evoked responses using pure tone stimuli. J. Speech Hear. Res. 9: 266-272, 1966.)

or absence of an evoked response from young, sleeping children to range from 59% to 75% agreement in consistency in the identification of an evoked response. The impact of the problem is reflected in a recent study by Rose et al. (1972) in which auditory thresholds were determined by five audiologists in 50 patients with evoked response audiometry and routine clinical audiometry. The results of the study showed significant differences between ERA results and routine audiometric results, and the authors urge caution in the clinical use of data obtained by the ERA technique. In essentially the same study reported in another journal, these authors (Rose et al., 1971) conclude that ERA lacks objectivity when conducted without specific objective criteria.

An important consideration in the use of evoked response audiometry is the time required for the tests, particularly for children. Rapin (1964) reports 2 or 4 hours as necessary for ERA administration; Davis et al. (1967) indicate an average time of 50 minutes to evaluate three intensity levels; Barnett and Goodwin (1965) report the need for approximately 90 minutes; McCandless (1967) reports testing time for five frequencies in one ear to take 1 hour. Obviously, disagreement exists as to the question of required time for ERA measurement. In calculations made by Stewart (1970), if 64 stimuli are averaged for each response, presented at a rate of one every 2 seconds, the minimal time required to average one response will take 2 minutes. She indicates that one should average two, or preferably three stimulus runs before deciding whether a response is indeed present or if a false positive has been recorded. Considering at least three intensity levels to determine threshold, these figures yield a minimal test time of 18 minutes per test frequency, not including the read-out time. Thus, a threshold test of four frequencies in one ear might realistically require 2 hours assuming no breakdowns or other problems.

Review of the literature indicates that although the majority of subjects yield satisfactory results, unfortunately those groups who are most difficult to test by conventional audiometry, the young and the mentally retarded, are precisely the groups who are most difficult to test with ERA. Reneau and Mast (1968) describe a telemetric EEG system for use with the profoundly retarded which permits the patient to be tested without restraint or sedation.

Clinical applications of evoked response audiometry continue to be developed including its use with speech audiometry (Feldman and Goldstein, 1967) and bone conduction testing (Liebman and Graham, 1967b). Current investigations are concerned with problems in evoked response audiometry during sedation (Suzuki, 1973). The ERA technique is more difficult and yields less reliable information than in the waking state, but for some young or hyperactive children, it is the only way ERA can be performed (Davis, 1973).

Rapin and Bergman (1969) studied 15 children who presented diagnostic problems with evoked response audiometry and typical behavioral audiometry. The judgments attained in both procedures were essentially in agreement. They conclude that the ERA testing, in spite of its length in time, the uncertainty in interpretation of tracings, and the lack of information concerning the child's ability to utilize his hearing for communication, constituted significant results in the uncertain diagnosis of these difficult cases. Goldstein (1973) states that ERA is really not an objective procedure for threshold audiometry, even though a physiologic-type of response is utilized, due to the subjectivity of interpretation of results. Evoked response audiometry will probably continue as a valuable testing technique for a few children who are seen by clinicians skilled in the administration and interpretation of ERA results. It seems unlikely that this procedure, so expensive to set-up and so time-consuming to utilize, will become a routine testing technique under today's test conditions. The potential for its usefulness still exists, but we need a more objective approach, a better testing technique, and equipment that is within the realm of reasonable time and expense.

Electrocochleography

Investigators have long been intrigued by the electrical potentials generated within the auditory system. Clinicians have made many efforts through the years to utilize these auditory potentials in some form of clinical procedure. These measurements were termed "electro-cochleography" by Lempert et al. (1947). The most important cochlear potential is the cochlear microphonic which originates from the hair cells in the organ of Corti, originally described by Wever and Bray (1930). The cochlear microphonic reproduces faithfully the waveform of the stimulating auditory signal, and is usually measured by an electrode from the round window niche. The cochlear microphonic has no "threshold," other than the lower limits of the recording apparatus; that is, the cochlear microphonic, or CM, is produced to any auditory signal, no matter how slight. Hence, it is very much like a microphone.

The electrical potential from the auditory nerve is the action potential, noted initially by Derbyshire and Davis (1935). The action potential consists of nerve impulses in the eighth nerve triggered by the cochlear micro-phonic. The action potential response consists of a well synchronized volley of impulses called N_1, which may be followed by smaller waves known as N_2 and N_3. Although initial clinical attempts to use auditory electrical potentials centered around the cochlear microphonic, the action potential response is currently proving most valuable in clinical use.

Davis (1957) pointed out that external electrodes were, in general, inadequate for analyzing intracochlear events, because the electrodes pick up a mixture of responses including the action potential, summating potential, and cochlear microphonic. Yoshie and Yamaura (1969) comment that during the measurement of human cochlear potentials, effects of the physiologic activities coming from other tissues and organs than the cochlea must be taken into account. They indicated that the three most common distorting factors in such electrophysiologic measurements are: (a) the subject's own physiologic noise, (b) reflex contractions from the middle ear muscles, and (c) the combination of the cochlear nerve action potentials. The effects of all these factors may vary with signal intensity, frequency, condition of the subject, and position of the electrode.

Fromm et al. (1935) were the first to detect cochlear potentials from the human ear. They tested patients with large perforations of the tympanic membrane and inserted an electrode, consisting of a fine wire with a cotton-wrapped end, in the niche of the round window. They reported good recordings of the cochlear microphonic signal from the round window niche, otic capsule promentory, the mastoid process, and even from the walls of the external auditory meatus.

Russian scientists soon attempted to replicate this recording technique in humans. Andreev et al. (1939) utilized the same technique in patients with large perforations of the tympanic membrane. They reported observing "small magnitude potentials" of less than 26 microvolts from round window electrodes even to "painfully loud sounds." When they moved their electrode placement to the bony capsule surface near the round window, the potentials were weakened even more. Perlman and Case (1941), using basically the same procedure, reported positive results in nine patients to signals within 20 dB of normal-hearing levels. They also reported that recording positions away from the round window site gave only feeble results or no results at all.

Concurrently, during this time period, Lempert's fenestration middle ear operation (developed in 1938) was being widely used by otolaryngologists as a treatment for oto-sclerosis. Lempert et al. (1947) stated that a need existed for an objective test to determine the "existing reservoir of cochlear function in deafened ears." They knew that the cochlear potentials were generated by the hair cells of the organ of Corti and, accordingly, were affected by the pathway between the origin of the potential and the electrode. That is, since the hair cells are spread out along the cochlear spiral, any specific electrode position cannot be equally effective for signals of various frequencies. They felt that the recorded cochlear potential had only "relative significance," and consequently did not provide a direct or absolute representation of cochlear activity. They felt that the cochlear potential is generated by a mechanical process, indicative of end organ response—but not related to responses of the auditory nerve or more central auditory processes. On the other hand, more medial auditory responses to the cochlea cannot be expected unless the cochlear potential is present.

Lempert et al. (1947) reported results of electrocochleography which they conducted at the time of surgery in 11 patients. They stated that the location of the active electrode was very crucial and that contact with the round window yielded the largest magnitude potentials. They used a hypodermic needle for the inactive electrode inserted in the skin near the patient's external ear. From the 11 patients, they obtained positive responses from four and faint responses from two others. They commented that good electrode contact with the round window was difficult to achieve because the typical otologic middle ear surgical approach provided only limited access to the round window niche.

A near devastating setback was afforded to electrocochleography in a follow-up report by Lempert et al. (1950). They concluded that recording the human cochlear potential was not a practical clinical procedure. They substantiated through 3 years of experience that the recording procedure was indeed objective, precise, and easily reproducible. They verified that the response of the ear over a large range of stimulus intensities could be measured. They felt that the peripheral sensory end organ could be evaluated without complication from the central nervous system, and the technique could be used to differentiate between sensory and neural deafness. These investigators attempted recordings from 32 human cases and 16 monkeys, with poor results. George von Békésy designed a special optical instrument to improve the view of the round window, but his effort did not solve the many problems. Although electrocochleography could be done at the time of surgery, the technique proved difficult to do through an intact tympanic membrane. Lempert and his associates tried nine cases with an electrode pushed through the tympanic membrane to the bony promontory, but observed positive results in only three cases. They filled the middle ear cavity with saline to improve electrical conductivity, but this did not help. In their concluding statements, Lempert et al. (1950) felt that a clinical procedure

should be routinely applicable and reliable. To provide the information they sought, electrocochleography needed to be accomplished prior to reaching a decision for surgery, and was not nearly so useful when conducted at surgery where the diagnosis had already been made. Since the technique was too difficult to do through the tympanic membrane, and results were too sporadic, they stated conclusively that the procedure was clinically impractical.

After a few dormant years, research with cochlear potentials was started again by Ruben and his associates at Johns Hopkins Hospital. Ruben, during surgery, placed an electrode on the round window of four patients and obtained good responses from two of them (Ruben et al., 1959). In 1960, Ruben et al. reported observations on 17 patients who showed good cochlear potentials in response to pure tones, and noted the presence of the eighth nerve action potential in the same recordings with an N_1 latency of 1.2 to 2.0 msec (Fig. 6.15). At this time, Ruben reported that the cochlear potential recording procedure had to overcome two major problems. First, the

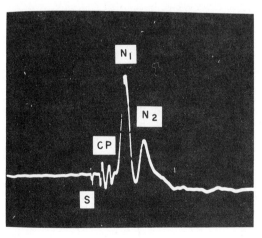

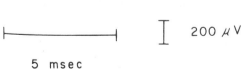

5 msec

Fig. 6.15. Oscilloscopic tracing by Ruben et al. (1960) showing presence of eighth nerve action potential, N_1 and N_2, in the same recording with cochlear potential (CP) and stimulus click (S).

technical aspects of the auditory stimulation, such as amplification of the small potentials in the poor environment of the operating room. Secondly, he pointed out, again, the difficulty in recording due to the adverse anatomy of the human ear for this procedure (Ruben et al., 1961).

Ruben and his colleagues, however, continued their efforts. In 1962, they reported obtaining cochlear potentials and action potentials from 50 patients. Their group included 15 children tested under general anesthesia. The children were grouped as having "serious difficulties with verbal communication," "seriously impaired speech," or "no evidence of hearing." The technique was validated on 12 adults with otosclerosis, 11 of whom gave good cochlear potentials and 7 showed good action potential responses. From the 15 children, 8 gave no cochlear or action potentials, 4 gave good cochlear potentials but no action potentials, and the other 3 showed good cochlear and action potentials. Ruben and his associates suggested that these latter three cases may be the first factual validation of central deafness since proof of a functioning cochlea and eighth nerve was evident in light of a picture of severe hearing loss. From this study, the authors concluded that auditory potential measurement is a good technique to teach us more about problems of childhood deafness.

In 1967, Ruben summarized his experiences with the use of cochlear potentials as a diagnostic test in deafness. He felt that the two types of responses, the cochlear potential from electrical activity of the hair cells and the $N_1 N_2$ action potential from the cochlear division of the eighth nerve, could be measured clinically, through a tympanotomy incision, with an electrode in the round window niche. He reported that the technique had at least three uses: (a) may serve as a basic research tool to relate physiologic phenomena to behavioral activity; (b) may provide clues to understanding various disease states of deafness which look similar in standard audiometry; and (c) can provide the physiologic area for the diagnosis of an individual's deafness, i.e., eighth nerve deafness, from cochlear or conductive deafness.

More recently, investigators have been working to find a technique for measuring auditory potentials other than during surgery. The technique utilized in cortical evoked response audiometric measurement provided the answer in the form of desk computers used to summate successive small responses to repeated, identical acoustic stimuli. In this manner, an "average" response is obtained to many stimulus presentations. The computer signal averages an evoked response from out of extraneous, random background activity. This "average response" method for electrocochleographic measurement has been used by Ruben and Walker (1963) and Ronis (1966), both studies done on patients at the time of surgery.

The use of signal averaging technique was very important to those interested in electrocochleography. Since this procedure now permitted recording of very small voltage responses, it was no longer necessary to place the electrode as close as possible to the organ of Corti. Thus, Yoshie and his colleagues in Japan have published several reports since 1967 concerning parameters of action potentials of the eighth nerve obtained from the external auditory canal; Sohmer and Feinmesser (1967) in Israel made action potential recordings from the lobe of the ear; Spreng and Keidel (1967) reported in Germany their recordings from the mastoid scalp area; Portmann and Aran, both Frenchmen, have reported several papers with data obtained directly from the promontory, Cullen et al. (1972) at Louisiana State University School of Medicine record action potential responses from an electrode placed against the lateral side of the tympanic membrane; while Coats and Dickey (1970) used the needle inserted in the ear canal described by Yoshie. Electrocochleography is apparently an international venture, and as might be expected, the various clinical team approaches and results are somewhat different and worthy of our review.

Yoshie et al. (1967) and others from the Otolaryngology Department of Shinshu University in Matsumoto, Japan, have contributed much toward improving recording techniques in human auditory responses and the development of the procedures into useful clinical tools. In their 1967 report, they describe the use of an average response computer to record action potential responses from patients with an electrode in the external auditory meatus. They use a local anesthesia to place a needle electrode in the skin of the posterior wall of the external auditory canal, 5 mm from the annulus of the tympanic membrane. The acoustic stimulus is 500 presentations of clicks at a rate of three or 10 per second. They described a typical action potential response, recorded through the average response computer, to clicks of moderate intensity, as an initial negative wave, N_1, followed 1 second later by a smaller negative wave, N_2, and followed occasionally by a still smaller negative wave, N_3 (Fig. 6.16). The latency of the wave N_1, defined as the time between arrival of the click at the eardrum to the peak of N_1, was 2 to 3 msec. The amplitude of the response as measured from the response baseline to the peak of the wave was a function of click intensity and click interval. The baseline for the action potential wave is an idealized line drawn through the tracing of spontaneous activity at the zero response level. The N_1 response also seemed related to the time interval following the previous click. At this time, Yoshie et al. suggested that new fields of audiometry may now be open, and that it may ultimately be possible to extrapolate results backward to zero amplitude of the action potential to estimate auditory threshold.

In 1968, Yoshie reported that changes in the latency of the action potential seemed closely related to the loudness of the clicks. The latency of N_1, in patients with conductive hearing loss was a very obvious clue to the nature of their hearing impairment. However, the amplitude of the N_1 response is a likely measure of the number of eighth nerve fibers that respond. Yoshie reported clinic behavioral auditory thresholds and conductive loss thresholds to be in "good agreement" with

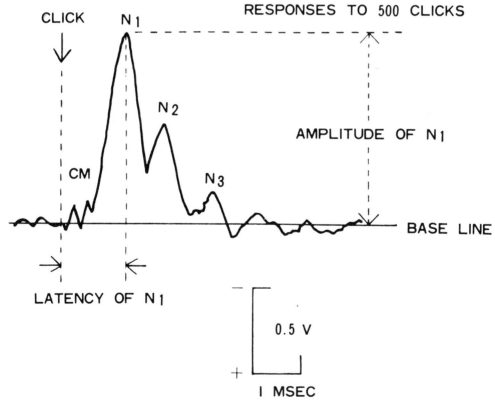

Fig. 6.16. Electrocochleographic averaged response as recorded by Yoshie and Ohashi (1969) from an electrode in the wall of the external auditory canal. The stimulus was 500 clicks at 100 dB peak equivalent SPL. This figure illustrates the definition of latency, N_1 amplitude, and the interpolated baseline.

their action potential records. A sample record showing average auditory nerve action potentials in response to clicks of varying intensities is shown in Figure 6.17.

Yoshie also examined input-output functions which plotted click intensity against amplitude of the N_1 wave in microvolts. He found that the curve rises rapidly at first from a threshold

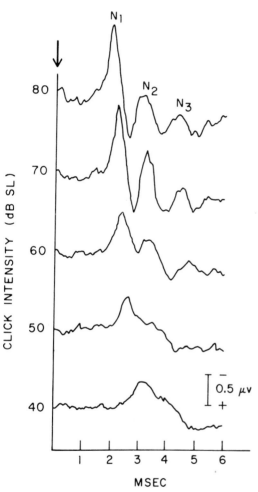

Fig. 6.17. Averaged auditory nerve action potentials to 500 clicks at a rate of three per second. Curves were obtained from stimulus presentations of various intensities. Note the increase in amplitude of N_1 as signal intensity increases, and the longer latency of N_1 as the signals approach threshold levels. (With permission from N. Yoshie, T. Ohashi, and T. Suzuki: Non-surgical recording of auditory nerve action potentials in man. Laryngoscope 77: 76-85, 1967.)

level of response to an initial hump and then rises again to a second hump which is the maximal level of output (Fig. 6.18). The curve shows an inflection point at which the slope changes in the click intensity region from 70 to 80 dB peak equivalent sound pressure level. Yoshie designated the names low and high intensity portions of the action potential response, or L- and H-curves, respectively.

Yoshie and Ohashi (1969) reported cochlear nerve action potentials from 25 patients including 8 normal-hearing subjects, 15 patients with sensorineural hearing loss, and 2 patients with conductive hearing losses. For the normal-hearing subjects, the N_1 curve showed the two distinct segments of the input-output function (L- and H-curve) which the authors suggest may each be generated by a different population of neurons stimulated by a different class of sensory cells. The patients with conductive hearing loss showed a latency shift for the N_1 wave and amplitude change that was proportional to the degree of hearing loss. Results from the patients with sensorineural hearing loss showed three points of significance: (a) an over-all reduction in the amplitude of N_1 which may be related to the reduced total number of neurons capable of firing; (b) the disappearance of the L-curve segment of the input-output function which may relate to a specific group of pathologic sensory cells; and (c) a prolonged latency of N_1 which might be attributed to neural delay from asynchrony of neural impulses.

Current clinical application of the electrocochleography technique has been largely due to the well publicized efforts of Portmann and Aran at the Phono-Audiology ENT Clinic in Bordeaux, France. They have been using the computer-averaging technique since 1967 to record auditory nerve and cochlear microphonic potentials by means of an electrode placed on the promontory through the tympanic membrane (Aran and LeBert, 1968). They report clinical ease of this procedure which is done on adults and children over 8 under local anesthesia. Younger children are tested under general anesthesia, primarily to insure quietness rather than reduction of pain. By placing the active electrode on the promontory, Aran (1971) reports the potential to be approximately 10 times larger than potentials recorded from the external ear canal. Although their measurement technique actually records the sensory response of the cochlea including the cochlear microphonic and summating potential as well as the neural response—the whole nerve action potential, they do not give consideration to the cochlear responses. Since the cochlear microphonic theoretically has no "threshold," has no latency interval to the acoustic stimulus, mirrors the same pattern as the eliciting stimulus, is of small amplitude compared to the action potential of the nerve, and may often actually be the result of electrode vibration rather than sensory process-

ing, at strong intensity levels only the whole nerve action potential is measured and interpreted. The cochlear microphonic is, in fact, eliminated from the recording procedure by a clever means of reversing the polarity of the stimulating signal and adding it to the picked-up cochlear microphonic in the averaging computer. The sum of these two signals in the computer is zero and they essentially cancel each other out of the recording. Meanwhile, the sum of the action potential is free of microphonic influence, and quickly presents itself in the recording apparatus, totally free of interference from the cochlear microphonic.

Critics of the Portmann-Aran technique

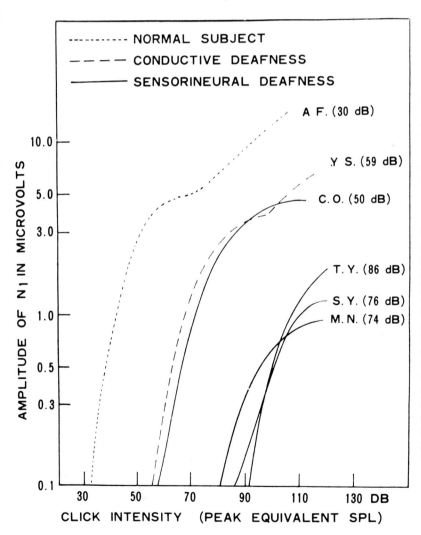

Fig. 6.18. Input-output functions of N_1 recorded from the promontory of patients with various types of hearing loss. The dotted curve represents a typical function from a normal-hearing patient; the dashed line was obtained from a conductive loss patient; the four heavy line curves are from patients with sensorineural hearing loss. The numbers in parentheses indicate subjective thresholds for clicks in peak equivalent sound pressure level. (With permission from N. Yoshie and T. Ohashi: Clinical use of cochlear nerve action potential responses in man for differential diagnosis of hearing losses. Acta Otolaryngol. (Suppl.) 252: 71-87, 1969.)

usually cite their criticism toward the use of the needle electrode of .2-mm diameter which is inserted through the tympanic membrane and positioned against the promontory. The apparatus is held in place under tension from a special headband as shown in Figure 6.19. The authors of the procedure state that the healing of the perforation created is almost always very rapid and without complications. They prefer this electrode position because of the stronger auditory system response, and the fact that artifact from the test tone is reduced when evaluating patients with profound hearing loss. They define electrocochleography as a test which notes, records, and measures the averaged electrical signals which are set up between the bony promontory of the cochlea and the lobe of the ear in response to very short

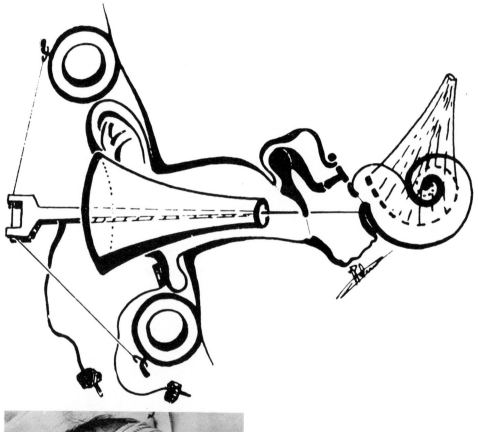

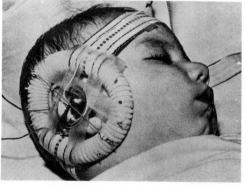

Fig. 6.19. The Portmann-Aran technique for positioning the electrocochleographic active needle electrode against the promontory, through the tympanic membrane. (With permission from M. Portmann and J. M. Aran: Electro-cochleographic sur le nourrissons et le jeune enfant. Acta Otolaryngol. 71: 253-261, 1971.)

acoustic stimuli (clicks and filtered clicks) of alternately opposite phases.

Aran (1971) indicates that they are most interested in the dynamic range of variation in the N_1 response rather than its absolute amplitude. He measures the peak-to-peak amplitude of the response and the latency of the first negative peak, N_1 as shown in Figure 6.20. He describes the typical pattern of his response to be diphasic (negative wave-positive wave) at low and medium intensities, and monophasic (negative wave only) at high intensities. The latency interval ranges between 4 and 5 msec at threshold. The latency interval becomes smaller and may approach 1.5 msec for clicks of 80-dB sensation level. These Frenchmen also record input-output functions as suggested by Yoshie (1968). Aran has an interesting technique of showing several types of results on the same clinic form including the threshold of the response to click, the pattern, or input-output function, of the click-evoked response at suprathreshold levels and the amplitude and latency pattern of several curves as shown in Figure 6.21.

In his 1971 paper, Aran summarizes results obtained from 29 children and more than 100 adults. Children as young as 1 month of age have been tested with his technique (Fig. 6.22).

No response was obtained from nine of the 29 children even to a click stimulus of 100 dB SPL; slight responses were obtained with three children at 100 dB; clear responses with threshold between 60 and 90 dB were obtained at least unilaterally in seven children. Six additional children had clear responses between 0 and 30 dB, although two of these children had no reaction to classic audiometric techniques which Aran suggests may be due to a disorder at a higher brain level. The last four children showed "abnormal" responses which were peculiar because of a sharp positive peak of very short latency (<1 msec), followed by a slow negative wave. Aran attempts to explain this abnormal response, which he also has seen in at least three adults, as an indication of a peculiar cochlear (sensory) disorder.

Portmann et al. (1973) published an interest-

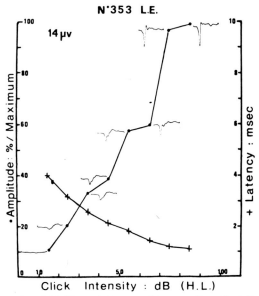

Fig. 6.21. Normal electrocochleogram from the left ear of a 3-year-old child who could not be tested with classic techniques. Normal features to be noted are (1) progressive decrease in N_1 latency curve (solid "x" line) as click intensity is increased; (2) the "L" and "H" parts of the amplitude curve with the initial hump around 50 dB HL; and (3) diphasic response of the averaged response near threshold and monophasic pattern around 85 dB HL. (With permission from Portmann et al.: Testing for recruitment by electrocochleography. Ann. Otol. Rhinol. Laryngol. 82: 36-43, 1973.)

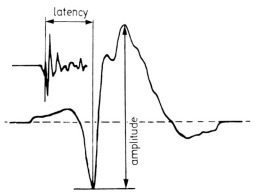

Fig. 6.20. A typical click-evoked peripheral response from the promontory of the cochlea by Aran. Note the differences in waveforms, latency, and amplitude measures from the Yoshie procedure as shown in Figure 6.16. (With permission from J. M. Aran: The electrocochleogram: recent results in children and in some pathological cases. Arch. Klin. Exp. Ohren. Nasen. Kehikopfheilkd. 198: 128-141, 1971.)

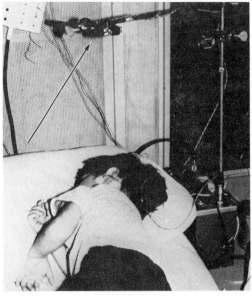

Fig. 6.22. Anesthetized youngster being tested with electrocochleography with the technique of Cullen et al. (1972). Arrow identifies test earphone. (Photograph courtesy of Charles I. Berlin, New Orleans, La.)

ing paper on testing for recruitment by electrocochleography. They describe the recruitment response to consist of three characteristics: (1) a short latency interval at threshold of about 2 msec which is always noted above 40 dB HL; (2) a diphasic response pattern at all sound levels; and (3) an amplitude which increases rapidly with increasing click intensity, and without a plateau. The amplitude catches up to the amplitude of a normal subject at the same level of intensity, although it is considerably closer to the threshold of the "recruiting" patient. Above threshold, the amplitude of the response may increase as much in 10 dB as it might in a normal subject in a 50-dB increase. In their study of 17 patients (22 ears), the majority of results presented by 12 cases showed positive correlation between classical pure tone tests for recruitment and electrocochleography. In the other five patients, the electrocochleogram was deficient in one of the three required characteristics of the recruiting electrocochleogram. The authors present a very concise discussion of the physiology of recruit-

ment from their own viewpoint which is recommended as worthwhile reading.

Sohmer and Feinmesser (1967, 1973) report dissatisfaction with the techniques of electrocochleography which require perforation of the tympanic membrane with an electrode, or the insertion of a needle electrode into the skin of the external auditory canal. They report good results obtained with an active earlobe clip electrode and a reference scalp vertex disc electrode. A third electrode forms the ground and consists of another disc electrode applied to the patient's nose.

The Sohmer-Feinmesser response is a series of five waves beginning 1.4 msec after stimulus presentation with the last wave appearing about 6 or 7 msec. Lower stimulus intensity gives rise to smaller amplitude responses with longer latencies. These investigators believe that each of their waves in the electrocochleographic response coincides to an auditory neuron level, with the first wave generated by first-order cochlear nerve fibers, second wave generated by the cochlear nucleus, third wave from the superior olivary complex and the fourth and fifth waves related to the inferior colliculus. These Israeli clinicians report good success with this technique in 57 infants and children with suspected hearing loss or uncertain diagnosis. In 22 cases, absence of the electrocochleogram response confirmed peripheral hearing loss; in 13 cases, normal electrocochleographic responses indicated that the behavioral hearing loss was not peripheral in origin. Abnormal responses with high thresholds, small amplitude or long latencies were found in 22 infants. In two subjects, electrocochleography produced hearing evidence prior to successful behavioral techniques.

Cullen et al. (1972) reported a nonsurgical method for recording human acoustic nerve action potentials with data from 18 normal-hearing subjects. Their procedure involves placing the active electrode against the tympanic membrane, held in place by a small strip of tape affixed to the electrode wire. A reference disc is attached to the mastoid with tape. A ground electrode is attached to the earlobe. The active electrode is placed as near as possible to the juncture of the annulus and the meatal wall near the posterior-inferior quadrant of the tympanic membrane. The active electrode is a fine silver wire, .5-mm diameter, sheathed in Teflon tubing, with a silver chloride ball electrode soldered to the tip of the wire. Potentials are amplified and fed into a summating computer.

These investigators report that clearly defined acoustic nerve action potentials in all their subjects were obtained at 50-dB sensation level relative to the average behavioral thresholds for clicks at 17 dB peak SPL. Their results are recorded in N_1 latency versus click stimulus level, and plotted against a normative regression line curve. The authors have chosen to disregard the N_1 amplitude, and study only the N_1 latency which is relatively insensitive to electrode position. Further, their initial studies indicate that the N_1 latency will suffice to distinguish between patients with normal hearing, conductive hearing loss, and sensorineural disorders. As example, preliminary data, reported by personal communication, shows that the latency-intensity function for patients with conductive loss or mixed hearing loss, shifts in the direction of longer latency (Fig. 6.22).

The facts are not yet all in regarding the best technique to use in electrocochleographic measurements. It seems sure, however, based on evidence accumulated thus far, that electro-cochleography does have strong clinical implication. Its international development will undoubtedly insure that this new technique is destined to survive and undergo further refinements. Electrocochleography seems to be particularly well suited for testing very young children, and may enable us to evaluate an infant's potential for hearing aid fittings or educational placement.

Ruben (1963) suggests a scheme whereby the anatomic diagnosis of sensorineural or nonconductive deafness might be made. The widespread use of such diagnostic tests could make the hearing loss description of "sensorineural" archaic—we could describe hearing loss as either "sensory" deafness or "neural" deafness depending on the outcome of the physiologic testing procedures. Ruben suggests that knowledge of the exact anatomic location of a child's deafness is very important to the over-all management of the individual. He adds that research into the prevention and treatment of nonconductive deafness must depend on our ability to diagnose the anatomical location of the disorder.

Presented in Table 6.3 is a summary of Ruben's suggested diagnostic rationale for the use of physiologic tests in anatomic specificity for locus of deafness. X-rays of the temporal

Table 6.3. Physiologic Diagnosis of Deafness*

Type of Disorder	X-ray Results	Cochlear Potential	Eighth Nerve Action Potential	Vestibular Response
Labyrinthine lesions				
Agenesis of labyrinth	Abnormal	Absent	Absent	Absent
Arrested development of labyrinth	Abnormal	Absent	Absent	Unknown
Total absence of membranous labyrinth	Normal	Absent	Absent	Absent
Partial absence of membranous labyrinth	Normal	Absent	Absent	Present
Types of deafness				
Total labyrinthine deafness	Normal/abnormal	Absent	Absent	Absent
Cochlear deafness	Normal	Absent	Absent	Present
Total eighth nerve deafness	Normal	Present	Absent	Absent
Partial eighth nerve deafness	Normal	Present	Absent	Present
Central deafness	Normal	Present	Present	Absent/present

* Modified with permission from R. J. Ruben: Anatomical diagnosis of non-conductive deafness by physiological tests. Arch. Otolaryngol. 78: 47-51, 1963.

bone can be used to identify agenesis of the labyrinth. Vestibular tests, such as electronystagmography, can be indicative of the function of the vestibular portion of the labyrinth, as well as the vestibular portion of the eighth nerve and higher pathways. Electrophysiologic responses of the cochlea, via cochlear microphonics, and the auditory portion of the eighth nerve can be evaluated with electrocochleography. The presence of cochlear potentials would indicate functioning hair cells in the organ of Corti. If the cochlear potential is absent, then there will be no eighth nerve action potential since there is nothing to stimulate the neurons. The presence of both cochlear potentials and eighth nerve action potentials in light of a deaf patient would lead the clinician to diagnose the disease to higher auditory centers in the central nervous system. As physiologic tests become more commonplace, clinic procedures for the accurate diagnosis of site-of-lesion deafness will become increasingly a more realistic goal.

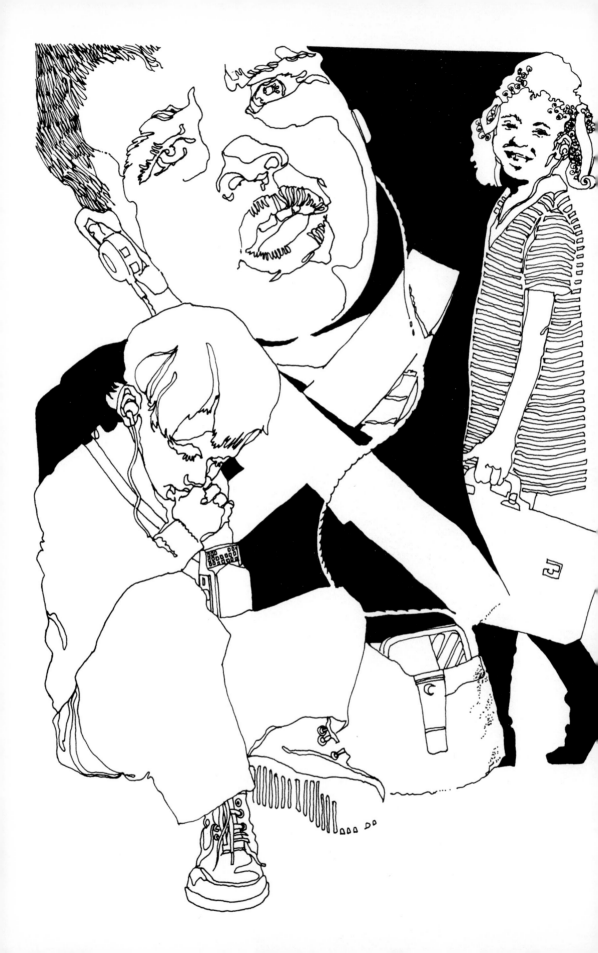

7 HEARING AIDS FOR CHILDREN

There is little doubt that the single most important invention to help the hearing-handicapped child is the electronic hearing aid. There is an old adage, " . . . as we hear, so shall we speak," and it is this very close relationship between hearing, speech, and language that is so important to the deaf child. Several electronic gadgets have been invented to help the deaf child learn to speak, including voice pitch indicators, speech timing equipment, vowel indicators, voice/nonvoice meters, speech spectrum displays, visible speech machines, etc. None of these inventions, however, is more fundamental to the deaf child's education, and his ability to learn speech, than a properly fitted hearing aid.

The task of selecting a hearing aid for a child is not to be taken lightly. Selection of a hearing aid for the hard-of-hearing or deaf child must not be undertaken by the inexperienced clinician or the nonprofessionally trained individual. The procedure involved in the process of selecting a hearing aid for a child involves many people including the otolaryngologist, the pediatrician, the audiologist, the hearing aid dealer, the speech pathologist, the teacher of the deaf, as well as other possible auxiliary professionals such as the public health or school nurse and the social worker. These individuals must work together closely, in a coordinated effort, to insure that the hard-of-hearing child obtains maximal benefit from amplification.

The audiologist is the most likely individual to coordinate and guide the hearing aid selection procedure, although in various clinics and circumstances it may be more appropriate for one of the other professionals to take charge. The audiologist, because of his extensive training, is able to identify the nature and degree of the child's hearing loss—which may in itself be an extremely difficult task. The audiologist insures that proper medical clearance is obtained prior to the hearing aid selection procedure. He is able to evaluate the performance of various hearing aids on the child, make an earmold impression if necessary, and work closely with the hearing aid dealer to obtain the best amplification available for the patient's hearing loss. As part of this entire process, the audiologist must counsel the parents about the new hearing aid, its care and use; he must arrange for therapy for the child and special training if necessary. And finally, he is able to devote the necessary time to follow-up the progress of the patient, and maintain an ever vigilant eye to be sure the hearing aid is in top operating condition. The audiologist must be careful not to use the hearing aid as a device to test a youngster's hearing, as it is no substitute for an accurate, knowledgeable hearing assessment. Do not confuse the problem by mixing the audiometric evaluation with the hearing aid evaluation.

Clinical hearing aid evaluations with children should include ample consideration for therapy. Many hours are involved in the pre-hearing aid workup for the hard-of-hearing child. Nearly as much time may then be necessary to select the proper hearing aid and earmold. Additional telephone calls and letters may be necessary to appropriate agencies to obtain financial assistance for the purchase of the aid. Communication with the hearing aid dealer is important to confirm proper fitting of the hearing aid itself. But the time consumed by these procedures is only fleeting seconds when compared to the long term therapy and follow-up programs that the child will need through the remainder of the school years.

Tremendous technologic advances in the hearing aid have been made over the past three decades. Only a few years ago, hearing aids were heavy, cumbersome units with large, unsightly battery requirements. The electronic hearing aid became a reality in the 1930's; the vacuum tube became part of the system in the 1940's; transistors permitted the hearing aid to be a much smaller unit in the 1950's. Today, tiny "solid state" electronic devices have reduced the instrument and its power source to a practical size and weight—with satisfactory cosmetic appeal to most consumers. Recent developments in the microphone component of the hearing aid have extended both ends of the frequency reproduction range. Microphones are now available that are truly directional—amplifying only sounds that are immediately in front of the hearing aid and at the same time attenuating sounds emitted from the sides or back of the listener.

Critics complain that we should not be satisfied with today's hearing aid, and that technologic advances must still be pursued. It is a mistake to accept a hearing aid that passes only a modicum of barely understood speech, at the same time denying children with hearing loss the full range of sounds and auditory experiences. To paraphrase J. D. Harris (1973), current hearing aid amplification is similar to eyeglasses that would just barely let you recognize one face from another at close range—or to read printing letter by letter. He suggests that the normal child is immersed from birth in an acoustic environment where every sound has meaning. Through an endless succession of aural cues, the child is shaped into the social process and becomes a full member of the household. Is it enough to offer the hard-of-hearing child three octaves of sound to one ear through a hearing aid amplification system that is immediately distorted through an earmold? How does a deaf child learn the sounds of anger, sorrow, gladness, content, or displeasure through a hearing aid that will not reproduce the sound of a fife, or the sibilant "s" sound? In short, even if we had achieved the maximum in terms of amplification, our state of knowledge about achieving optimal use of the hearing aid with children is alarmingly sparse. Add to this picture the fact that the typical hard-of-hearing or deaf youngster listens to his own voice, as well as the speech of other deaf youngsters, through a hearing aid, and one cannot help but wonder how the speech of normal-hearing parents and teachers must sound to him?

The operation of the hearing aid may be likened to a miniature hi-fi set designed as a group of tiny components, which picks up sound wave vibrations from the air and converts them into electrical signals. The signals are passed through an amplifier which increases the electrical strength of the signals. A battery supplies power to the system, and a tiny loudspeaker, known as the receiver, changes the amplified electrical signals back into sound waves and directs them to the eardrum through an earmold which is fitted into the external ear canal (Fig. 7.1). The hearing aid has a volume control so the user can increase or decrease the intensity of the sound as it enters the ear. Readers interested in a technical discussion of the development of hearing aids and their operation principles are referred to Berger (1970), or to educational materials provided by hearing aid manufacturers such as Zenith's book, *Hearing Aids and Their Components* (Zenith, 1965).

According to Ross (Libby, 1973), our most important task is to insure that the hearing-impaired child gets the most effective signal at all times. His hearing aid is more important to his scholastic endeavors than paper, pencils, and books. When systematic checks of hearing aids and auditory training units are made, they are often found to be performing poorly. Even if the amplification units are functioning properly, chances are that the acoustic environment of the classroom is too noisy to make the use of personal amplification even tolerable. Ross prepared a most informative chapter on classroom acoustics and speech intelligibility in Katz' *Handbook of Clinical Audiology* (1972). The problem seems to be that classroom acoustics, including optimal reverberation, noise, and microphone distance, have well known solutions, but the solutions have almost total nonapplication in our schools and classes for the hearing-impaired. In addition, further problems are created by the lack of understanding of amplification instrumentation by the classroom teacher.

Very few formal studies had been reported on the status of hearing aids worn by children until recently. Persons working with children who use hearing aids are familiar with the "maple syrup syndrome," in which the hearing aid catches all sorts of debris and quits working.

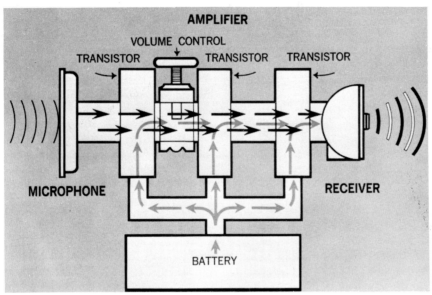

Fig. 7.1. The components of a modern hearing aid. (With permission from E. Corliss: Facts about Hearing and Hearing Aids. A Consumer's Guide from the National Bureau of Standards, U.S. Dept. of Commerce. Washington, D.C., U.S. Govt. Printing Office, 1971.)

Gaeth and Lounsbury (1966) interviewed 134 hard-of-hearing elementary school children and their parents as part of a longitudinal evaluation program. The results confirmed that the parents, as a group, were poorly informed about the hearing aid, its operation, and its use and care. Electroacoustic measurements were made on 120 hearing aids and showed that only 16% of the children were wearing hearing aids that could be considered adequate, and only 50% of the children, by the most lenient standards, were obtaining adequate hearing from the aids.

Zink (1972) reported results from a 2-year longitudinal electroacoustic hearing aid program of analysis of aids worn by children. He warns that just because a child wears his hearing aid faithfully, the assumption cannot be made that the aid is functioning adequately. In the evaluation of 92 hearing aids in use by children, only 55% were found to be acceptable. Zink recommends that each amplification unit in regular use receive regular longitudinal electroacoustic analysis. Often, a child's difficulty in adjusting to amplification or his reluctance for continued hearing aid use can be traced to poor function of the hearing aid (Zink and Alpiner, 1968).

Northern et al. (1972) sent a survey questionnaire to 50 residential schools for the deaf in the United States to ascertain the status of their hearing services. Responses were obtained from 44 schools. Only nine schools indicated that all the students who could benefit from the use of a personal hearing aid actually owned one. The responses from the other 35 schools suggested that an estimated 1,557 additional students need hearing aids. The children who currently had personal hearing aids composed 81% of the preschool population, 67% of the elementary student population, 56% of the secondary student group, and 46% of students older than 18 years. One can surmise that increased awareness and improved identification of hearing impairment in young children accounts for the large proportion of preschool children using amplification.

Types of Hearing Aids

Modern technology provides a variety of sensory aids for the hard-of-hearing or deaf child. The basic principle is to provide as much useful amplification as possible, taking best advantage of whatever residual hearing exists.

Innovative experimenters have attempted to transform certain acoustic features into other sensory modalities such as vibrotactile or visual stimuli, or to change the physical acoustic properties of the signal into other auditory characteristics. There appears to be agreement that a more efficient and widespread means of providing maximal benefits of amplification among hearing-impaired children may help alleviate some of the present burdens of deafness (Levitt and Nye, 1971; Libby, 1973).

Basic to the concept of hearing aid recommendations is a realistic understanding of what the aid can do for the patient. No hearing aid will enable a hard-of-hearing youngster to perform normally in *all* situations. The primary reason for recommending the use of personal amplification is to enable the child to communicate better with a hearing aid than without it. Such improvement may be possible in only a few select conditions for a child, but he will ultimately learn, with good teaching, to utilize the aid to its maximal benefit. In the words of Mark Ross, an acknowledged expert in the area of hearing aid utilization by children, "merely because one can 'get along' without a hearing aid is *not* an adequate reason to discourage its use" (1969).

The Earmold

The earmold itself is an essential feature of the hearing aid system. It provides support for the aid, directs the amplified sound into the ear canal, and prevents acoustic feedback if fitted properly. If the earmold does not fit properly, it will cause feedback in the form of whistles, squeals, or produce local irritation and soreness. Ready-made standard size earmolds are available, but to achieve a good fit and lasting earmold it is worth the trouble and expense to have a custom earmold made to fit the exact shape of the patient's ear (Corliss, 1971).

Ross (1972) points out that the earmold is an integral part of the electroacoustic events that begin with the hearing aid and end with the patient's ear canal. Northern and Hattler (1970) have shown that variations in earmolds can alter the electroacoustic characteristics of the hearing aid as shown in Figure 7.2. Accordingly, it is important to evaluate a

hearing aid with the earmold which is to be used with it. This may mean two visits with the child, one to take the earmold impression, and an additional session after the permanent custom earmold has been fabricated. It is particularly difficult to conduct hearing aid evaluations with children using stock earmolds, since they often do not fit well in the child's ear canal and most certainly do not represent how the hearing aid will perform and sound to the child when he has his own earmold. The pinna continues to grow in size in children until about 9 years of age. Thus, earmolds may have to be remade every 3 to 6 months in the child's early years, or once a year after age 5 to insure adequate fit.

The earmold can be crafted in many ways to enhance the hearing aid, with open vents, various tubing, filters, etc. The material of the earmold is relatively nonsignificant, as long as a good tight fit of the mold is achieved in the ear canal. Lybarger has long been regarded as one of the foremost experts on earmold acoustics, and interested readers are referred to his report (1972) for additional information.

Classification of Hearing Aids

Hearing aids may be classified in several ways. One system of classification is based on the place where the hearing aid is actually worn—body-type hearing aids or ear level hearing aids. The on-the-body model of hearing aids has a relatively large microphone, amplifier, and power supply enclosed in a case which is attached to the clothing, placed in a pocket, or carried in a harness around the chest. An external receiver attaches directly to the earmold and is driven by power supplied through a thin flexible wire from the instrument case. Body-type hearing aids usually provide greater gain and power output than ear level instruments. Since the microphone and receiver are separated by considerable distance, the probability of acoustic feedback (or squeal) from amplified sound that leaks out around the earmold and "feeds back" into the microphone of the hearing aid is reduced. Acoustic feedback is usually caused by an ill-fitting earmold.

Body-type hearing aids are often recommended for children. In spite of their size, bulk,

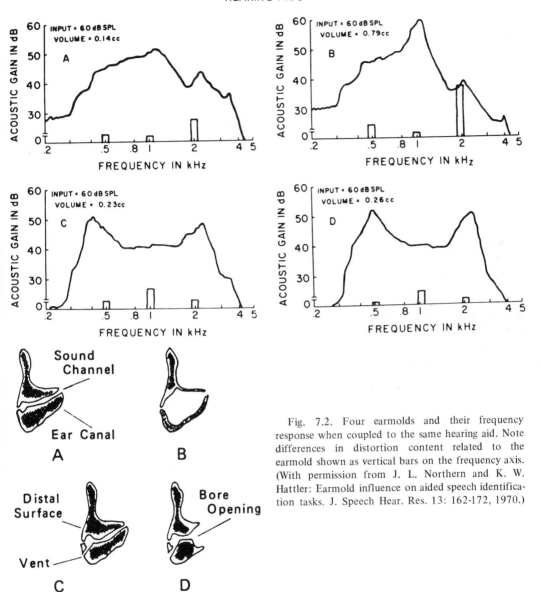

Fig. 7.2. Four earmolds and their frequency response when coupled to the same hearing aid. Note differences in distortion content related to the earmold shown as vertical bars on the frequency axis. (With permission from J. L. Northern and K. W. Hattler: Earmold influence on aided speech identification tasks. J. Speech Hear. Res. 13: 162-172, 1970.)

and cord, body aids can be firmly carried by young children in garment-type carrier harnesses. The body aid is more durable and less likely to be broken than ear level instruments. The external controls are easier to adjust, although this often creates problems with children who play with the aids or inadvertently turn the hearing aid volume down or shut it off. Some clinicians believe that body aids are too often recommended for children and not enough consideration is given to ear

level instruments. Sometimes, body aids are too powerful and may create temporary threshold changes in children with sensorineural hearing loss as discussed elsewhere in this chapter.

Problems with body-type hearing aids for children are not uncommon. Parents complain that the aids are too bulky for the youngster to carry on his chest; we recommend turning the harness around and putting the aid on the youngster's back until he is old enough or large enough to use it on his chest. Receivers are famously fragile, and crack far too easily when dropped or bumped. The receivers are often too large for small children and may pull the earmold out of the ear.

The body-type hearing aid case breaks when children fall on it, and it seems remarkable to us that industry cannot find more substantial and hardy materials to use for the hearing aid case and receiver. External controls need snap-on plastic covers that cannot be removed by children, or recessed controls that can only be adjusted and set by parents. We are amazed that manufacturers cannot find a thicker, or stronger, receiver cord that does not break so easily or one that cannot be bitten in half with one chomp! Manufacturers have attempted to reduce amplification of clothing noise by placing the microphone on top of the hearing aid instead of on the front face of the unit. In theory, this is an improvement, but in practice the top microphone is open to spilled food and drink, or sand, dirt, and maple syrup!

In spite of these many problems, the tradition of using body aids for children, even youngsters with moderate hearing loss, will undoubtedly continue. The advantages of the body aid with children, especially younger than school age, still outweigh the disadvantages.

Ear Level Hearing Aids. Ear level instruments include behind-the-ear models, eyeglass models, or all-in-the-ear aids. The all-in-the-ear instruments fit directly into the ear canal. They have no external wires or tubes and are very lightweight. They are generally used only for adult patients with mild hearing loss and are seldom used to provide amplification for children. The all-in-the-ear instrument is too small and fragile to be used with children.

The behind-the-ear model hearing aid has all its components housed in one curved case which fits neatly behind the pinna and rests against the mastoid surface. A short plastic tube connects the earmold to the hearing aid case. Ear level hearing aids are generally not as powerful as body-type aids and deliver about 55 to 60 dB of gain and 125 to 130 dB maximal power output. Since the microphone and receiver are in the same case, and in very close proximity to the earmold, increased opportunity exists for acoustic feedback.

Ear level hearing aids have been the most popular type of amplification instrument since the early 1960's according to 1972 statistics from the Hearing Aid Industry Conference. The reasons for the success and popularity of the ear level hearing aid are many. This type of aid is less conspicuous than the body hearing aid; it does not amplify clothing noise since it is worn on the head; and most important, from the audiologist's point of view, hearing is restored to the more natural level of the head rather than on the body which is somewhat similar to having an ear on your chest! Our success with the behind-the ear hearing aid with children has been very good and we tend to recommend this type of aid whenever possible. We have fit ear level instruments on youngsters as young as 3 years of age with little problem.

The eyeglass-type of hearing aid was quite popular when it first appeared on the commercial market in the late 1950's. The eyeglass unit is essentially the same aid as the behind-the-ear type except that the plastic case that encloses the components is part of the eyeglass temple piece. These units have become less popular in recent years, and we seldom recommend eyeglass aids for children. The major problem is that when repairs are necessary on either the eyeglass set or the hearing aid, both units are lost to the user while service is performed.

As children grow older they become more concerned about the cosmetic appearance of their hearing aid. As they reach those trying "teen" years, they often find excuses for not wearing their body-type hearing aid. Many of these patients can use powerful ear level instruments, and we are always happy to make this recommendation when possible. Difficulties arise, however, when a youngster obviously desires an ear level instrument, yet the hearing loss is too severe to permit the satisfactory use of the smaller ear level instrument. The clinician must use his ingenuity to sway the patient's opinion and make him realize that the body aid does a better job of providing the necessary amplification. By this age, most experienced hearing aid users can appreciate and understand the comparative performance information of the ear level and body-type instruments. In such circumstances, one can only hope that the patient will realistically understand his need for the stronger body aid. However, if it becomes obvious that the body aid has been rejected, we feel that recommendation of a powerful ear level instrument that will be worn regularly is a better solution than turning the patient away and insisting that he stay with the body-type instrument. Better to underfit the patient with a hearing aid that will be willingly used, than to force the use of an unwanted hearing aid that will not be worn.

Monaural-Binaural Hearing Aids. Monaural hearing aid systems are those which provide amplification for one ear only. A binaural hearing aid system consists of two complete hearing aids including microphones, amplifiers, and receivers—one complete stystem for each ear. Some manufacturers house both systems in one case with two separate cords and receivers plugged into the sides of the unit. Generally, binaural fittings are accomplished with two separate hearing aid units of the same make and model.

A long controversy has existed among professionals concerning the benefits of the binaural hearing aid system over the monaural system. Obviously, the binaural system is twice as expensive as the monaural systems. However, hard-of-hearing adults will often state that the binaural system increases the directional sense, helps separate wanted sounds from annoying background noise, and is well worth the additional expense. Other adults choose to use only a monaural hearing aid for their listening problems.

Children are unable to make judgments regarding monaural versus binaural hearing aid use, and the decision falls to someone else. The clinical evaluation procedure is typically hard-pressed to show superior performance with binaural hearing aids over a monaural hearing aid, and this single fact has stoked the monaural-binaural controversy for years. Initial studies that were published produced contradictory results (Jerger and Dirks, 1961) with no clear-cut evidence that binaural fittings were indeed superior to monaural aids. Clinicians and the hearing aid industry quickly lined up on opposite sides over the monaural-binaural issue. The Federal Trade Commission issued a statement in 1969 that contrary to the advertisments, the use of two hearing aids, one in each ear, for those suffering from bilateral hearing impairment is not, in most cases, more beneficial than the use of only one hearing aid in one ear. Newby (1964) wrote that audiologists are being more conservative in recommending binaural instruments because of the lack of evidence that such aids are superior to monaural fittings.

Common sense, however, as well as patient preferences (Haskins and Hardy, 1960; Kodman, 1961; Dirks and Carhart, 1962), supports the view that two ears are better than one. More recent research reported by many investigators including Koenig (1950), Carhart (1958, 1965), Belzile and Markle (1959), and Harris (1965) has matched binaural hearing aid performance against monaural hearing aid performance, often through the delivery of speech discrimination test materials in simultaneous competing noise signals, substantiating the superiority of binaural listening. According to Hirsh (1971) the principal advantage afforded by binaural listening is the improvement of discrimination in noise due to the ability to localize the sound source. Ear level binaural aids are especially advantageous since the microphones are at the level of the head, shielded by the head, resulting in improved time-intensity parameters of the wanted signal.

In the fitting of hearing aids for children, Briskey (1972) states that audiologists have revised their thinking and many now recommend a hearing aid for each ear. Although two body-type instruments may not provide improved localization ability over a single body aid because of the close proximity of the two microphones in the binaural system, they are recommended because the child is receiving additional information through binaural stimulation. To enhance directionality of the signal, the two body instruments may be placed so that one is on the child's chest and the other is on his back. Another factor in favor of binaural aids for children is that the critical listening situation is often in a noisy classroom with poor acoustic properties, so that the child's head movements will naturally favor the desired signal.

The best candidates for binaural hearing aids are those children with bilateral, symmetrical hearing loss. Ross (1969) advocates the use of binaural aids in children with severe hearing losses, based on his experience that children fitted with two body aids seem to make better progress than those fitted with just one hearing aid. The clinical and experimental evidence of binaural fittings with children support Ross' viewpoint (Bender and Wig, 1962; Fisher, 1964; Ramaiya, 1971). A survey of over 1000 cases treated with binaural hearing aids in Scandanavia reported by Jordan et al. (1967) led to a conclusion that binaural hearing aids should be the standard treatment in every case of binaural hearing loss. These authors recommend that ear level aids should be tried with all hearing losses up to, and including, 80 dB HL; two body aids should be used for patients with hearing loss exceeding 80 dB HL.

The Y-Cord Hearing Aid. The Y-cord hearing aid provides a means of supplying an electrical signal to two receivers, one in each ear, from a single monaural body-type hearing aid. The advantage to the Y-cord hearing aid is that amplification can be provided to both ears of the user, with very little increase in cost over a straight monaural system, and considerably less expense than a binaural system. "Bilateral" listening is thus possible with a Y-cord hearing aid, but not true binaural listening since the user will have little ability to localize sounds.

Y-cord hearing aids became popular in Europe in the late 1950's and early 1960's. Reports by Groen and Hellema (1960) and Whetnall (1964) indicated that children performed better with Y-cord hearing aids than with one hearing aid for one ear. The American literature has a paucity of material concerning the use of Y-cord amplification. There seems to be agreement among clinicians that, whenever possible, a binaural hearing aid system is preferable to the Y-cord hearing aid. The real question seems to be, when can a Y-cord aid be of benefit?

Black and Hast (1962) concluded that Y-cord dichotic listening has no advantage over monotic fitting since the Y-cord merely amplifies the signal at each ear. Smith (1967) indicated that the use of a Y-cord arrangement on a conventional monaural hearing aid is rarely an acceptable practice which cannot be justified in the hearing aid evaluation procedure. Kinstler (1964) concluded that the Y-cord is

utterly useless when binaural fitting is indicated. The truth of the matter is that our lack of empirical evidence precludes reaching such conclusions.

Lybarger (1973) published an essay on the electronic problems, advantages, and disadvantages of the Y-cord hearing aid. He cited advantages of the Y-cord as follows:

"(1) Both ears of the user are receiving sound and are thus receiving sound 'education.' This may be much more important than is generally realized. Our experience is that auditory training of one ear does not fully transfer to the other ear.

"(2) The experimental evidence is that better discrimination is obtained with the 'Y' cord than with a monaural system, although the performance cannot be expected to be as good as with a binaural hearing aid with good separation (8″ to 12″) between the microphones.

"(3) The cost is very low in comparison to a binaural hearing aid.

"(4) Battery cost is significantly lower than for two aids."

He felt that certain limitations also exist with the Y-cord hearing aid:

"(1) Not all hearing aids work well with the 'Y' cord arrangement. Only hearing aids specifically designed for good 'Y' cord performance should be considered.

"(2) The balance range in output that can be obtained, without more distortion than is generally desirable, is limited. The 'Y' cord therefore works best where the average hearing threshold levels in the two ears is within 5 or 10 dB. The use of an acoustic filter in one earphone permits the extension of this difference to perhaps 15 dB. Rheostat devices in the 'Y' cord have been found to cause quality deterioration in the hearing aid performance and cannot be recommended.

"(3) There is a small loss in gain and output in a well designed 'Y' cord arrangement of about 3 dB. In aids not designed properly for 'Y' cord use, the losses may be much greater."

In one of the few experimental studies that actually used a Y-cord system in the examination of monaural and binaural reception of speech, Harris (1965) showed an average of 4% improved discrimination abilities in 89 normal listeners for a comparison of Y-cord condition and monaural condition. With 36 listeners who had asymmetrical hearing loss (clinically poor candidates for Y-cord fittings), their intelligibility score for speech in the better ear averaged 29.1% and in the poorer ear was 14.6% in the monaural testing mode. The average discrimination score for these patients rose to 31.8% with the Y-cord fitting which is an increase of about 3% over the better ear monaurally.

Y-cord hearing aids may be wired electrically in "parallel" or "series." although most Y-cords in use today are of the parallel type, which unfortunately increases hearing aid distortion, sometimes dramatically. Hearing aid gain drops when a Y-cord is used on a conventional aid from between 6 to 17 dB. The maximal power output will also drop from 3 to 6 dB with a Y-cord arrangement. The frequency response of the aid usually changes only slightly when a Y-cord is used. Table 7.1 shows the effects of Y-cords on three different hearing aids.

In order to evaluate improvements in Y-cord design of one manufacturer's instrument, Northern et al. (1973) undertook an electroacoustic and audiometric experiment. We did a "blind" study with two seemingly identical, Y-cord hearing aids. One receiver of each hearing aid unit was enclosed in a black bag with a dummy 2-cc cavity attached to the receiver. In reality, only one hearing aid was a true Y-cord; the other aid was actually performing as a straight monaural instrument, although the Y-cord was attached to the instrument. The question was basically, could we differentiate the real Y-cord aid from the dummy Y-cord either through electroacoustic analysis or behavioral measures using only the exposed receiver? The results of the electroacoustic study indicated that the characteristics of both hearing aids were identical. Behavioral responses from four normal-hearing subjects to speech discrimination materials in competing noise were also identical for the two hearing aids. We concluded that electroacoustic characteristics and behavioral responses of a properly designed hearing aid, showed no differences regardless of whether the aid was used in a monaural or Y-cord mode.

Although the use of a Y-cord on a properly designed hearing aid does not necessarily degrade its performance, we have observed significant changes in hearing aids for which the manufacturer supplies a Y-cord, but the aid is not designed properly to handle the Y-cord arrangement.

In conclusion, we see no contraindication to the use of Y-cord hearing aids, when binaural fittings are not possible, provided certain considerations are met. The clinician must be cautious to select only hearing aids for Y-cord recommendations that have been evaluated to perform properly with such an arrangement. Be aware that gain and output of the hearing aid may drop slightly, or change drastically with the Y-cord addition, and such changes in performance are not necessarily consistent among models and makes. We do not think the Y-cord fitting should be used in children for whom auditory thresholds have not been adequately established. The Y-cord should be

Table 7.1. Y-Cord Effects on Three Models of Hearing Aids*

Instrument	Arrangement	Gain at 1000 Hz	MPO	HAIC Distortion
		dB	*dB*	
Model A	Single receiver	65	133	2%
	Y-cord: parallel	48	128	6.8%
Model B	Single receiver	70	134	1%
	Y-cord: series	65	131	2%
Model C	Single receiver	58	134	1%
	Y-cord: parallel	49	128	31%

* Courtesy of Vicon Instrument Company, Colorado Springs, Colorado.

reserved for patients with established symmetrical hearing loss. Beware of Y-cords with variable rheostats or potentiometers in the Y-cord since adequate "balance" of output in the two receivers is nearly impossible to achieve. The Y-cord fitting can be clinically useful, and is not necessarily a detrimental instrument.

The CROS Hearing Aid. In 1965 a new concept in hearing aid fittings was reported by Harford and Barry of Northwestern University. They fitted 20 subjects with severe unilateral hearing loss with a special instrument that utilized a microphone on the side of the head with the bad ear, and transmitted sound electrically as picked-up by this microphone to the good ear through an open-type earmold. They named this special instrument CROS, or Contralateral Routing Of Signals. This simple procedure has opened up many new applications of amplification for hearing-impaired persons.

The basic premise of this amplification system is to improve hearing by eliminating the "head shadow effect." This arrangement of placing the microphone beside the patient's poorer ear and feeding the amplified sound to the better ear, prevents the head from blocking sounds, directed to the bad side, from reaching the better ear. The most common arrangement for this apparatus is in an eyeglass frame as shown in Figure 7.3. Some patients, who do not wear glasses, use a wire or a thin plastic tube draped around the back of their head, often under their hair, to connect the microphone to their good ear. In some designs, the sound is directed into the better ear by only a plastic tube without an earmold. The open-type earpiece is an essential part of the CROS system, since the good ear when left unoccluded allows normal reception of sound directed to the better ear.

While the CROS-type hearing aid is undoubtedly a great help to persons with unilateral hearing loss, it quickly turned out that this type of hearing aid would be very useful to the large group of people who have bilaterally symmetrical high frequency hearing loss. These persons may have normal hearing up to 1000 Hz, but then show significant hearing loss for the higher test frequencies. In the past, these persons were often told that a hearing aid would not benefit them because although it would amplify the high frequency sounds that they were missing, the aid would also amplify the low frequency sounds too much to be useful to them. It has been long recognized that these persons do have difficulties in hearing. Fletcher (1929) wrote that elimination of frequencies in communication above 1500 Hz reduces only 10% of the energy available, but reduces discrimination ability by 35%.

The use of an open-type earmold, or the use of a tube without an earmold enhances speech discrimination for persons with high frequency hearing loss (Dodds and Harford, 1968, 1970; Green, 1969; Hodgson and Murdock, 1970). Lybarger (1968) explained that the success of the open canal fitting is due to a reduction in gain and maximal power output so that even very loud sounds in the low frequency spectrum do not produce discomfort to the patient.

The success of the CROS aid was immediate. Some 10 versions of the CROS principle have now been incorporated into various designs and applications, including localization for blind persons with unilateral hearing loss (Rintelmann et al., 1970). The most common variant of the CROS aid is termed the BICROS system (Fig. 7.4). The BICROS consists of two microphones—one above each ear—which send electrical signals to a single amplifier. The output from the amplifier goes to a single receiver which delivers sound to the better ear through a conventional earmold.

CROS instruments were specifically not recommended for children by Harford and Barry (1965) and Harford and Dodds (1966) since they believed unilateral hearing loss children could not appreciate the benefits from CROS fittings. Matkin and Thomas (1972) verified that children do benefit from CROS hearing aids. They report the need for careful consideration of CROS aids in youngsters with unilateral hearing loss only, or new hearing aid users in their teenage years. Children with bilateral high frequency hearing impairments do very well with CROS fittings.

In our experience, the CROS fitting can be very beneficial to children when their motivation to hear is good, and the interest of their parents in the handicapping condition is evi-

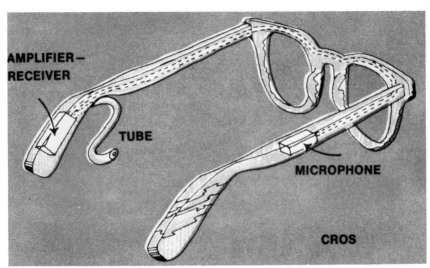

Fig. 7.3. The CROS hearing aid with the microphone located on one side and the amplifier-receiver on the opposite side. This hearing aid system picks up sound on the "bad" ear side, transmits it electrically, and amplifies the signal to the "good" ear. (With permission from E. Corliss: Facts about Hearing and Hearing Aids. A Consumer's Guide from the National Bureau of Standards, U.S. Dept. of Commerce. Washington, D.C., U.S. Govt. Printing Office, 1971.)

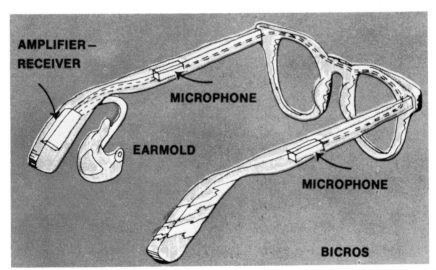

Fig. 7.4. The BICROS hearing aid. This amplification system is a variation of the CROS aid consisting of two microphones which deliver sound to a single amplifier and to one ear. (With permission from E. Corliss: Facts about Hearing and Hearing Aids. A Consumer's Guide from the National Bureau of Standards, U.S. Dept. of Commerce. Washington, D.C., U.S. Govt. Printing Office, 1971.)

dent. Our successful fittings of CROS instruments are enhanced if the youngster already wears glasses. The local hearing aid dealer is a most important ingredient in the CROS aid for children, and the clinician must work closely with him. Rental trials with CROS aids may be of benefit to allow the parent an opportunity to judge how much use the youngster obtains from the aid. CROS fittings can be so rewarding that the clinician must be cautious to not overfit hearing-impaired persons with this system.

Extended Frequency Hearing Aids. Conventional hearing aids attempt to provide optimal amplification for the speech frequency range between 300 and 3000 Hz. For years, however, attempts have been made to produce amplification systems which can provide supplemental speech cues for the profoundly hearing-impaired. The frequency response of the hearing aid has been under consideration by several researchers. In general terms, results have shown that the majority of adult subjects respond to test materials best when they are amplified with a flat or gently rising frequency response over the 300 to 3000 Hz range, or amplification which is a "mirror image" of the audiogram configuration (Knight, 1967; Jerger and Thelin, 1968). An interesting study by Reddell and Calvert (1966) reported that hearing aids custom-made to conform to the patient's threshold configuration produced better speech discrimination scores than conventional hearing aids.

In recent years, special amplification systems have been developed to enable the deaf with residual hearing in the low frequencies to use amplification. The history of these attempts was reviewed by Erber (1971). These special hearing aids provide greater low frequency acoustic stimulation than does the conventional hearing aid. Initial evaluation of these amplification systems by their proponents were reported to be favorable, but later studies have produced conflicting results.

One system extends the lower frequency limit of amplification with a special wide range microphone, in several research projects. Ling (1964) has reported that the use of low frequency hearing aids increases the awareness of deaf children and improves their voice and speech patterns. Briskey and Sinclair (1966) corroborated these findings in their study of extended frequency range hearing aids with several deaf children who received special auditory training.

A second low frequency emphasis system developed by a Swedish engineer, Bertil Johansson (1961, 1966) is the transposer hearing aid. The aid was designed to transpose or change high frequency information as present in the spectra of phonomes [s] and [ʃ] into low frequency energy. It was felt that since many persons with profound sensorineural hearing loss have residual hearing in the low frequencies only (below 1.5 kHz), this new transposed information could be processed as cues for high frequency phonemes.

The transposer aid described by Johansson is basically a two-channel system in which channel one can be operated alone in the conventional mode, or both channels can be used simultaneously in the transposition mode. Channel two provides the frequency transposition and cannot operate alone. When both channels are utilized, high frequency (above 4 kHz) information is split and passed normally through channel one, and filtered simultaneously in channel two. This filtered energy is modulated with a 5-kHz tone, and the resulting difference tones are passed through a low pass filter. The output of channel two is mixed with channel one prior to the receiver. The final outcome for a phoneme [s] for example, is its normal spectrum as well as the added low frequency burst. Phonemes without strong high frequency energy are unaffected by frequency transposition.

Early studies on performance with the transposer hearing aid involved hearing-impaired children and normal-hearing adults having simulated losses. These studies produced some conflicting results. Wedenberg (1971) and Johansson (1966) showed significant improvement in speech discrimination for nonsense syllables and monosyllabic words, using the transposer hearing aid. They noted the greatest improvement was for the high frequency phonemes such as [s] and [ʃ].

Ling (1968) conducted several studies using Johansson's transposer as well as other transposing devices. Again his subjects were hearing-impaired children. He found that while significant improvement in discrimination of monosyllabic words was evident for the transposed mode of amplification, this improvement was also noted for conventional amplification. His conclusion was that intensified training rather than transposition accounted for the improvement.

In another experiment, Ling and Druz (1967) used a hearing aid that transposed sounds from the 2000 to 3000 Hz range down into the 750 to 1000 Hz range. This frequency range was selected to avoid superimposing the transposed sound on the low frequency spectrum, and instead adds to it. Results were negative. Ling and Maretic (1971) attempted to use the transposer as an aid to speech rather than auditory discrimination. Two groups of children were trained, an experimental and control group, but results were essentially the same for both groups. Ling (in Levitt and Nye, 1970) indicated that his results from several years work on extended low frequency aids has not been very encouraging and that he was clearly doubtful about the value of frequency transposition.

A recent study by Foust and Gengel (1973), involving hearing-impaired adults, revealed that some showed significant improvement in speech discrimination for monosyllabic words using the transposer hearing aid. They did report, however, that group data were misleading, as no specific group per se can be considered eligible candidates for frequency transposition. The individuals in this study who did show improvement with the transposer aid had several different configurations of hearing loss, including residual hearing through 4 kHz. These investigators concluded that while frequency transposition can be of value to some persons, it is very difficult to determine, without extensive training, which individuals are best suited for this form of amplification; consequently, at the present time the conventional use of the transposer hearing aid is questionable. However, there are implications for its use as a special auditory training device, particularly for teaching the discrimination of [s] and [ʃ] as well as a speech training device. It seems unlikely that fitting a frequency transposition hearing aid on a school age child will produce observable successful result. An evaluation is needed of frequency transposition hearing aids on infants who can use these special hearing aids from prelanguage acquisition age.

Figure 7.5 illustrates spectrograms for the syllables /si/ (upper portion) and /pi/ (lower portion) in conventional and transposed hearing aid modes. Spectrograms give a graphic display of speech. Frequency is represented on the

vertical axis, time on the horizontal axis, and intensity is characterized by the shading of the display, i.e., darker indicates greater intensity. Since most of the spectral energy for the phoneme /s/ is high frequency, there is a marked difference in the spectrograms from (a) to (b). The voiceless stop phoneme /p/, has little spectral energy in the high frequencies and is virtually unchanged in the spectrograms from (a) to (b).

Principles of Hearing Aid Fitting for Children

The selection of a hearing aid for a child is the exclusive responsibility of the audiologist. It challenges the ultimate skills of even the most experienced person. One of the requisite experiences in fitting very young children is practice with the fitting of current models on adults. Even a little on-going exposure to the way current hearing aid models perform on various adults with hearing losses is helpful. Extrapolation can then be made from the adult who is easily testable to the child who is not easily testable!

When the child has both receptive and expressive speech and language sufficient for speech reception testing, the selection of an aid is fairly simple. It is the nonverbal child who poses the greatest problem—either the infant and very young hearing-impaired child or the older, profoundly deaf nonverbal child. No specific rules can be formulated to direct the hearing aid selection, but a few general principles can be proposed, plus the always present exceptions that accompany them.

Table 7.2 gives a general guide to hearing aid fitting at various age levels and when different levels of hearing prevail in children. There will always be exceptions to these categories, of course, for it is not possible to specify an exact fitting in each case. A discussion of the philosophies behind this categorization will help in interpreting the table.

Hearing Loss

As indicated in Table 7.2, hearing aid fitting begins with a 20-dB loss. It is not quite accurate to state that at this level a hearing aid fitting

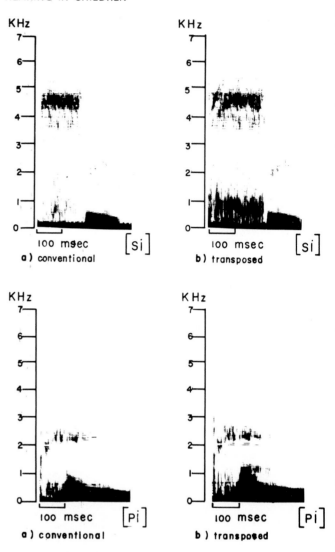

Fig. 7.5. Spectrograms for the syllables /si/ (upper portion) and /pi/ (lower portion) in conventional and transposed hearing aid channels. Since most of the spectral energy for the phoneme /s/ is high frequency, there is a marked difference in the spectrograms from a) to b). The voiceless stop phoneme /p/ has little spectral energy in the high frequencies and is virtually unchanged in the spectrograms from a) to b). Spectrograms show a graphic display of speech. Frequency is represented on the vertical axis: time on the horizontal axis: and intensity is characterized by the shading of the display, i.e., darker indicates greater intensity. (With permission from K. O. Foust and R. W. Gengel: Speech discrimination by sensorineural hearing-impaired persons using a transposer hearing aid. Scand. Audiol. 2: 161-170, 1973.)

should be made. In our experience successful results have been obtained from hearing aids on 15-dB average losses, and unsuccessful fittings have been made on 25-dB average losses in children. In this borderline area all that can be said is that hearing aids should be considered for a child, and sometimes tried out, before a decision is made. The successful fittings at 15 dB have been in the child, dull-normal in intelligence, who needs every bit of hearing he can get in the educational situation. The unsuccessful fittings at 25 dB have been in the child whose intelligence or superior listening strategies allow him to function well without an

aid. Occasionally behavior problems preclude successful fittings at this level.

When considering an aid for slight losses in the 15- to 25-dB range, consultation should be requested with the teacher, parents, and managing physician. If a trial of an aid is attempted, reports should be requested from everyone dealing with the child. Only in this way can a meaningful decision be made.

There are special cases in which a hearing aid may be recommended even when normal hearing prevails at a given time. These are the children whom we call "recalcitrant otitis media" cases, and there is a series of over 50 of them in our files. They originally present, at 6 months to 6 years, with serous otitis media and hearing losses of 30 to 40 dB. Myringotomies are performed, and the hearing returns to normal. However, in a short time there is a recurrence of ear disease, the tubes may be extruded, and the hearing drops again. Myringotomies are performed again, and after a period of normal hearing the children present with 20- to 30-dB hearing losses. These episodes may be repeated four, five, six, or seven times and the hearing will be normal only for short periods. Over a space of 1 to 3 years, it can be seen that as much as two-thirds of the time the children are functioning with below normal hearing levels of 15 to 30 dB.

In such recalcitrant cases, consultation with the otolaryngologists managing the cases has produced the decision that hearing aids should be obtained for the children. The aids will be used at such times as the hearing is reduced, and parents and teachers are counselled as to the indications of when the aids should be used. No child should be without adequate hearing for any period during his formative and educational years. Eventually the tendency to ear disease may be outgrown, and normal hearing will be present. In the meantime, the child is protected against periods of inadequate hearing.

The kind of hearing loss also makes a difference in the judgments of whether to fit with a hearing aid. Strangely enough, the conductive hearing loss may be in greater need of an aid with slighter hearing level averages than the sensorineural loss. The reason is that at above threshold levels the loudness sensation in a conductive loss is less than in the sensorineural loss. The latter is most generally accompanied by recruitment, giving a louder sensation at above threshold hearing levels. It is also more difficult to keep a hearing aid on a child with mild sensorineural loss than on one with a mild conductive loss. Many times the child with 25- to 30-dB average sloping sensorineural loss will actually function better without an aid. In such cases, trials with aids over a period of time will have to reveal how this particular child functions. Arbitrariness in recommending aids is to be avoided when dealing with such cases. The otolaryngologist, the parents, and the teachers should be a part of all decisions that are made.

At what upper level should a hearing aid *not* be recommended? It can be argued that a child with aplasia of the cochlea would get no use from a hearing aid, but it is not known whether that is true. The tactile sensations from a bone conduction receiver or even those from an air conduction receiver may give the infant or young child an opportunity to use the sensation of sound or no sound to some limited advantage. Very limited, yes, but we have found such a child who appears to want to wear the hearing aid, for some reason as yet undetermined. Until it is known just what the addition of some tactile sensation in sound detection does for the child, it behooves us to give him the opportunity to use it. The vibration from the aid may not be as valuable as other kinds of tactile stimulation such as an arm vibrator, and there is no reason why other techniques such as this should not be attempted. Particularly if started at a very early age, the cues that are learned from such vibration may be useful beyond our present expectations.

At this point of time, then, it must be said that no child should be denied the opportunity of "hearing" what he can with even the most minimal of sound input. Not until the child himself rejects the amplification at an older age should it be given up. It may be visionary to set down this principle, but it is in the best spirit of child advocacy that it is done.

The Hearing Aid

Wherever possible an ear level type is the aid of choice for a child. We have placed the cut-off point at 3 years, arbitrarily, but the exceptions will be numerous. For some very active children of 3 or 4, the parents may not be able to maintain an ear level aid. The behavior levels of other older children may not permit such an easily accessible aid. On the other hand, a quietly behaved 2½-year-old may be given consideration for an ear level aid. Parents should be warned that a great many such aids end up either flushed down a toilet or chewed up by the family dog or thrown out of a window or used as a pacifier. The parents can

Table 7.2. General Principles of Hearing Aid Selection for Children

Age	Loss			Hearing Aid				
	Kind	Average 500–2000 Hz (ANSI) *dB*	Slope	Type	Ear Fitted	Gain *dB*	MPO (SPL) *dB*	Frequency Distribution
0–3 yr	Sensorineural	20–50	Flat	Body, or ear level	Better, or both if equal	25–45	95	High fidelity—small high frequency emphasis (3–8 dB)
			Falling	Body, or ear level	Same as above	20–35	90	High frequency emphasis: 5–12 dB/octave*
		50–75	Flat	Body, or ear level	Same as above	40–50	110–120	High fidelity—small high frequency emphasis (8–16 dB/octave)*†
			Falling	Body, or ear level	Same as above	40–50	105–110	High frequency emphasis: 8–15 dB/octave
		75–100	Flat	Body, or ear level	Same as above	50–65	115–120	High fidelity—small high/frequency emphasis
			Falling	Body, or ear level	Same as above	50–65	110–115	High frequency emphasis: 8–15 dB/octave
		100+	Fragment in lows	Body	Same as above	60–65	120–135	Low frequency emphasis: to 100 Hz
	Mixed	50–75	Flat	Body, or ear level	Same as above	45–65	115–125	High fidelity—small high frequency emphasis (3–8 dB)
			Falling	Body, or ear level	Same as above	40–60	110–120	High frequency emphasis: 8–16 dB/octave
		75–100	Flat	Body	Same as above	55–70	125–135	High fidelity—small high frequency emphasis (3–5 dB)
			Falling	Body	Same as above	50–65	120–130	High frequency emphasis: 8–16 dB/octave
		100+	Fragment in lows	Body	Same as above	65–75	130–150	Low frequency emphasis: to 100 Hz
	Conductive	20–40	Flat	B/C where necessary	Worse ear	20–30	110	Flat curve, very slight high frequency emphasis
		40–65	Flat	B/C where necessary	Choice of either	40–60	120–135	Flat curve, very slight high frequency emphasis

Age	Type	Hearing loss (dB)	Audiogram	Placement	Ear	Gain (dB)	Max output	Frequency response
3–16 yr	Sensorineural	20–50	Flat	Ear level if possible	Better, or both if equal	25–40	95	High fidelity—small high frequency emphasis (3–5 dB/octave)
			Falling	Same as above	Same as above	20–35	90	High frequency emphasis: 8–15 dB/octave*
		50–75	Flat	Same as above	Same as above	40–50	110–120	High fidelity—small high frequency emphasis
			Falling	Same as above	Same as above	40–50	105–115	High frequency emphasis: 8–15 dB/Octave*†
		75–100	Flat	Same as above	Same as above	50–65	115–120	High fidelity—small high frequency emphasis
			Falling	Body	Same as above	50–65	110–115	High frequency emphasis: 8–15 dB/octave
		100+	Fragment in lows	Body	Same as above	60–65	120–135	Low frequency emphasis: to 100 Hz
	Mixed	50–75	Flat	Ear level if possible	Same as above	45–65	125–135	High fidelity—small high frequency emphasis
			Falling	Same as above	Same as above	40–60	120–130	High frequency emphasis: 8–16 dB/octave
		75–100	Flat	Body	Same as above	55–70	125–135	High fidelity—small high frequency emphasis: 3–5 dB/octave
			Falling	Body	Same as above	50–65	120–130	High frequency emphasis: 8–16 dB/octave
		100+	Fragment in lows	Body	Same as above	65–75	130–150	Low frequency emphasis: to 100 Hz
	Conductive	20–40	Flat	Ear level if possible (B/C where necessary)	Worse ear only	20–30	110–120	Flat curve
		40–65	Flat	Same as above	Choice of either	40–60	120–135	Flat curve

* Consideration of open mold or acoustic modifier.
† Consideration of acoustic modifer or vented mold.

make the decision whether they can handle the problems of the ear level aid. They will then assume the responsibility of seeing that it is cared for.

Bone conduction aids have been advised for those children who have atretic canals, microtia, or recurrent ear disease. It is not necessary, however, to place a bone conduction aid on an older child who has had myringotomies and polyethylene tubes. An ear-level instrument with a vented earmold functions quite satisfactorily in such cases.

There is no objection to a child's wearing bone conduction aids at any age. We have placed them on infants 1 month old who have stenotic canals or microtia, with excellent results. No obvious misshaping of the head has occurred, but special padding should be applied to the end clip and sometimes to the entire headband. Soft felt material or Styrofoam can be used to pad the band. The transmitter can be placed in back, if the baby lies on his stomach, or in front when he lies on his back.

The only provision to make in placing bone conduction aids on children is that it be understood that this type will not be worn permanently. Experience with older people who have always worn bone conduction aids is that when a decrease in the sensorineural hearing renders the bone conduction reception inefficient, it is very difficult for them to change to air conduction. It is like learning a new language and they neither like it nor do well with it. Although it is impossible to speculate on what the chances are of a decrease in sensorineural hearing, at some point a decision should be made to change to air conduction aids where possible. It should be done with a child before the time that a change will be strongly resisted.

In the case of a very young child with a mild to moderate loss, as small a body aid as possible can be selected for him. Unfortunately, small body aids are in short supply, and it is hoped that with the increasing need for such instruments, manufacturers will produce them.

The cut-off point for ear level aids has been placed at 75 dB. This point is an arbitrary one, and may vary with individual needs. The level may also become higher with new developments of tightly fitting earmolds and new

hearing aid design. The ideal would be for all hearing-impaired children and adults to wear ear level aids, regardless of degree of loss. Hearing aid manufacturers are actively researching these new designs, and may soon meet this challenge. Also, with the new trend toward lower outputs in hearing aids for even severe losses, the 75 dB cut-off should not be considered a fixed rule.

Another exception to the 75-dB loss criterion is for the adolescent child. At the age of 12 or 13, the child who has worn a body aid all his life will suddenly become self-conscious about it and begin to reject wearing it. The young boy suddenly feels that the obvious cord and receiver of the aid draw attention to him as a handicapped person. It impugns his masculinity. The young girl whose breasts are developing finds it difficult to wear two body aids inconspicuously, and even one hearing aid is bulky. She also wants to wear swimming suits in the summer, and dislikes the attention that is drawn to the aids. These are normal, legitimate complaints that should be given careful consideration. The old adage, "the best hearing aid is the one that is worn," should be remembered. If it can be shown that an ear level aid gives performance reasonably close to that of the body aid, it should be recommended. Often the youngster will make his own decision after a trial of the head-worn aid; many have admitted that their hearing reception is not as good, and have gladly gone back to the body aid. Others have taken to the ear level aid eagerly and well. As in all other factors, the individual's special needs must be evaluated.

Which Ear to Fit?

It has been our philosophy that whenever possible, two separate hearing aids should be fitted on a child. The observations made by teachers, families, and the children themselves over many years have convinced us that in general it is a sound approach. The criterion for binaural fittings has been the presence of identical or fairly similar losses in each ear. Occasionally, however, real advantage has been demonstrated through fitting a moderate loss in one ear with a moderate hearing aid and a

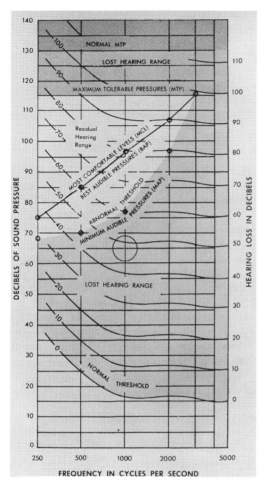

Fig. 7.6. Victoreen's hearing aid fitting table. (With permission from J. A. Victoreen: A Guide to Applied Otometric Procedures. Colorado Springs, Vicon Instrument Co., 1973.)

In summary, Tables 7.2 and 7.6 can be used as a starting point in making judgments on hearing aid selection for the individual child. It is assumed that accurate electroacoustic frequency analyses, gain, power output, and harmonic distortion will be available on the instrument which will be recommended for the child—not on that general model of instrument, but on the instrument which he will wear. Only then does the selection have any fairly respectable validity.

Hearing Aid Selection Procedures

The Preverbal Child, Birth to 2 or 3 Years Old

The initial choice of those hearing aid brands from which to select an aid for the preverbal child should be made on the basis of principles that will include dealer criteria:

1. Dealer Service. Is the dealer who sells the particular brand of hearing aid known to be reliable, to be available at all times, and to handle children well? Is he willing, if requested, to make some sort of trial/rental arrangement? In case of damage or malfunction of the aid, will he offer a temporary loaner aid as a substitute while the repairs are made? Are warranties adequate, or does he have some type of insurance program? Does he offer a reasonable time payment plan? Is he able to make an adequate earmold, and if it is not adequate at first, will he remake it at no extra cost? Does he communicate well with you, offering his ideas freely and listening to yours? An experienced hearing aid dealer with whom one has a relationship of mutual confidence can be of great assistance in offering suggestions as to the improvement of the fitting or ways of making the wearing of it mechanically better. Any audiologist who refuses to enlist a responsible dealer's suggestions and advice is missing one of the most valuable adjunct guides he can obtain. No audiologist knows everything that is to be known about the performance and wearing variations of a given aid. You will find most dealers sincerely interested in a child's welfare and eager to do a good job.

2. Appropriateness for Children. Is the hearing aid known to be sturdy and long lasting? Are heavy duty cords available? Does the transmitter minimize clothing noise, in the case of a body-worn aid? Is the aid able to be worn so that food and liquids will not spill into the microphone? Are the controls sturdy and not easily breakable? (Wheel controls are better than levers.) Are the prong inserts at both ends of the cord strong? Is the size the most convenient that can be selected for this loss?

3. Pretested Approval. If a public or private agency is purchasing the aid for the child, is the aid on their approved list of pretested models? After a few general brands have been selected, the aids within these brands which furnish the approximate gain, power output, and frequency response shown in Table 7.2 for a specific kind of loss can be chosen for further consideration.

A further narrowing down of the list is made by specific application of the dynamic range principle described previously. To do this, fair approximations of threshold levels and tolerance limits should be known. Attempts should be made to observe tolerance limits under earphones. If possible, an audiometer with higher outputs than the standard levels should be used, up to 120 or 130 dB. An infant may cry or start when his maximal tolerance level is reached. Using this level in relation to the threshold levels obtained by observations or objective techniques, the desired gain and maximal power output may be estimated from the graph in Figure 7.6.

The list at this point will be narrowed down to three or four aids. Now, subjective observations will begin. Wearing each aid, the child should be given various levels of gross speech through a loudspeaker. Thresholds of awareness should be obtained, plus observations of reactions to louder levels. The instruments which produce evident discomfort at low speech levels can be eliminated. "Reasonable" levels can be estimated in relation to the degree of hearing loss. An approximation of what should be expected is as follows:

Degree of Loss	Reasonable Level of Awareness
100 dB HL+	45-55 dB HL
75-100 dB HL average	35-50 dB HL
50-75 dB HL	20-35 dB HL
25-50 dB HL	10-25 dB HL

A greater gain can be tolerated by the child with a conductive or mixed loss than by one with a sensorineural loss. For example, a child with a conductive loss of 60 dB HL average can easily tolerate a gain that brings his awareness level to 20 dB HL or even less. But a sensorineural loss of that degree will not allow the child to tolerate receiving such thresholds; 25 to 30 dB HL may be the best that can be expected for him. It is simply not realistic to

expect normal or near-normal thresholds of awareness on children. They will not wear an aid giving those levels, despite all our ambitions to bring them to normal levels.

The Nonverbal Child, 2 or 3 to 16 Years Old

The child 2 or 3 years and older who can be play-conditioned or taught hand-raising responses to sounds can be given a satisfactory hearing aid evaluation. The principle of such an evaluation is to compare the unaided audiogram and the speech awareness levels with similar measures using hearing aids. The initial choice of which hearing aids to try may be made on the basis of the principles listed in Table 7.2. In addition to these can be added the three initial criteria described above.

On the basis of those principles and criteria, no more than three aids need be selected for trial on a young child; more might exceed the attention limits of a child for a testing session. In fact, it may be necessary to schedule more than one testing session for the 2-, 3-, or 4-year-old. His tolerance for testing has a limited time span and it is fruitless to try to extend it. Some bright 2- or 2½-year-olds are able to learn play-conditioning techniques for speech or pure tones and sustain their interest for very short periods of time. A 2-year-old may surprise you by learning simple play-conditioning long enough to give a speech awareness level or a threshold at one frequency during short periods of time. Two or three frequencies are sufficient to place the loss: 500 and 2000 Hz, or 500, 1000, and 2000 Hz. This is the major frequency range of hearing aid amplification.

Given a threshold audiogram, plus observed tolerance limits obtained from observation or acoustic reflexes, the following is a suggested procedure for hearing aid selection.

On each hearing aid selected for trial, obtain the five measures listed below. (The approximate volume setting can be estimated from the hearing aid analysis charts in relation to the mid-point of the dynamic range.)

1. Using gross speech, obtain a speech awareness level through play-conditioning techniques or hand-raising. The simple word "now"

is as good a speech signal as any.

2. Using warbled pure tones, obtain an aided free field audiogram on each aid. Use intermediate frequencies in addition to the standard frequencies (750, 1500, 3000 Hz) if possible.

3. Test the tolerance limits of the aid on the child by raising the speech level gradually until the child evinces discomfort.

4. Evaluate the aids first on the basis of the best speech awareness in relation to tolerance levels. The measure of highest tolerance limits should be given precedence over the lowest speech awareness levels. An aid giving a 15- or 20-dB speech awareness level but producing tolerance limits at 65 dB should be eliminated in favor of one with a 25- to 30-dB awareness level with a tolerance limit of 75 or 80 dB.

5. The next evaluation of aids should be made on the basis of the aided pure tone thresholds. The threshold at 2000 Hz is the most critical, and the aid showing the best threshold there should be given preference. The contour of the audiogram should be fairly even, without high peaks at any frequencies.

This procedure should allow a selection of one or two acceptable aids which can be recommended. If there is any question, a trial of the finally selected aids can be suggested. During the trials, observations of the child's performance with each aid can be made by parents, teachers, or clinicians. From these observations the ultimate selection can be made.

The Verbal Child, 3 to 16 Years

When receptive language is present in the child, some gross discrimination testing can be accomplished with hearing aids; when in addition there is expressive language present, finer discrimination tests are applicable, with varying degrees of sophistication.

The initial choice of which aids to test are made on the basis of the criteria and principles previously described. A minimum of three and a maximum of five should be selected for trial. In the descriptions of testing at various age levels which follow, there will be overlapping in the ages at which children can perform the tests. The variable factors are the degree of hearing loss, the level of language skills, and the

intellectual function of the child. A mentally retarded child of 9, for example, may have to be handled like a 3-year-old. Previous audiometric testing should have determined the level of testing that can be used on each child.

3 to 5 Years of Age. It will be unusual for a hearing-handicapped child of this age to attend long enough for detailed discrimination tests. He will require motivational techniques, even for speech reception testing. Therefore, toys or pictures of objects should be used to sustain interest in the test. The steps that can be followed are:

1. Set the level of the first aid at one-half to two-thirds volume, as indicated by the predetermined gain and volume charts. An aid should never be tested at full volume, as some distortion may occur at high levels.

2. Obtain a speech reception threshold using the toys suggested in Chapter 5, or the picture tests described. Work as fast as possible, foregoing the standard three-out-of-six-words criterion for threshold. Select as threshold the last word repeated on a descending threshold starting at 40 dB and proceeding rapidly downward in 5-dB steps. Express pleasure or clap your hands at each response. Record the level.

3. Starting at 40 dB, sweep upward in 5-dB steps, giving a "buh-buh" at each step. Observe carefully the first sign of discomfort the child shows. He may wince, or put his hand to his ear, or grimace, or even remove the receiver. Record this level.

4. Repeat steps 1 through 3 on each aid chosen.

5. Use as criteria for selection the combination of the best SRT and highest tolerance level, giving more weight to the tolerance level. No aid with a tolerance level much under 65 dB should be chosen, nor an aid with an SRT higher than 30 dB. These general criteria can be set because the child of this age who has receptive language probably has a mild to moderate hearing loss. He should be expected to hear speech comfortably loud at 40 dB HL with an aid. He need not be expected to have a 10- or 15-dB HL threshold, unless it can be obtained with a high tolerance level. This last condition often obtains in cases of conductive loss, but rarely is found in sensorineural losses.

6 to 10 Years of Age. The cooperative child at this age can be given more sophisticated speech reception tests. Always determine which of the children's spondee words he is familiar with, and if he will at least try to repeat the discrimination words. These steps can be followed:

1. Set the first aid at the indicated level between one-half and two-thirds volume.

2. Obtain a speech reception test using 8 to 10 children's spondees, giving them to him first in the sound room. Start at 40 dB HL and descend in 5-dB steps, giving one word at each level. Bracket the threshold level with no more than three words around threshold. Keep the child's interest by smiling with pleasure at each response, and praising him when he is through.

3. Give a half-list of PB-K words at 40 dB HL maintaining his attention with praise. The 40-dB level is selected because the goal for the child should be to hear normal conversational speech level. Some people prefer to use 45 dB as the criterion for normal speech level, and the choice of either is an arbitrary one. Verbal children of this age most likely have moderate to moderately severe losses at worst, and should be expected to understand normal conversational speech with an aid. His responses may not be clear enough on any words to be correct, but you should set up a mental criterion of what he is probably hearing correctly, even if he cannot pronounce it correctly. A consistent criterion will produce meaningful results. Another useful criterion is the latency of his responses. One aid may provide the child with a signal that permits immediate response; another aid may produce hesitation on each word. This observation should be noted.

4. Starting at 40 dB HL, ascend in 5-dB steps giving a spondee at each level. Watch for the first sign of discomfort. If he has sufficient understanding, he can be instructed to tell you when it becomes too loud. In this case, make three presentations of the ascending levels, and record the average level of the three discomfort responses.

5. Repeat steps 1 through 4 on each aid.

6. Use as criterion for final selection of the aid, the combination of the best discrimination score, the best SRT, and the highest tolerance level. Speech discrimination is given the greatest weight, tolerance level follows closely, and SRT is of the least importance.

10 to 16 Years of Age. Depending on the language level and capacity of the child, standard or slightly modified adult techniques can be used at this age range. The six steps are:

1. Turn the aid to a setting between one-half and two-thirds volume that seems most comfortable. Speaking normally at a distance of 3 or 4 feet, ask him, "Do you like it this loud?" . . . " Is it better this loud?" Often he will indicate a quite definite preference for one volume setting, if he understands.

2. Obtain an SRT with 12 or 15 spondees that have been previously presented to him. Standard speech reception threshold technique can be used, but should be shortened in the case of poor attention span.

3. Give a one-half list of PB words at 40 dB HL or of PB-K words if it appears indicated. In the case of poor articulation, again set up mental criteria of what you will accept as correct. Consistency is the essence in these judgments. Knowledge of the kinds of logical substitutions that are commonly made by hearing-impaired children will help decide on the criteria. The judgments must be made rapidly, and comprise another skill in the art of audiology.

4. Instruct the child to tell you when your voice becomes "too loud" for him, and give spondees in 5-dB ascending steps from 40 dB HL. Repeat three times and take the average of the response levels.

5. Repeat steps 1 through 4 on each aid to be tried.

6. Use as criteria for the final selection the best discrimination score, the highest tolerance level, and the best SRT, in that level of importance. At this age the child may voice a preference for one aid over the other. If it is not the aid that performed the best, determine on what basis he made his choice. If it is on size, shape, or color, try to point out better features of the aid that performed best. Assure him that he will hear the best with the selected aid. Letting him listen again with both aids may persuade him. Rarely, an extremely obstinate child will refuse the aid selected. In this case it is well not to make an issue of it. One should

always keep in mind the audiologist's adage: "The best hearing aid is the one that is worn." Occasional compromise is better than a permanently uncooperative hearing aid user.

Can Hearing Aids Damage Hearing?

Clinicians are often asked, "Can hearing aids cause further damage to the hearing of my child?" This question has been tossed around for many years. Review of the literature identifies scattered articles dealing with this problem, mostly case reports and a few experimental efforts to answer the basic question, can hearing aids cause traumatic injury to residual hearing?

Kasten and Braunlin (1970) presented a case study in which they could create deterioration in a patient's hearing through the use of a hearing aid. Their patient was a 10-year-old girl with bilateral, moderate sensorineural hearing loss. She wore a body-type hearing aid satisfactorily in one ear for 14 months and then began to complain that the aid was not helping as much as it did previously. An audiometric evaluation showed marked worsening of the hearing in the aided ear and no change in the hearing of the unaided ear. The young girl was scheduled for a subsequent hearing aid evaluation and advised not to use her present aid. Re-evaluation of her hearing 7 weeks later showed a 20- to 30-dB improvement in the previously aided ear. Kasten and Braunlin were able to show temporary deterioration in the aided ear, regardless of which ear wore the hearing aid. The aid in question had an average gain of 39 dB and average saturation sound pressure level of 120 dB. They recommended a less powerful hearing aid of 30-dB gain and 100-dB saturation sound pressure level. (Incidentally, the authors caution clinicians to carefully evaluate fitted hearing aids and cite the fact that at least three hearing aids were delivered by the dealer and the manufacturer with considerably different characteristics than were ordered.) Finally, when the less powerful hearing aid was fitted to the patient, and worn alternately between ears, evaluations verified that the temporary deterioration of hearing was no longer present. Their conclusions included recommendations that all chil-

dren, and their fitted hearing aids, be carefully re-evaluated shortly after initiating hearing aid use. They also suggest that clinicians have some means of verifying the electroacoustic characteristics of each hearing aid.

The question of traumatic hearing loss from personal amplification was raised as early as 1940 by Holingren who affirmed that in his experience hearing aids never affected hearing adversely. Divergence of opinion on this issue is reflected by two national conference groups on two continents in 1967. While the World Health Organization stated that no evidence existed to support contentions that use of a hearing aid could cause deterioration of hearing, the American Speech and Hearing Association indicated in 1967 that the question of whether amplification can endanger residual hearing had not been adequately resolved.

Harford and Markle (1955), Ross and Truex (1957), and Sataloff (1961) present case studies which link temporary hearing loss to hearing aid use. In each case, removal of the hearing aid permitted the hearing of the aided ear to return to its preaided level. Placing the hearing aid in the opposite ear created deterioration of hearing in that ear also. Roberts (1970) presented a case study of a youngster who showed a 40-dB decrease in hearing level in the aided ear which did not recover even though the aid was removed. Roberts, as well as Barr and Wedenberg (1965), suggest that the use of amplification in children with progressive sensorineural hearing loss may cause acoustic trauma and thus accelerate the hearing deterioration in the aided ear.

Rojskjaer (1960) reported an evaluation of 390 cases of all types of hearing loss treated with hearing aids for 5 years or more. He found nine cases with additional hearing loss in the aided ear. No cases were noted where hearing deteriorated in nonaided ears. Griffiths (in Davis, 1965a) states that when normal-hearing infants are exposed to amplified sound from a hearing aid, they will respond by crying within 30 seconds. The infant with non-normal hearing does not cry, but in fact, "tolerates the aid with pleasure."

Details of several experimental investigations regarding use of amplification and its effect on residual hearing have been summarized expertly by Ross and Lerman (1967). Naunton (1957) reviewed charts of 120 patients selected from a population of 1480 cases. He compared thresholds from the nonaided ear with the aid ear of these patients, and concluded that changes in hearing due to hearing aid use are statistically and clinically nonsignificant. On the contrary, in a similar study by Kinney (1961) with 178 patients, sufficient numbers of unilateral traumatic hearing losses were attributed to amplification that he recommended that aids fitted to children with sensorineural deafness be limited to less than 40 dB of gain. Kinney also recommended frequent audiologic follow-up visits for children who wear hearing aids.

Macrae and Farrant (1965) evaluated changes in the aided and unaided ears of 87 children and concluded that (a) individuals with sensorineural hearing loss should be fitted with limited maximal power output hearing aids; (b) frequent audiologic follow-up of aided children should be required; (c) children should alternate use of the aid in each ear whenever practical; and (d) users should be cautioned about wearing hearing aids in high ambient noise environments. Macrae (1968a, b) found substantial temporary threshold shift in the aided ears of children with senorineural deafness following use of powerful hearing aids. He measured the hearing levels of four children from a school for the deaf on Friday afternoon after the youngsters had worn their hearing aids all week. He then kept the aids, and deprived the children of amplification for 66 hours, until the following Monday morning. Hearing levels in all four children showed improvement on Monday morning which again deteriorated after four hours of hearing aid use.

The evidence for powerful hearing aids causing threshold changes in the aided ear certainly seems, to us, to confirm this unfortunate circumstance as a real possibility to be considered by clinicians. It is our hope that the attention of additional researchers and hearing aid manufacturers will be drawn to this problem. Further developments will hopefully assist in identifying children, in advance, who might suffer trauma from hearing aid use. There is much we still do not know about some basic psychophysical facts related to hearing loss and hearing aid use. Danaher and Pickett (1972)

noted in subjects with profound hearing loss that their most comfortable hearing level may actually be 125 dB SPL, with a loudness discomfort level of 128 dB SPL. Many patients with profound hearing loss have no loudness discomfort at any level, while other patients, with seemingly similar hearing loss, have loudness tolerance problems so severe that they cannot tolerate any type of amplification.

We wholeheartedly make the following recommendations, supported also by Ross and Lerman (1967), to alleviate, or lessen, the possibility of inadvertent traumatic hearing loss related to over-amplification.

1. Additional hearing loss is most likely related to use of extremely high levels of maximal power output which exceed 130 dB SPL; hearing aid recommendations for children with sensorineural hearing loss should include only hearing aids with less than 130 dB SPL MPO.

2. Although we recognize that traumatic hearing loss may be related to hearing aid use, the incidence seems quite small, and our concern is by no means to be interpreted as contraindicatory to amplification. In fact, we believe that denying a child a hearing aid during the critical language years may only be saving his hearing for no good purpose. If the aid is fitted too late, it won't help anyway.

3. Frequent follow-up audiometric and hearing aid evaluation is an absolute must for all children with sensorineural hearing loss who wear hearing aids. We re-evaluate our aided children twice a year.

A Primer for Parents of a Hearing-Aided Child*

Let's Start with the Hearing Aid

Your audiologist has fitted your child with the best hearing aid available. It may be one aid or two—one for each ear. Whichever it is, trust the audiologist's judgment that it is the best fitting for your child.

Think of the hearing aid as you would a pair

---

* Much of this material is taken from pamphlets prepared by M. Downs and D. Pollack between 1951 and 1961 at the University of Colorado Medical Center.

of glasses. Both are something that a child must learn to wear during all his waking hours. He will put the aid on in the morning just as he puts on his clothes.

It may take a little time for your child to get used to wearing the aid. It isn't easy to suddenly hear a lot of loud noise after having lived in a quiet world. That is why a special program of gradually getting him used to the aid is being outlined for you. Some children can get used to the aid very quickly; others take more time—and much patience.

Decide right now that you are not going to be embarrassed or apologetic about the aid. If adults or other children show interest in the aid, make a point of explaining that some people cannot see very well and wear glasses which help them to see more clearly; your child cannot hear well, and must wear a hearing aid. If he cannot talk, explain that because he can hear more clearly, he will learn to talk. Parents have noticed that other children like to hold the receiver to their ears and listen—they may call it a little "radio" and they feel the hard-of-hearing child is very fortunate to possess something they do not have.

Another thing you must be clear about is what you should expect from the aid. Even at best it will take some time before the sounds that are heard through the aid become meaningful. It takes a newborn baby a full year of just listening to speech before he, himself, can produce even one word. If your child has not heard speech before, he will be like a newborn baby in relation to learning what sounds mean. It may take him more than a year or it may take him less to develop the understanding of what speech means.

The Home Program

Usually children will become accustomed to wearing aids if you follow the very simple kind of program outlined in this section. The next section discusses problems which may arise.

The First Week. *Short Periods Only.*—For 10 minutes if you can retain his interest, increasing gradually to 30 minutes per period.

1. Wear the aid in a quiet room at home, preferably occupied by only two or three people. Do not take the new aid when you visit friends or are in a movie theatre.

2. Set the aid at a low volume, saying "Hello ___, isn't this fun," etc., gradually increasing the volume until your child shows a slight awareness of your voice.

3. During the first week you might put the aid on while he is eating, so that he has a pleasant association with it.

4. Turn off the aid and remove the ear insert *before* the child becomes tired or restless. Do not show any impatience or anxiety if the child rejects the aid—you can always try again later. If the aid is persistently rejected, seek expert advice from an audiologist.

Prepare activities for these periods so that they are really enjoyable: You might read stories; make a scrapbook together, cutting out pictures and talking about them; model clay (but don't build blocks: it's too noisy!); play games like Picture Lotto or dressing paper dolls; draw or crayon, talking quietly about the colors, etc.; look out of the window—talk about the things you can see; or follow any activities that are being given by his therapist: color matching, nursery rhymes, etc.

The Second Week. *Two or Three Periods a Day for Approximately 1 Hour per Period.* Continue with the games and activities enjoyed before and add phonograph records, television, or musical programs on the radio. Adjust the volume and teach your child to adjust the volume of the aid—if the music is soft, the child will increase the volume until he can hear it, and vice versa. Very young children will enjoy watching you sing, dance, march, etc., to music or will tolerate rhythmic activities to music, such as Looby Lou, Mulberry Bush, etc. They do not usually enjoy just sitting and listening to music for some time.

Add Sounds around the House. Using low volume, introduce your child to the sounds made by the telephone, vacuum cleaner, water running, clock, etc. Exaggerate, with a pleasant expression, your own reactions to these sounds.

If your child is receiving *speech training*, use the aid for the exercises, etc., to be practiced at home, whenever this is specifically recommended.

Go outdoors and take a walk (after turning the volume fairly low); listen carefully and identify all the sounds you hear—children's voices, dogs barking, horns blowing, etc., always drawing your child's attention to them and indicating who or what made these sounds. If your child will not wear his aid for any length of time, postpone this until later.

The Third Week and Later. Now is the time to encourage the idea that wearing the aid is as necessary as wearing shoes! Put it on when your child is dressing and try leaving it on for 2 or 3 hours at a time—that is, *if your child has already made a successful adjustment to the aid.*

Your child may now start to wear his instrument for a longer time, wherever he goes, so that he will eventually be in a hearing world all day. Arrange for these experiences: turning the volume fairly low, go outdoors and take a walk if you have not tried this before; go to the movies, sitting 8 to 15 rows from the front, as close to center as possible; play outdoors (if the play is not too boisterous or noisy), gardening, sandbox, swings, etc.; go to the zoo, the band in the park, etc.

Children with moderate losses often enjoy games at this time in which they have to depend on hearing. For example, cover your face and ask your child to point to certain toys or perform certain actions. (Color the dog black, make your doll dance, ring the bell, etc.) You, and your child, may be surprised how much he is now hearing and understanding. Very young children enjoy sound discrimination games: indicating whether you blew a horn or rang a bell, knocked on the door, etc.

Children with a hearing impairment have great difficulty in locating sound, and will enjoy games to overcome this. For example, they close their eyes and point to the corner of the room in which you ring a bell or call their names.

Problems in Hearing Aid Use

If you are having trouble keeping the hearing aid on your child, it may help to know that other parents have had the same troubles. Here are some of the problems and complaints others have had, with suggestions as to what to do about them (Downs, 1971c and Downs 1967c).

Complaint: THE RECEIVER AND EAR-MOLD WON'T STAY IN THE EAR—THEY KEEP COMING OUT.

Remedy: In the case of a very young infant, the whole outer ear and ear canal may be too small to allow both the earmold and the receiver in it. To remedy this, the audiologist may recommend that the receiver be attached to a short tube leading to the earmold. The receiver can then be positioned just behind the ear flap, and the tube strengthened with wire so it will hold its conformity to the ear. This is a compromise that should only be used when necessary.

After a year or 18 months of age, the ear should be large enough to hold both the receiver and the earmold. If they still keep falling out, ask to have another earmold made, preferably of soft plastic material. Experiment several times if necessary to see if a perfect fit can be obtained. Remember that whenever you have an earmold fitted, you should demonstrate to your child what is going to happen: Take a large doll, lay it on its side, and put a piece of clay or cotton into the doll's ear. Show the child that this is what will happen to him. Lay him on his side and put cotton in his ears very gently. Praise him for lying still. A little preparation now saves a lot of screaming later.

Sometimes the cord keeps getting in the way of small hands, and the receiver is accidentally pulled out. Try placing the aid on the back instead of the front, and anchor the cord on the back of the shirt collar with a safety pin. Slip the cord through the safety pin, rather than piercing it.

If the earmold still keeps coming out, you may have to devise a knitted band for him to wear on his head to hold the receiver in place. Or, in the case of a girl, a ribbon or a little bonnet can be used.

Complaint: JOHNNY CONTINUALLY PULLS THE RECEIVER OUT OF HIS EAR, SO THE EARMOLD MUST BE HURTING HIM, OR THE AID MUST BOTHER HIM, OR PERHAPS HE DOESN'T NEED AN AID AND IT DOESN'T DO HIM ANY GOOD.

Remedy: You've probably let Johnny get the upper hand, Mother. But just to be sure, check the aid carefully.

1. If there's some real irritation from the earmold that is hurting him, there's a way to find out: make an appointment with your ear doctor, and put the earmold in Johnny's ear for

an hour before you see the doctor. He will then examine the outer ear and ear canal for evidence of irritation. If there is, the mold can be remade with special attention to the spot that is irritating, or the "high spot" on the mold can be ground off and repolished.

2. If the aid is "bothering him," the audiologist can tell by doing tolerance tests at different volume settings of the aid. If certain levels of sound cause Johnny to blink, or to jerk, or to cry, then the audiologist will make the proper adjustment in the aid.

3. If you feel Johnny "doesn't really need the aid," you should ask the audiologist to make another evaluation. He will show you the levels at which Johnny hears, and where he doesn't hear. Often, after a child has worn an aid for a while and has learned to identify sounds in his environment, he will respond to some sounds even when he is not wearing the aid. He is responding to "reduced cues"—that is, once he is aware of the importance of sounds, he will attend to some that are loud enough just to reach his threshold. He may be hearing only a part of a sound, very faintly, but he now pays attention to it. This does not mean that his hearing has improved or has become normal, much as we would like that to happen. It is very exciting to know that he is making use of every bit of residual hearing he has, and it is a good sign for his future functioning with the aid.

If you continue to have trouble keeping Johnny from taking off the hearing aid, you can work toward training him never to touch the receiver or to take it off. The following program may take 3 or 4 days of your time, but it will suceed in convincing Johnny that you mean business.

First Week. The first thing in the morning, show the child the earmold and aid, and set them near the clock. Point out that at 9:00 you will put the aid on for 5 minutes, and then you will take it off. He need not understand the time concept, but he will get the idea that you know what you're going to do and that you intend to do it consistently. When 9:00 comes show him the time and put the earmold in without turning the aid on. If he does not object to the mold, play quietly and lovingly with him for 5 minutes, and then remove it. If

he protests actively, hold his arms and legs, placing him sidewise on your lap so his feet can't kick you. Do not let him take the mold out. After 5 minutes, remove the aid and put it back near the clock. Point out the next time of application.

Apply the aid in this way four times a day, showing him what you are going to do, and *do it*. He must learn that you are in control of the situation, not he. By the end of the fifth or sixth day of this routine he will tolerate wearing the mold, you may be sure.

When he has tolerated the mold, at the next session turn the aid on to one-fourth volume and talk quietly into it, "Hello, isn't this nice? How's Johnny?" Then put it into his pocket or harness, and leave it on for 5 minutes. Play with a favorite game or toy during that time. If necessary, again hold down his arms and legs, avoiding flying feet!

Second Week. Apply the hearing aid as above four times a day for 15 minutes, turning the volume to one-third position. (Place a small piece of adhesive tape over the volume wheel to hold it at that position.) Play quietly or read for the first 5 minutes, then take him around the house to investigate various noises. Point out the door bell and listen to it ring; show him the vacuum cleaner, the refrigerator, the washer, and listen for their noises. Each time, point to your ears and say "I hear it—it's a BIG sound" (or a little one)—and demonstrate big and little with your hands.

Third Week. Apply the hearing aid as above four times a day for 30 minutes, turning the volume a little above one-third. After 5 minutes of quiet play with him, go about your household tasks, placing him near you in a crib, playpen, or on the floor. As you work, call his attention to all the sounds you make in your work: banging pans together while washing dishes—"Listen, Johnny, what a BIG sound"; clinking glasses together—"What a LITTLE sound"; shaking out towels from the laundry—"What a funny noise." Whenever a dog barks, a truck goes by, or someone knocks at the door, call his attention to it and imitate the sound.

Fourth Week. Apply the hearing aid as above four times a day for 45 minutes, turning the hearing aid almost to the prescribed level.

Fifth Week. Apply the hearing aid as above

four times a day for 1 hour, turning it to the level that has been prescribed, e.g., one-half, two-thirds, three-fourths volume. It is a good idea to put a dab of nail polish on the wheel at a point that will tell you where the prescribed level is. As long as necessary, place a strip of adhesive over the wheel so the child can't turn it.

If the aid squeals, or feeds back when the volume is placed at the desired level, try some Vaseline around the canal piece. If this doesn't prevent feed-back, go immediately to have a new earmold fitted. Never allow the feed-back to dictate where the volume control is set, even though it may be necessary to have new earmolds made every 3 or 6 months.

Sixth Week and Thereafter. Increase the time of wearing the aid gradually until by the second month he is wearing it all day long with the following exceptions: (1) three 10-minute rest periods a day (turn the aid off; you needn't take the mold out); (2) rough play outdoors; and (3) nap time.

There may, of course, be other problems which you, as a parent, will have to overcome. Consult with your audiologist whenever you need help in solving a problem situation; chances are it isn't the first time he's heard the problem. More than likely, he'll have some helpful suggestions for a remedy.

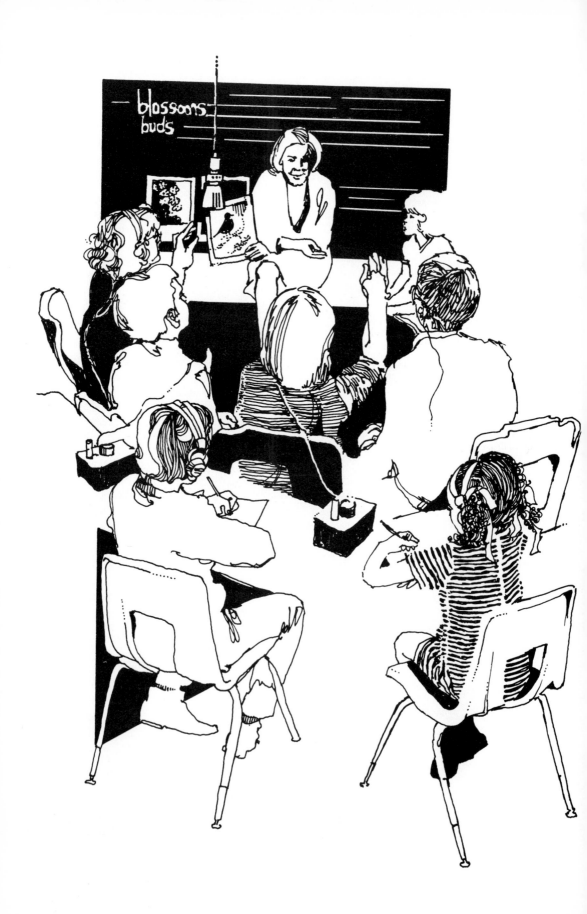

8 EDUCATION FOR HEARING-HANDICAPPED CHILDREN

Audiology and Education of the Deaf

The audiologist is often hard put to maintain the distinction between himself as an expert and himself as an advocate. When he expresses an objective judgment within the field of his expertise, he is on safe ground; but when he advocates a chosen position on questions of general policy not directly related to his expertise, he should recognize his tenuous position.

In this book we have described objective measures that have been fairly adequately standardized, and we have also outlined subjective assessments that lend themselves to some measurable degree of judgment. Here we are under a fair amount of control. However, in the field of directing hearing-impaired children into educational channels, the audiologist becomes an advocate of a cause. No audiologist has had at his fingertips a complete familiarity with all training methods and what they can do, an understanding of all the variables that will affect the child's functioning in a given training method, nor does he usually have an exhaustive collection of all the objective measures obtainable on the child. He has almost been forced to advocate a cause, not to make an objective judgment. In order to rectify these inadequacies, we point out that the audiologist, in addition to his own empirical testing, must seek the judgments of various physicians, educators, psychologists, sociologists, and others. With these people he must evolve a decision concerning the direction of management of the child—one that is flexible enough to change with the further accumulation of information. When the audiologic clinician makes such a judgment, he is still an advocate—but one without a "cause." He has become an informed advocate utilizing the information gathered from many disciplines which, however far from the ideal, is still the best anyone can know for the child.

It is our philosophy that the audiologist can become an "advocate without a cause" in the field of educational management for the child. He should not be biased in the direction of any training method or philosophy. He should consider only what will best ensure the child's maximal ultimate development. In this book we try to give the audiologist the tools with which he can arrive at a working construct concerning the direction of management for a child.

But, in another sense, the audiologist can espouse advocacy for principle or cause alone. This is in the sense of fighting for the child's right to be given a chance to show what he can do, despite contrary evidence. We would be something less than human if we failed to let hope play a part in judgments of multiple handicapped children. We also would be less than human if we failed to glow with satisfaction when a child who was scheduled for institutionalizing becomes trainable with a hearing aid and hearing therapy, upon our insistence—or when an infant who was thought to be incapable of developing useful auditory perceptions becomes in every way a hearing person with adequate speech and language abilities.

So many disciplines address themselves to consigning children to hopelessness that it may be the audiologist whose stance should be as advocate for the child. No matter how small the potential for learning seems to be, let us beg for a chance to see whether the child will be able to achieve a slightly higher status in life than had been predicted. In his own limited field the audiologist has the challenge of standing up as an advocate for decency and compassion to his small fellow human beings.

Among the fundamental rights that we as surrogates for children should demand from society is a child's right to achieve his maximal potential communication abilities. Even if a child be deaf, or blind, or crippled in any way, we should demand of society that special provision be made to help him over-ride the disability and become as "normal" as his limitations will allow. The world-famous child psychologist, A. L. Gesell, said in a 1956 publication, "The . . . aim should not be to convert the deaf child into a somewhat fictitious version of a normal hearing child, but into a well-adjusted non-hearing child who is completely managing the limitations of his sensory deficit." This is the audiologist's charge—and a hard one it is. Other disciplines solve their problems more easily.

The Educational Controversy

Any professional person who works with hearing-impaired children will undoubtedly, sooner or later, find himself in a position of offering advice about the educational future of the children with whom he works. Unfortunately, many professionals who come into contact with hard-of-hearing or deaf youngsters are by no means qualified to offer such advice. Yet, poor qualifications seem little reason for these persons to hold their tongues. We have many "armchair" experts who are physicians, audiologists, speech pathologists, or parents of deaf children. These "experts" have little or no formal orientation to deaf education and often base their comments on hearsay evidence. They often ignore the vital consideration of deaf adulthood, or have never come into contact with deaf adults.

Certainly there is a definite need for a variety of experts in the field of deafness. The difficulty comes from the fact that few "experts" have the important ingredient of objectiveness when it comes to evaluating the field of deaf education. The professional groups who know most about this area are the teachers themselves or program administrators. Yet these people are often limited in number and relatively isolated from new parents of a deaf child.

In the place of real experts, parent groups often arise in the larger metropolitan areas. These groups are formed of parents of deaf and hard-of-hearing children who have joined together for mutual support. They often eagerly accept new parents and proceed to share their experiences, good and bad, and happily offer sage advice about various educational approaches, school programs, etc. Although parent groups can be very strong organizations, too often they harbor a point of view totally immersed in emotions.

This emotional contingency may be the most serious problem in the education of the deaf. No other area of special education continues to promote controversy that has existed for hundreds of years. Even the teachers themselves are not in agreement about the best approach to education of hearing-impaired children. And in the final scene, the new parent has no place to turn for an "unbiased" opinion. In fact, an "unbiased" opinion is so rare that one is immediately suspicious that the opinion must be from someone who really doesn't know anything about education of the deaf!

The major area of controversy boils down to differences of opinion between those who advocate oral and manual approaches to deaf education. According to Moffat (1972), proponents of both views agree that when severe hearing loss exists, learning to talk with your hands is easier than learning to speak aloud. The supporters of the oral system feel that the child who uses the manual system will ultimately be forced into a "deaf society" because of his limited communication abilities (Rupp, 1971). Proponents of the manual system feel that deaf children learn more easily when taught primarily through the "visual" mode, and thus develop a wider base of knowledge for future use.

This controversy is so appealing to the public that daily newspaper editorials often contain letters regarding deaf education, and lay magazines become jousting grounds for opposing educational factions. *Harper's Magazine* some years back published as essay (Kenny, 1962) advocating reconsideration of the common lip-reading system in deaf education and proposing use of the sign language in more schools. A few months later, the Editors of *Harper's* indicated that they had received "a flood of mail" within 3 weeks of the article from 22 states and Europe! Opinion reflected in the letters was reportedly evenly split for and against the Kenny point of view, but the fact that so many took sufficient interest to express an opinion shows the tremendous overlay of emotional concern.

Current Status in Education of the Deaf

The current status in education of the deaf is reflected by the Babbidge report (1965) produced by a national committee sponsored by the Department of Health, Education, and Welfare which stated that "the American people have no reason to be satisfied with their limited success in educating deaf children and preparing them for full participation in our society." The Babbidge report cites the underlying cause of this poor result as a failure to launch an aggressive assault on the basic problems of language learning by the deaf, and lack of progress in the development of improved systematic and adequate programs for educating the deaf at all grade and age levels. Since the initial contributions of early deaf educators such as Abbé de L'Epée, Thomas Hopkins Gallaudet, and Alexander Graham Bell, education of the deaf is almost exactly where it was 150 years ago. Except for innovations in medical technology and sophistication in psychology and linguistics, the educational establishment is still graduating the deaf from high school with a fourth to sixth grade reading level, and a very crude command of the English language (Babbidge, 1965).

McClure (1973) blames the "Ostrich syndrome" demonstrated by certain deaf educators as one of the reasons for failure in deaf education progress. The "Ostrich syndrome" is manifested by (1) an inability to accept change; (2) an inability to recognize the educational implications of modern research on deafness; (3) a tendency to do little research and to castigate investigators who depart from the traditional approaches; and (4) an overwhelming desire to bury their heads in the sand hoping that current trends will disappear or that contradictory research will suddenly appear to maintain the status quo.

Where are today's deaf students? Each year the January issue of *The American Annals of the Deaf* is devoted to a directory of information concerning all deaf education programs in the United States. The 1973 Directory issue indicated that nearly 50,000 deaf children were enrolled in 807 schools and special education classes. Approximately, 20,500 of these pupils were located in only 74 public and private *residential* schools. The 650 day classes and day school programs, public and private, accounted for 14,580 deaf students. An additional 1,757 students were listed in 82 multihandicapped or specific handicap facilities.

An interesting fact of note in these figures is that the majority of deaf students attend residential-type programs. Traditionally, residential schools are aligned with manual education while private, day school programs are oral in nature. Such dichotomy, however, is currently not so specific. Additional statistics from the Directory indicate that one-fourth of these residential school students attend as day pupils. Thus, some 32,000 pupils can be categorized as day students, while only some 17,000 can truly be considered residential or "live-in" students. Obviously, the family prefers for the deaf child to live at home in spite of the fact that he attends residential school classes.

Every deaf child has the right to the best possible education, which may be in a public or private school. The residential school concept is here to stay much to the dismay of many who are usually unfamiliar with the facts. In many states, there are not enough urban areas sufficiently populous to support local deaf education programs. Parents often go to extremes to seek local special education classes or insist on establishment of supplementary teaching in regular classrooms so as to avoid enrollment of their child in an "institute" or the "deaf and dumb" school. Such special placement often results in insurmountable educational, psychologic, and social damage to the child.

The residential school recognizes the residential aspect of their program as their major deficit. The approach has been to make the residential dormitory an asset in terms of social education, complementary language and speech experiences, leadership development, and involvement in extensive extracurricular programs generally denied to the day school student. On the other hand, residential deaf school employees must endure annually the first few weeks of homesickness with the deaf child and cope with the grief of the parents. Of special interest is the fact that over 40% of the professional deaf educators in the residential schools are certified by the Conference of

Executives of American Schools for the Deaf or the Council on Education of the Deaf. Only 17% of the professionals in day programs are equally certified.

All educators would agree that the most vital aspect of any child's intellectual development is language. Upon the child's successful handling of language skills hinges his progress in school and in life. His ability to communicate his thoughts, wants, and needs to others, and in turn his understanding of thoughts and feelings of others, depend on crucial language skills. It is not by chance that these skills have been immortalized as the first two of the three R's.

The deaf child's problems have been clearly summarized by Louie Fant (1963) of the Department of Education at Gallaudet College and we are indebted to him for the following discussion. He believes that hearing plays a vital role in language development to build concepts and clarify them. The deaf child lacks this valuable input channel and accordingly throughout life has trouble developing and clarifying concepts. The entire process is slowed down and becomes laborious.

Language and concept developments, according to a scheme developed by Fant, clearly proceed hand-in-hand with communication. For the hearing child, the early states of communication are primarily via speech and hearing, and may be categorized into five components:

1. Reception: Sensory data are fed into the brain via the senses.

2. Symbols: Words, signs, gestures which are used in *Reception.*

3. Encoding: Meaningful arrangement of symbols.

4. Transmission: Meaningful sending of encoded material to someone else.

5. Decoding: The receiver's mind now utilizes the message and extracts meaning from it.

Fant states that for smooth, free-flowing communication, all five components must be operating efficiently. There must be a sufficient number of symbols to represent the message (vocabulary). There must be sufficient skill to encode the symbols (grammar). There must be sufficient mechanisms for transmission such as speech and writing. The process of decoding involves understanding vocabulary and grammar which form the very basis of the most important factor, the substance or content of the message itself. Incomplete communication and frustration result from a breakdown anywhere along the line.

So the educator of the deaf faces the problem with every deaf child. The deaf child is stuck at the very first element of the communication process. His mind is deprived of the rich sensory data supplied normally through the auditory mechanism. He often has a meager supply of symbols to use for labeling, categorizing, and storing. New symbols are difficult to come by. The deaf child functions on the concrete level of mental operations and, thus, abstract operations are most difficult for him because they are performed with words—the very commodity of which he never has enough. Abstract operations demand precise encoding and decoding and mastery of "word" concepts. Deaf children seldom attain sufficient language skills to master abstract operations even after arduous effort.

And finally, Fant points out that the usual process of trial and error learning—or teaching for that matter—is seriously hampered for the deaf child. The deaf child cannot hear his errors of vocabulary or grammar. Attempts to correct the deaf child's errors are chancy undertakings. Because of the often indistinct transmissions (speech), the listener cannot be certain that the child made an error in his use of words or grammar or whether the listener just did not understand his speech. Suppose the listener thinks an error was indeed committed; imagine his task in trying to correct the error. Or suppose an error was committed, but the listener is unsure and because of problems in trying to correct the error situation, is content to deduce an answer and let the error go. Thus, the child's error is reinforced and will surely be perpetuated.

One is never really sure what the deaf child is thinking because of difficulties in communication. Consider this example relayed to us by a teacher of the deaf. In her classroom of hard-of-hearing preschoolers, when some object would drop accidentally on the floor with a loud noise, the concept was conveyed to the children by the teacher who quickly held her hands over her ears and showed exaggerated facial expression of disdain. The children could see the situation clearly and quickly followed example with similar behavior each time an object was dropped. A few days later following this lesson, a pencil was dropped on a soft carpet accidentally. As expected, the preschoolers clapped their hands over their ears and made exaggerated faces! To what were they reacting? Surely not "noise" as the teacher thought she was teaching a few days previously. And so every concept must be carefully considered by the deaf educator from the eyes and mind of the hearing-impaired child.

Today the problems of teaching the deaf are further complicated by the fact that a greater proportion of our deaf young people were born deaf, or were deafened before the acquisition of language than was the cause 25 years ago. In fact, today, with medical achievements creating more control over the various etiologies of deafness, the communication dilemma is even more of a problem, for there are fewer adventitiously deaf children who might have some language acquisition prior to their deafness, entering our deaf education programs. Today's deaf child is usually congenitally deaf, and exhibits many more difficulties and frustrations in meeting language needs and speech skills than his predecessor who may have lost his hearing after the critical language age of 2 years. Further, many of today's deaf children, if born 20 years ago, might not have lived to enter school. Today they live, often exhibiting multiple handicaps and creating very special problems for the educator of the deaf to solve. Perhaps, under such circumstances, the fact that the achievement level upon graduation day continues to be the same as shown by their deaf predecessors may be cause to commend deaf education!

Kohl (1966) expresses a different view concerning the problem of education for deaf youngsters. He notes that the deaf child, who 90% of the time has two hearing parents, experiences rejection through dislike, pity, and misunderstanding from the hearing world as soon as his deafness is discovered. It is thus not surprising that the deaf children of deaf parents seem to be much happier and better adjusted than deaf children who have hearing parents. Kohl believes that most deaf children thus have social problems which complicate their language disability. Accordingly, the frustrated deaf child is noted to show outbursts of anger and rage which accompany him throughout his school years. In schools run by hearing teachers, the deaf children probably develop strong emotional ties and loyalties to each other which prepare them to enter an exclusive and excluded community of the deaf as adults (Northern et al., 1971).

McClure (1973) believes the problem is not so much the development of better teachers and of greater skills, although these are desirable, as to put into effect that which we already know. The deaf child learns primarily through vision, so we must make the imperceptible become perceptible. We need to find better ways to utilize the deaf child's vision in developing language mastery and improving school achievement. When we instill in deaf children the desire to communicate and provide the necessary language skills to do so, teaching speech will become a far easier task.

THE METHODOLOGIES

Many claims have been made for success of education of the deaf. Most of the claims, however, are from teachers of the deaf who have a personal belief in their own teaching techniques. Most claims, furthermore, are mere testimonials supported by a demonstration from one or two deaf children who have performed exceedingly well under the advocated, or advertised, method. Closer scrutiny seldom turns up any objective scientific evidence to support the proposed case. Few new systems withstand the test of time. In this section we will limit our discussion to the oral, manual, and total communication philosophies of deaf education and a few of the most significant variations of these three major categories. Although virtually volumes of material have been written on the methodologies in education of the deaf, we can only provide a basic, and necessarily shallow, synopsis in these few pages.

The Oral Method

Essentially three methods of oral education for deaf children are in use in the United States today. The traditional approach is to use them in the order described below. If the first method does not seem to do the job, then the second approach is attempted, and finally the third method is utilized. All three oral methods have the commonality that they essentially depend on lip reading, and wholly exclude the use of any natural signs or gestures. The greatest appeal of the oral methodology is to hearing parents of deaf children, since the main aim of the system is to make the deaf youngster a part of the hearing society through good speech and lip reading.

Silverman and Lane (1970) report that at the present time 85% of children enrolled in schools for the deaf are reported to be instructed by the oral method, at least in their early years. The fundamental assumption of the oralists is that every deaf child should be given an opportunity to communicate by speech. They prefer that children taught by the oral method not be mixed with manually communicating children, even in living dormitories, because these oral "speaking" children must adjust to the child who cannot talk, and thus valuable practice in oral communication is lost. Advocates of this method indicate that an employer is more inclined to hire a deaf person to whom he can give oral instructions over an equally capable deaf person to whom he must communicate in gestures and writing. Oralists feel that orally trained children do very well in life and that training in speech and lip reading permits an earlier adjustment to a world in which speech is the chief means of communication.

The first and primary oral method may be termed *pure oralism* or *auditory stimulation.* It developed in America at the Clarke School for the Deaf during the late 19th century. All sign language is discouraged, and the child is exposed to sounds and spoken language at every opportunity. He is fitted with a hearing aid if possible, and every excuse for auditory stimulation is utilized. In theory, the deaf youngster is to "hear" everything that a youngster with normal hearing might be exposed to, only the auditory stimulation must be conducted with more deliberate action and intensity than usual circumstances might dictate. The method starts with visual attention to lip reading and includes isolated sound elements, sound combinations,

words, and finally, speech. Much of the work must be done at home, and if a nearby preschool for the hearing-handicapped is not available, a home-study course is offered by the John Tracy Clinic in Los Angeles.

When auditory stimulation alone or lip reading is not sufficient to initiate satisfactory speech and language development, the second oral method known as the *multisensory/syllable unit method* is called into use. It is essentially the same as the pure oral procedure with lip reading, except that reading and writing of orthographic forms of English are included. Sight and touch are utilized as well as sound. This system is probably the most widely used oral method. A program emphasizing the reading aspects of this approach has been reported by Krug (1968).

Everything in the deaf child's environment is labeled and his attention is drawn to the relation between the written form and the object, as well as the relation between the written form and the spoken word. The teacher may use the motokinesthetic approach to learning speech, where the child mimics speech production by feeling the teacher's face and reproducing the same breathing and vibration effects.

The third oral method is called the *language association-element method or "natural language" method.* It was proposed and developed by the long time principal of the Lexington School for the Deaf in New York City, Mildred Groht, who felt that the deaf child should learn to speak through activity (Groht, 1958; Hart, 1964). This type of program is developed around activities, and teachers continually talk to the deaf children and encourage them to ask questions with speech. Activities are supplemented with specialized instruction in lip reading and speech.

At times it is difficult to separate these three oral education approaches and some eclectic programs choose to utilize the best from all three methods. It would seem that the children who do best in such programs are those with good residual hearing. Every oral teacher, however, has examples of children with total hearing loss who have also done well in such educational programs. Oralists prefer the use of amplification with personal hearing aids, yet do not feel that inability to use a hearing aid is just cause for abstaining from oral education.

Opponents of the oral method cite several objections to the approach. In general, their complaints are against lip reading itself, and the fact that the oral method depends too heavily on lip reading as the primary mode of reception. Lip reading is too ambiguous because (a) many sounds and words look alike on the lips (homophenous words such as mat, pan, and bat); (b) too many sounds are not visible because they are made in the back of the throat such as k, g, ng; and (c) too many people do not speak clearly and distinctly and speaking styles vary tremendously.

Lip reading is an art mastered by very few—regardless of the motivation or training involved. Those who have the talent may do very well and serve as demonstration students. However, the opponents claim, the majority of orally trained deaf pupils never master lip reading. It depends on acute vision, good lighting, and exposure of the lips and is extremely limited by distance between speakers. Lip reading is almost totally useless in dimly lit environments, within groups of talkers, or for speaker-audience formats.

Lip reading provides an inadequate means for the deaf child to monitor his own language. What is more frustrating than two oral deaf pupils, both encumbered by language disabilities and speech articulation errors, attempting to lip read each other? The intense concentration required for lip reading may place too much emotional stress on the child's personality and may produce inordinate anxieties.

And finally, strict use of the oral method is too time-consuming. Because of the difficulties encountered in lip reading, the teacher and pupil must repeat, repeat, and repeat. Motivation is dulled. Time spent on lip reading and speech is better spent on providing knowledge and instruction to the deaf pupil as he is always too far behind his hearing peer.

Arguments against the oral multisensory approaches have been summarized by Stewart et al. (1964). They state that children cannot effectively handle several simultaneous sensory stimuli at the same time. They cite previous reports that use of a combined multisensory system may actually reduce the efficiency of performance, and that success in such methods demands that all sensory systems operate in a normal manner and that one sensory input system is not always the same as other sensory input systems in deaf children.

This well recognized variant of the oral method is the so-called "unisensory" or "aural approach" to education of the deaf (Pollack, 1970; Rupp, 1971). Rupp cites the features of an auditory emphasis program as (a) audition is the most suitable perceptual modality by which a child learns speech and language; (b) it develops the impaired hearing modality to its fullest by focusing attention on audition; (c) the unisensory approach has applicability to the very young child; and (d) normalcy of environmental contacts at all levels is necessary for success of the method. The unisensory approach is dependent on very early identification, early parental guidance, early amplification, and total exposure to normal language stimulation.

The unisensory approach to deaf education has numerous advocates, and is practiced throughout the United States, but few data are available by which to judge its impact on the field of deaf education. Pollack (1971) states that much is to be gained from a unisensory, or acoupedic, approach for a child whose major deficit is congenital hearing loss. She feels that the youngster becomes more fully responsive to his environment, has a more natural voice quality with fluent speech, learns language more easily and naturally, and becomes a better lip reader. The stated goal of the acoupedic approach is the successful integration of children with hearing impairment into a hearing world.

A final, but major objection to the oral approach has been voiced by physiologists, otolaryngologists, and other students of temporal bone pathology. Temporal bones from children with profound deafness have been reported with total absence of the cochlear structures or eighth nerve tissue. Any sort of hearing in such a child is absolutely impossible. Amplification can provide no benefit except possible tactual cues. Such a child is not a good candidate for the oral method and certainly has no business in a unisensory or totally aural stimulation program (Fig. 8.1).

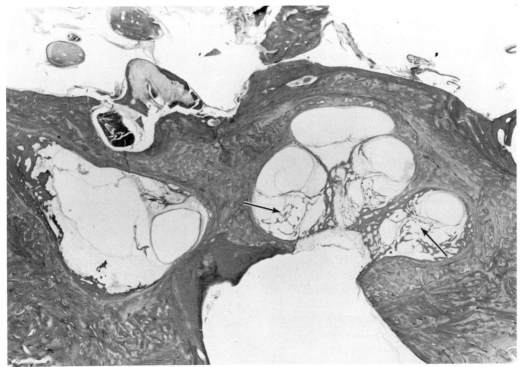

Fig. 8.1. Midmodiolar section from the temporal bone of a patient whose deafness was caused by meningitis. Note the partial ossification that has taken place in the scala vestibuli portion of the cochlea (arrows), and the lack of eighth nerve fibers and spiral ganglia. This patient had no measurable hearing. The absence of essential sensory and neural structures makes amplification with a hearing aid useless. (Courtesy of I. Sando, M.D., University of Colorado Medical Center.)

Yet, oralists continue to believe that every child has some usable hearing even if it is beyond the capabilities of the audiometer to measure it (Silverman and Lane, 1970).

Evidence is beginning to grow concerning the widespread inability of the oral method to live up to its expectations. In spite of efforts of the Alexander Graham Bell Association of the Deaf to publicize the oral deaf education methods, some of the advocators of the oral system are beginning to be vocal about their plight. Even Eric Greenway, the well known British educator of the deaf, recently indicted oralism with this quote:

> "... for almost a century we have witnessed the great oral experiment ... In theory it is ideal and there are essential virtues in its principles. In many respects it has been a courageous attempt to bring the deaf into the world of the hearing by simulation of the normal means of communication. But an honest appraisal of the results shows plainly that it has not met with the overall success that teachers hope for or that the deaf themselves desire and demand ... It cannot be denied that there have been some outstanding successes with an exclusive oral system, but for the majority it fails because it is unable to provide the fullest and most congenial means of communication." (From E. B. Greenway: The communication needs of the deaf child. In Report of the Proceedings of the International Congress on the Education of the Deaf, pp. 433-439. Washington, D. C., Gallaudet College, 1964.)

All educators of the deaf would agree that every child should learn speech. As youngsters, the profoundly deaf children seem to dislike speech lessons, but as they grow older and realize the importance of speech in every day society living, they show renewed interest in learning good speech skills. Most educators of the hearing-impaired support the statement that if the child's deafness is detected early enough, if he can use a hearing aid, if he comes from a good family environment, and if he is exposed to good teaching, he should learn as well through the oral method as the manual method (Moffat, 1972).

The Manual Method

It is said by many, including the vast majority of deaf adults, that the sign language is the common, natural language of the deaf. The signs have concrete meanings. Words can be spelled on the fingers to connect the signs into sentences. According to Ridgeway (1969), ". . . the sign language with deaf children is part mime; it is beautiful to watch, highly expressive and receptive."

Education of the deaf has not always been dominated by the oral methods. Some 100 years earlier than the advent of the oral method, L'Abbé de L'Epée, a French priest, undertook the education of two deaf sisters in the year 1750. Fingerspelling had been used earlier to teach language to the deaf in France, but to it L'Epée added a "natural language of gestures." He established a school to teach the deaf in Paris in 1860, and was later succeeded by his equally famous pupil, L'Abbé Sicard.

In 1815 an American named Thomas Hopkins Gallaudet, a minister from Hartford, Connecticut, met a young deaf neighbor girl, Alice Cogswell (Fig. 8.2). Gallaudet was deeply taken by Alice's plight of mutism and the fact that she had no place to go to school. He sought support from families of other deaf children and ultimately went to Europe to study methods of teaching the deaf. He visited London and was refused access to Watson's Asylum, where secret and expensive educational methods were jealously guarded (Stokoe, 1960). However, he met L'Abbé Sicard and was invited to Paris to learn L'Epée's system of sign language. From this warm welcome in France, he returned to America with a young deaf teacher, Laurent Clerc, and established the first school for the deaf in the United States in 1817, the American School for the Deaf in Hartford. The school was replicated throughout

the United States, and L'Epée's sign language was fused with the natural gestures used in America and became the basis for our present day sign language (Stokoe, 1960).

Years later, Thomas Hopkins Gallaudet, enjoying the success of establishing schools for the deaf across the United States was still not satisfied. As an old man he passed his vision of visions onto his son, Edward Miner Gallaudet, and his dream was realized with the establishment of Gallaudet College in 1864, the world's first college for the deaf in Washington, D.C. The last decade has seen the establishment of the National Technical Institute for the Deaf associated with Rochester Institute of Technology in New York as a second college program for the deaf—more than 100 years following the dedication of Gallaudet College.

The language of signs has been subjected to systematic analysis by several investigators including Stokoe (1960) and Tervoort (1964). Their conclusion is that sign language is an independent language that is neither a translation of oral language nor a poor imitation of it (Kohl, 1966). Natural gestures and fingerspelling depend on situational understanding; when a sign has a tendency to become repeated and understood by more than one person the sign is "formalized" and no longer a natural gesture. The manual alphabet and samples of sign language from David Watson's fine book *Talk with Your Hands* (1964), are shown in Figures 8.3 to 8.5.

Louie Fant, one of the finest interpreters for the deaf in the United States, and author of the book, *Say it with Hands* (1964), points out the importance of facial expression as one communicates with the sign language. The face, in fact, carries most of the meaning and many of the subtleties needed to enrich the communication. The limitations of sign language are also recognized and acknowledged by the experts. It is limited in scope and expressive power when compared to oral language. The sign language is bound to the concrete, and limited in expression of abstractions, metaphor, irony, and humor. However, Schein (1973) announced that two schools within New York University, the Graduate School of Education and the Graduate School of Arts and Sciences, have accepted the American Sign Language, or

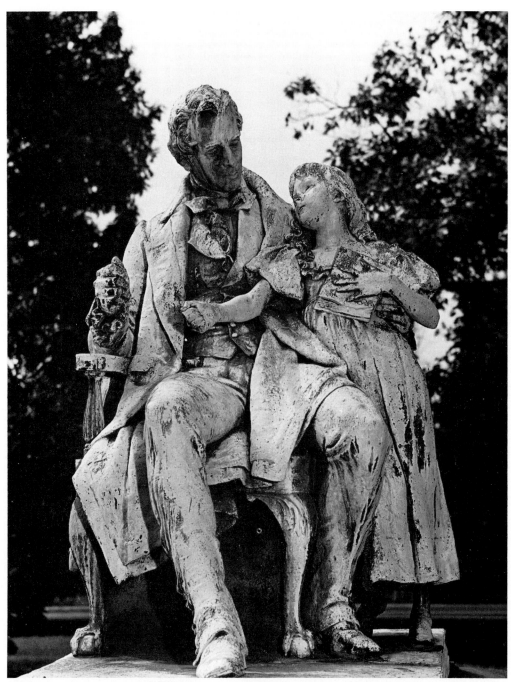

Fig. 8.2. Statue of Thomas Hopkins Gallaudet teaching a young deaf girl, Alice Cogswell, the letter "a" from the manual alphabet. This statue is symbolic of manual deaf education in the United States, and currently stands on the campus grounds of Gallaudet College, Washington, D.C. (Courtesy of the Public Relations Department, Gallaudet College.)

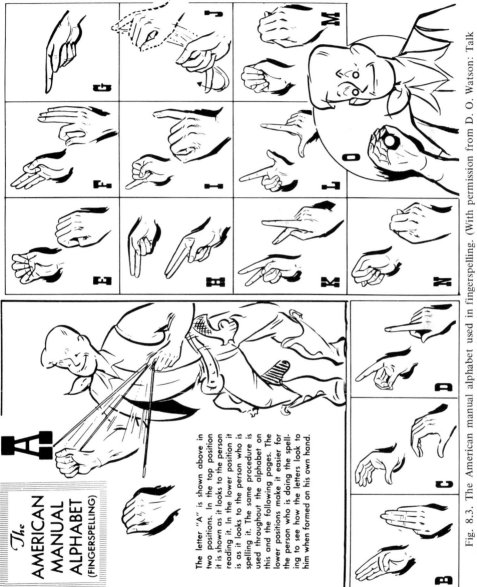

Fig. 8.3. The American manual alphabet used in fingerspelling. (With permission from D. O. Watson: Talk with Your Hands. Winneconne, Wis., 1964. © 1963.)

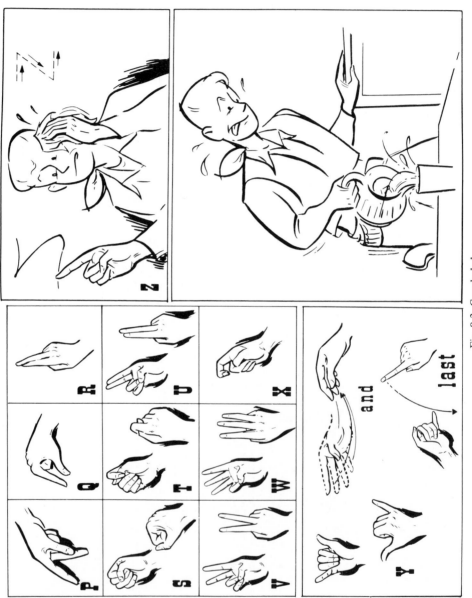

Fig. 8.3. Concluded

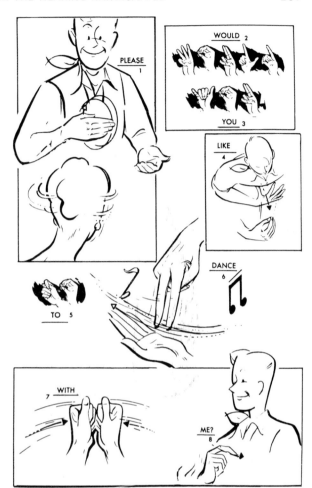

Fig. 8.4 Signs and fingerspelling used in the sentence, "Please, would you like to dance with me?" (With permission from D. O. Watson: Talk with Your Hands. Winneconne, Wis., 1964. © 1963.)

"Ameslan" as it is now commonly known (Fant, 1972), in fulfillment of the doctoral requirement for proficiency in a foreign language. American University and the University of Minnesota have each permitted the use of Ameslan in lieu of the doctoral foreign language requirement.

Two important facets of Ameslan have contributed to the standardization of American Sign Language: the valuable contribution of Stokoe's *Dictionary of American Sign Language* and secondly, the establishment of a National Registry of Interpreters for the Deaf (RID), with three levels of certification according to interpreting skill based on standardized tests administered by expert hearing and deaf interpreters.

The argument of the manualists is a relative one. They define the role of an educational program as that of providing an education to the deaf child which is equitable to the education of a hearing child. The manualist questions the implementation of speech and lip reading into the curriculum to the diminution of the three R's. He differentiates between language skills and speech/lip reading and submits that language skills are paramount to speech both educationally and socially.

Garretson (1963), a respected deaf educator and long time advocate of the use of fingerspelling and signs in spite of the fact that he was brought up in the oral tradition, cites the following factors as assets for the manual method:

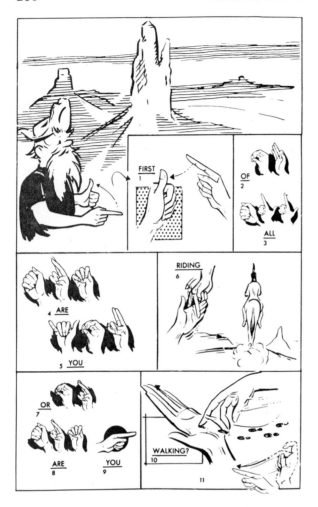

Fig. 8.5. Signs and fingerspelling used in the sentence, "First of all, are you riding or are you walking?" (With permission from D. O. Watson: Talk with Your Hands. Winneconne, Wis., 1964. © 1963.)

1. Denying a child the right to use his hands along with speech and lip reading creates anxiety and emotional stress on the pupil.

2. With the use of fingerspelling, signs, and speech, there is no doubt as to what is being communicated.

3. Signs on the hands are considerably larger and clearer than lip movements.

4. Fingerspelling and signs do not discriminate against anyone and all have equal opportunity to participate and learn from classroom activities.

Garretson concludes that during the last 75 years of education of the deaf, signs and fingerspelling have never been made compulsory for the student, while speech and lip reading are usually taught in special sessions in schools for the deaf. The fact that the manual system has persisted among deaf adults, and is the preferred method of communication by the majority of the deaf, speaks for the value of the manual system.

Mention should be made of two early variants of the manual system known as the combined method and the simultaneous method. Fant (1963) defines the combined method as utilization of speech, speech reading, hearing aids, and fingerspelling. The simultaneous method is essentially the same as the combined method with the addition of the language of signs. Fant stated that in his opinion the combined method represented a reasonable compromise between the pure oral and pure manual systems of communication.

One of the major drawbacks to Ameslan is that its crude syntax is not conducive to the development of acceptable English. With the Ameslan system it is difficult to express pronouns; verb tense is indicated by context; signs follow each other according to convenience and not necessarily accepted English order; and what is acceptable for communication is the *general concept,* not the *specific intent.* Proponents of the oral methods use this syntax problem as their major objection to manualism.

The Rochester Method

The New York state deaf residential school staff questioned the educational validity of signed English (siglish). They noted that deaf children who had been taught in the oral method during elementary school years and then introduced to "siglish," still were not acquiring educationally acceptable English. There arose subsequently the Rochester method which is the simultaneous use of speech and fingerspelling—a sort of "writing in air" technique superimposed on normal speech (Scoaten, 1964). This technique is also known as "Visible Speech" because the teacher is able to face the class and synchronize what is said and shown on the lips with a more visible form of English as spelled on the hands. This system is under close scrutiny now and is used in at least three state residential schools with promising results.

The more visible approach of the Rochester method is the best supplement to an otherwise oral method because it is a pure, visible, English medium (McClure, 1973). It represents a multisensory visible oral-plus approach to language development. This method is said to continuously emphasize the traditional oral approach, supplemented by simultaneous and very visible fingerspelling. Actually, Kohl (1966) considers the Rochester method a fourth method of oral education for the deaf.

Total Communication

Comparatively recently, in terms of deaf education tradition, a philosophy termed total communication has arisen. The proponents of total communication recognized the educa-tional advantages of visible speech, yet they also noted certain difficulties. The manual dexterity of the preschool child limits his ability to fingerspell quickly, and his limited attention span makes it difficult to attend intensely on "flying fingers and fleeting flexible faces" for an all day instruction session.

Total communication, as it is stressed by its advocates, is indeed a philosophy and not simply another method for teaching deaf children. The basic premise is to use every and all means to communicate with deaf children from infancy to school age. No particular method or system is to be omitted or stressed. The student is exposed to natural gestures, Ameslan, fingerspelling, facial expression, body English, all accompanied simultaneously with speech heard through a hearing aid. The idea is to use any means that works to convey vocabulary, language, and idea concepts between the deaf child and everyone to whom he is exposed. The important concept is to provide an easy, free, two-way communication means between the deaf child and his family, teacher, and schoolmates. When the teacher is able to establish which technique works best with the particular child, this method will be the principal method used throughout the remainder of the school years. In some environments and educational facilities, total communication is practiced continually with all pupils throughout their school years.

The concept of total communication appealed very quickly to the manually oriented observers, since it really involves little in terms of compromise on their part. The orally oriented faction, however, have seemingly been more reluctant to join the total communication movement. To agree with the total communication philosophy means utilizing signs and fingerspelling which for so many years have been totally outlawed and forbidden in the oral deaf tradition. The Alexander Graham Bell Association of the Deaf has been openly opposed, and even antagonistic, toward public displays of manual communication (Ridgeway, 1969).

According to Moffat (1972), opponents of total communication complain that if a teacher of the deaf really favors one method over another, the teacher will unwittingly move the students in the direction of that approach under the guise of teaching total communication. Some educators believe that it is not possible to evaluate the effectiveness of any one approach while using all the approaches at the same time. These arguments, however, seem to miss the main concept of total communication which says that it is paramount to communicate without regard for which "method" is really doing it. The total communication approach has been criticized because it is too much of a shotgun approach to education of the deaf. Critics argue that the overstimulation of the deaf child is actually detrimental to communication.

For years, the approach to deaf education was to start all children in an oral-type program for their early years of school. At some point in time, second or third grade or age 7 or 8, the child would be evaluated in regard to his educational progress and the oral method. If he was doing well, he would be continued in an orally oriented program. If he was not doing well he would be transferred into a manually oriented class. For most children, this timing of selecting their educational method so long after the critical years of language and speech development makes education prognosis very poor. Total communication in the early years seems to be an important new concept in behalf of the deaf child, and should add years of head start toward his formal education. The concept of total communication has caught on and spread quickly in the United States until our current status is such that school programs are unfashionable if they do not profess to be supporters of total communication. On the other hand, this rapid philosophical propagation has created little or no similarity among these programs. Time has been too short and growth too rapid to permit agreement and standardization concerning the application of total communication. The progress, thus far, is encouraging and the change in attitude from stressing a particular "method" to over-all concern for the deaf child's needs to be immersed in two-way communication, may turn out to be the most significant change in deaf education for over a hundred years.

Current Sign Systems

During the past few years, several manual sign systems have been developed as improvements to Ameslan since their design is such that they represent English. It is too early to judge the merits or impact of these new sign systems on the deaf consumer and user, but their presence is certainly creating attention and controversy. The new systems are described here to orient readers to the basic philosophies, approaches, nomenclature, and differences, since these approaches have been developed to overcome apparent inadequacies of the American Sign Language or Ameslan. An excellent essay regarding these current sign systems has been published by Bornstein (1973). The new systems have as their premise that Ameslan, with linguistically generated variations, can be the visual equivalent of spoken English. Furthermore, they share the idea that if this type of system is introduced to the deaf child at a very early age, the language skills, total experiences, mental health, and communicative abilities will be improved over our traditional approaches.

The new sign systems discussed below have several principles in common as described by Cokely and Gawlik (1973). The basic premise is that deaf children need a visual symbol system to develop their language competency to its fullest potential. They assume that the more syntactically correct the symbols, the more it will aid in development of language in the deaf child. Apparently, all argue that although the American Sign Language is an adequate communication tool, its syntax is such that it is not necessarily related to the grammatical structure of English. And finally, with exception of "cued speech," each believes that a visual symbol system can be developed to incorporate basic Ameslan signs with modifications that encourage the use of meaning through context that is consistent with the form of spoken English.

Cued Speech

Cued speech is a method of communication developed by R. Orin Cornett for the hard-of-hearing in which eight hand configurations and four hand placements are used to supplement the visible manifestations of natural speech. Cued speech was hailed in 1967 as a possible answer to the oralism versus manualism controversy. The 12 cues described above are used around the chin, cheek, and neck, drawing attention to the speaker's face and lips. The cued speech system follows natural English spoken language (Cornett, 1967).

Actually, the cues are not intelligible without proper mouth motions. Because "cueing" is completely dependent upon spoken language and lip reading, it satisfies the oralist's demand that emphasis be placed on learning to communicate with those who don't know sign language (Miles, 1967). It reportedly takes about 30 hours for a hearing person to achieve fairly fluent use of cued speech, but critics of the system complain that the cued speech system is too complex for easy learning. Cued speech has been under widespread evaluation in several institutions, but results of data gathering have not yet been reported.

Seeing Essential English (SEE)

This sign system, originated by David Anthony in 1962, and developed in Southern California, uses modifications of Ameslan to resemble English. SEE is intended for use by all age groups, and now has as its basis an impressive two-volume manual which includes an introduction to the system, how it is used, grammar and syntax guidelines, and over 3000 vocabulary entries (Anthony and Associates, 1971). The SEE system has the largest vocabulary of any of the new systems.

SEE signs represent word forms or word parts such as roots, prefixes, or suffixes. The signs are used in combinations to form any desired word. To reflect English syntax, SEE emphasizes complete English word order. Verb tense is clearly indicated and irregular verb forms have signed representation. In general terms, English words are represented by the traditional American sign word plus a suffix and/or prefix. English compound words are often made up of elements different from the single sign element often used in Ameslan. As a result, SEE words often do not closely resemble the original source sign in Ameslan. SEE is similar enough to Ameslan that American Sign Language users can almost read it in context, but may not be able to identify specific SEE signs without previous exposure or explanation.

Signing Exact English (SEE₂)

This sign system was developed in 1972 by a group of former members of the Seeing Essential English group, headed by Dr. Gerilee Gustasan. It is perhaps unfortunate that the new group did not select another name for their system that did not mimic Anthony's SEE system. Cokely and Gawlik (1973) use the notations, SEE_1 and SEE_2 to differentiate the two systems. According to Bornstein (1973), the reasons leading to the development of Signing Exact English is that SEE_1 utilized too many signs that were too distant from Ameslan, was too radical in its use of the root word, and too complex for the needs of parents and teachers. Accordingly, SEE_2 uses signs which represent words rather than roots, as well as basic affixes as needed. Signing Exact English has a vocabulary of some 2000 words published in booklet form.

Signing Exact English is also intended to be used by young children. It is readily apparent, then, that a situation can develop whereby parents and children who interact with persons trained in another system will use different signs for the same word. According to calculations reported in the Bornstein essay, 61% of the SEE_2 vocabulary is based on traditional Ameslan signs, 18% are modified Ameslan signs, and 21% were entirely new signs. When SEE_2 signs were compared with SEE_1 signs, some 80% of the traditional sign group were identical in both systems. Bornstein concludes that difficulties created by these sign word differences will be relatively minor.

Linguistics of Visual English (LOVE or LVE)

This sign system, developed in 1971 by Dennis Wampler, is intended for use by preschool and kindergarten deaf children. The system is based on hand positions that represent morphemes, the smallest meaningful unit in the English language. The morpheme may be "bound"—meaningless unless connected to another morpheme—or "free"—significant and meaningful by itself. LOVE distinguishes morphemes on the basis of similarity in sound, spelling, or meaning. LOVE signs are also designed to represent speech rhythms. The

LOVE system obviously resembles Ameslan less than SEE$_1$ or SEE$_2$. Additional information on the LOVE system is available in three booklets: *Questions and Answers on LVE, An Introduction of the Spatial Symbol System Used by LVE,* and *Morpheme List One* (Wampler, 1971).

Signed English (Siglish)

This system uses 2500 words to aid the language development of the preschool child. Some 1700 of these signs can be represented by existing Ameslan signs. Siglish was developed by Bornstein and his associates at Gallaudet College (Kannapell et al., 1969). Signed English substitutes American Sign Language words for English words without changing the English syntax structure. Complex English words are represented by natural Ameslan words in whatever form they exist. The authors of this technique indicate in Bornstein (1973) that they are not convinced that an altered form of the sign word actually facilitates learning of the English word form.

Signed English incorporates some 14 sign markers used after the sign word to denote plurals, verb tense, possessive forms, gerunds, etc. In an interesting project, a number of children's classic stories such as "Goldilocks and the Three Bears" and "Little Red Riding Hood" (Bornstein et al., 1972) have been illustrated in color, with line drawings of sign words in Signed English form (Fig. 8.6). Signed English has the unofficial endorsement of the National Association of the Deaf, and is used in many state residential schools for the deaf as well as at Gallaudet College.

The new sign systems are in a state of flux and transition. Incongruities and contradictions may be seen within the systems. To judge the systems today would be imprudent and unfair, and decisions, as of yet with no data, must be based only on personal intuition. The advent of the systems reflects dissatisfaction with the American Sign Language as a basic language instructional tool. Final judgment must be reserved until the results can be examined objectively.

What about Parents?

For perhaps too many years, attention of professionals has been devoted solely to the hard-of-hearing or deaf child, and little consideration has been given to the parents. We believe that the parents of the deaf child may be the key to one of the most significant factors in the deaf youngster's development. And fortunately, during the past few years, parent-oriented habilitation programs for children with hearing impairment have emerged.

As an example, a parent program is currently under development at the University of Denver, Department of Speech Pathology and Audiology. Sponsored by funds from the Bureau of Educationally Handicapped, U.S. Office of Education, their Project Parent-Child, is a program of "prescriptive intervention," designed to provide for the parents of hearing-handicapped children emotional support, education, participation in program planning, and guidance in parent-child interaction. This program is by no means the only approach to actively involve the parents of deaf children, but it conveys elements and concepts that might be included in any habilitation program for children.

The major objectives of Project Parent-Child include emotional support for the parents by helping them recognize, realize, accept, and understand the implications of their child's hearing problem. This increased awareness should help reduce anxiety and worry often expressed by parents of handicapped children. Education for the parents is included so that they might fully understand the nature of their child's hearing loss with realistic ramifications of the educational future for their youngster. The parent is taught to understand child growth and development as well as the need for communication skills, social contact, and emotional expression.

One of the unique aspects of the University of Denver approach to "parent therapy" is to offer the parents a choice in the communication system provided to the child. The goal is to help parents capitalize on the natural means of interaction with their children—either through a predominately aural approach or total communication approach. An interesting conclusion reached by Amon (1972) based on her experiences with this program is that parents must be the ones to choose the communication system the family wishes to use with the hearing-handi-

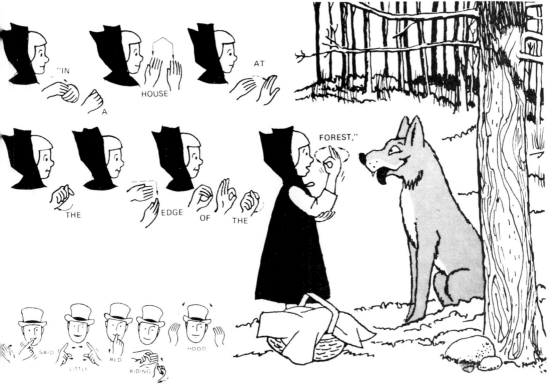

"In a house at the edge of the forest",
said Little Red Riding Hood.

Fig. 8.6. An example of one of the classic children's stories in Signed English produced by the Gallaudet Pre-School English Project. (With permission from H. Bornstein et al.: Signed English Basic Dictionary; *Little Red Riding Hood.* Washington, D.C., Gallaudet College Press, 1972.)

capped child. She states that the choice between communication systems is secondary to the desirability of the parents being in agreement, enthusiastic, and committed to the system of their choice. Professionals can provide guidance, exposure, and background to the parents, but the final choice, according to Amon, should be reached by them. She suggests that imposing the use of signs on parents who lack confidence in their ability to interact with the child is a common cause for failure. If the parents choose to use signs, the entire family must develop fluency with this means of communication.

A final objective in the Project Parent-Child is to teach the parents how to utilize and adapt daily activities of the home as experiential teaching events for the preschool child. Hopefully, the result is a stimulating home environ-

ment for the hearing-impaired child, where auditory, speech, and language development is a daily, ongoing, and natural activity for the youngster. The University has a mobile home completely furnished and operational with kitchen, bathroom, bedroom, playroom, etc. The home is stocked with typical utensils and furnishings. Parents spend time with the parent-training supervisor to learn how to develop a repertoire of experiences and activities to stimulate interaction with their children. Video tape is used extensively to observe parent-child interaction with immediate feedback to the parents in order to increase their abilities with their children. An active rural program, in addition to the metropolitan area program, actively seeks to identify children with hearing loss in their own homes and community. A home study course for parents is under development, and the parents may use a special telephone line to the Project staff to call for advice, support, or information whenever necessary.

A few other major cities and large clinic programs also have parent-centered projects underway, and it would appear that the deaf child will be the ultimate beneficiary of support and education aimed at his parents during the initial stages of discovery of the hearing loss. This concern for parents of hearing-handicapped children is an exciting trend which deserves further development and wider application.

Language as the Goal in the Selection of the Appropriate Rehabilitation Program

"The mystery of language is that it uses man as much as man uses it" (Ciardi, 1973).

Words trigger in us emotional signals that have been conditioned from early childhood; the way the words are put together triggers our judgments of fellow humans. It has literally taken an act of Congress for many people to recognize that responses to the word "black" or "Negro" have been inappropriately conditioned in us for 100 years; or to admit that the word "woman" does not denote a second-class citizen. We humans exist at the deep level of the language that we learned when very young. It is to our eternal credit that occasionally we are able to use language to reverse at least overtly our responses to emotionally learned language signals. But such civilized behavior is pure intellectuality, and it is probably impossible to submerge entirely what Ciardi calls the evolutionary depths of the rituals of our language.

All the progress that man has made, if one can call a highly technologic society progress, is due to sophistication in the manipulation of language. The symbols used for physical events, when placed in logical relationships to each other, produced $e=mc^2$. No amount of serendipity can accomplish the incredible results of a human mind thinking "If A, then B–." For man to conceive of reaching the moon, and soon the planets of our solar system, required a highly advanced ability to manipulate symbols. The symbols may be words or they may be mathematical concepts, but the manipulation of them is language. Man seems compelled by a primitive force to continue to expand the complexities of these manipulations.

It follows that language deprivation is the most serious of all deprivations, for it robs us of a measure of our own human-ness. Whether caused by sensory deprivation, by experiential deprivation, or by central disordering, in some degree it keeps one from the complete fulfillment of one's powers.

Language is the desideratum that we most wish for the hearing-impaired. For too long we have been misled into placing oral speech as the primary goal for all of these children, never realizing that the enrichment of their lives may be sacrificed for the ability to mouth words. What words?—and in what relationships? If one is not able to think in highly complex language symbols, does it matter whether he is able to vocalize any of them? And, most important, how can he verbalize adequately unless he has an adequate symbol system to utilize?

The premise of our proposal for the management of the hearing-impaired child rests upon language as the primary goal to be sought for the child. Whatever route will lead the way through his neurologic labyrinth to reach language understanding, that route must be taken. We must be ruthless in discarding methods and methodologies, entrenched techniques, and individual philosophies. We hold no brief for any established method or educational technique—nor any not yet established. Any, or all, should be selected for use when the need warrants. What is important is that an approach be selected on the basis of what is best for the child, not for the institution. For too long the child has been forced to be tailor-made to the program; we must now tailor-make a program for each individual child's needs. The primary goal is always to tap the innate language skills by whatever means possible. Secondarily only will we aim for intelligible oral expression of that language—a skill that itself depends upon the acquisition of a high degree of language competence.

Not only speech, but reading and writing skills are also dependent upon language skills.

One forgets that the sequence of development of language skills is first, listening; second, speaking; third, reading; and fourth, writing (Mackintosh, 1964). A foundation of competence in the input of language (listening) is requisite to the expressive skills of speaking and writing. Likewise, a firm basis of language input is requisite to capability in reading, which is the secondary receptive input skill. These facts are basic to the organization of a therapeutic and educational program for a hearing-impaired child.

It is the deficiency in language skills which is the spectre that haunts the clinician who sees a generation of hearing-impaired children grow to adulthood. Fully half of all the children in our clinical experience with severe to profound losses who were started at a very early age in an auditory-oral program did not develop language commensurate with their potential intellectual level. Their language levels are typified by the results of a recent demographic survey conducted by Gallaudet College (Reis, 1973a). This study reported the results of standard achievement tests in 19,000 deaf and hard-of-hearing children in the United States. Both oral and manual educational techniques were represented. The graph shown in Table 8.1 represents one of the most significant test results. This table indicates that the highest average score in paragraph meanings, which represents language comprehension, was obtained by the 19-year-olds and was equivalent to normal fourth grade level!

Preschool oral programs have not seemed to be successful in raising the level of language, lip-reading, and reading skills. Vernon and Kóh (1970) reported well controlled studies demonstrating that by age 9, no differences existed between deaf children who had had oral preschool programs and those who had not had such training.

Such studies do not refute the hypothesis that early language training can raise the level of language of the deaf; they do demonstrate that oral training at the preschool level is not effective for many children. What does seem to be effective is exposure to manual language patterns at a young age. A large number of studies show that the deaf children of deaf parents have a significantly higher level of

Table 8.1. Weighted Grade Equivalent Averages By Age and Battery Level for Hearing-Impaired Students, Paragraph Meaning Sub-Test, Stanford Achievement Test—Spring 1971

Age	All Batteries Combined	
	Number	Average
	16,815	3.02
Under 6	27	1.96
6	323	1.61
7	445	1.77
8	690	1.90
9	964	2.09
10	1,290	2.24
11	1,594	2.40
12	2,305	2.58
13	1,546	2.95
14	1,566	3.18
15	1,452	3.54
16	1,314	3.85
17	1,239	4.02
18	1,152	4.23
19	637	4.36
20	220	4.12
21 and over	51	4.23

language than all other deaf children, that they have equivalent speech development, that they achieve academically at a higher level, and that they tend to be better adjusted than all other deaf children (Vernon and Koh, 1970; Quigley and Frisina, 1961; Meadow, 1968; Stuckless and Birch, 1966). The plethora of reports confirming these facts can hardly be controverted by even the most zealous auditory-oral advocates.

It follows logically that structured infant and preschool programs teaching a syntactical form of manual language would capitalize on the time-locked nature of language learning and result in a higher level of language in the deaf. Whether this is a valid proposal cannot be demonstrated for many years. The problem with advocating any new educational approach is always that it may be done on the basis of logical deduction, on reports of successes in a few uncontrolled projects, or on an emotional basis. But the proof remains where is always has been—in the ultimate success of large numbers of children.

However, the lack of proof should be no

deterrent to developing new programs when a deep and urgent need can be shown to exist. Such a need is present in the education of the deaf, and calls for innovative methods.

The total communication program which has been described meets the criterion of logical deduction from the facts that are known: the time-locked nature of language; the critical periods for language development; and the proof that the earlier some form of language can be presented to the child, the better will be his ultimate skills.

The evidence is already accumulating that combining manual, auditory, and oral methods in no way detracts from the oral communicative abilities of hearing-impaired children. In fact, it appears that the learning of language through manual approaches strengthens speech, lip reading, and reading skills.

Schlesinger and Meadow (1972b) have made the most telling demonstration of the value of a total communication approach for the child with severe hearing loss or deafness. In a study on four children with losses over 80 dB whose families used signs and fingerspelling along with oral speech, they found that both the number of spoken words and the lip-reading facility of the children increased with sign language acquisition. The children's language developed in the same pattern as that of normal-hearing children. One-word utterances were being used holophrastically by one of the children by the age of 15 months, i.e., the word would have an adult sentence equivalent. This child quickly progressed through the other milestones of language acquisition of the normal child: two- and three-word combinations soon appeared that expressed complete sentence meanings in signs just as the normal child expresses them in words.

Another of the children with an excellent foundation in sign language in Schlesinger and Meadow's study was given a lip-reading test (Butt and Chreist, 1968) at the age of 3 years, 10½ months. Her score on the test was 60, as compared with the average score at age 4 of 27, and at age 5, 34. This unusual facility at lip-reading corroborates our contention that language must be present before lip reading can be acquired adequately, and that the better the language skill, the better the lip-reading ability.

To attempt to teach language through lip reading will never be productive of satisfactory results.

Another of the children showed a gradual increase in the use of speech alone and a decrease in the use of signing alone, by the age of 3 years, 3 months. It was apparent that the use of signs was in no way discouraging her oral communication development. This child had a signing vocabulary of 604 words at age 3 years, 4 months.

Perhaps the most significant finding by Schlesinger and Meadow concerns the parent-child relationship. The reciprocal communicative events between parents and child are described as happy and playful, because of the development of communication interchanges that resemble those of the normally hearing parent and child. "We find that these interchanges are characterized by early reciprocal understanding and are permeated with genuine enjoyment. Understanding of early meaning and enjoyment in mother-child communicative events may well represent one of the necessary features of normal language development." To anyone who has seen the often joyless efforts of mother and child to communicate when only auditory and oral modes are used, this statement offers a refreshing solution.

To demonstrate the theoretical advantage of early signing of language, it is interesting to relate problems encountered by the deaf to a few studies of language in animals.

Deaf children have difficulty creating a mental image of an object that is divided into separate parts. They also have problems in mentally seeing the other side of the object (Rozanov, 1973). Such tasks require that the child can carry in his mind the symbols for the parts or the sides of the objects, and that he can also use language constructs to put the parts mentally where they should be. For example, he must be able to think, "On the opposite side of that _____ was a _____." "Opposite" and "side" are both abstract symbolic terms in this case—terms which must be carried in the mind in order to recall them. The verb "was," in its use as "was—is still" becomes an even more difficult concept.

Such problems of deaf children are reminiscent of the research on chimpanzees who were required to pile boxes on top of each other in order to reach food suspended from the ceiling. So long as all of the boxes were in the visual field of the animal, he was able to pile them up and reach the food. However, when one of the boxes was behind him, he was not able to carry in his mind the concept "A *box was*—(is still) *behind me.*" And so he was not able to obtain the food (Langer, 1957).

The difference between the animal and the human child is that the human can learn such intricate symbols providing that an input of abstract language constructs is given in the first few years of life when the human organism is programmed to process them. The input must consist of complete syntactical language in order for the structures to be implanted in the developing brain.

To further illustrate the significant difference between the animal and the human, the studies of Gardner and Gardner (1969) demonstrated that a female baby chimpanzee could be taught to sign words and to use them to express her wants. Starting with an approximately 8-month-old chimpanzee, the Gardners trained her to form American Sign Language signs for nouns, verbs, adverbs, and adjectives. Thirty such word signs were used and understood by the chimpanzee after a period of 22 months of intensive training. Such words as "more," "hurry," "hear-listen," and "flower," were used by her correctly. Not only that, but such words as "flower" did not remain specific to the original referents, but were transferred spontaneously to a wide class of appropriate referents.

Further language learning of chimpanzees has been reported by Premack and Premack (1972) who utilized plastic chips to stand for words. Their chimpanzee was also able to learn 130 symbols, and could transfer her knowledge to symbols and situations outside the context of her training. Fleming (1974) states that these chimpanzees demonstrated basic criteria for language: (1) they learned an extensive system of names for objects in their environment; (2) they sign or signal about objects that are not physically present; (3) they use signs for concepts, not just objects, agents, and actions; (4) they invent semantically appropriate combinations; and (5) they use proper order when it is semantically necessary.

This kind of behavior is a high order of communication for a primate. Yet, at the present stage of research it does not yet resemble those aspects of language that we deem to be exclusively human.

What is deemed exclusively human in the area of language? Whichever modern psycholinguistic theory one ascribes to, Lenneberg (1966), Chomsky (1966), or Neisser (1967), all point to a genetically predetermined ability for syntactical language structure. The human infant and the primate infant both can learn to use symbols for objects, actions, and concepts. What the human infant alone seems programmed to do is to manipulate those symbols in a variety of logical relationships through the complex structure of syntactical language and to manipulate them without being specifically taught, in unlearned conceptual organizations.

It would seem that if a baby chimpanzee can learn to sign words, a baby human who is deaf should be able to, and that in addition he should be able to learn structural language forms if they are made available. Evidence is accumulating demonstrating that indeed they can, not only from Schlesinger and Meadow, previously cited, but from our own observations of very young children who have been placed in total communication programs. It is fortunate that there is available to such children logical syntactical language systems which, in combination with speech training, amplification of any residual hearing, and other methods of input, can give them the world of language constructs. The questions which remain are: Where does profound deafness end and adequate hearing begin? How does one select the child who can learn language through an auditory input, and also designate the child who requires the heroic measures described above? Auditory learning of language may be the most desirable system, as it is the natural one. One must avoid, if at all possible, placing a potentially auditorally adequate child into an unnecessarily structured program.

The major problem confronting us is how to separate in infancy those who will best learn language through a total communication program from those who can best learn via auditory and oral approaches. The audiologist, working with a team of otolaryngologists, educators, pediatricians, social workers, and psychologists, must take the responsibility for making this determination. At the present state of the art we can begin to devise formulae that will ultimately allow us to make such predictions.

The following discussion is intended to provide a point of departure for audiologists, from which we can begin to evolve the suggested kind of formulae. These consist of weighted scales which take many aspects of the child and his environment into consideration. Table 8.2 shows the "deafness management quotient" (DMQ), weighted on a 100-point scale, with a score of 81 or better necessary to an auditory and oral program (Downs, 1972a). Note that 10 points are added for conductive elements such as are found in about 50% of the rubella deafnesses. The central factors range from those readily diagnosed by physicians at or near birth, to those concomitant with other symptomatology and to the less obvious factors that developmental scales or auditory behavior can suggest. Expertise in language disorders, family-social psychology, and socioeconomics is needed to add structure to this formula. The difficulties of applying this scale may gradually be overcome as evidence is collected

that will give us the guidelines to apply the scale more effectively. Although it is impossible to evaluate the success of deaf children to whom we apply the scale now, it is possible to apply the scale in retrospect and observe results of our young adult deaf patients.

Figure 8.7 shows a 21-year-old girl's audiogram, who had been fitted with binaural hearing aids at 15 months of age and placed in an auditory program. She attended an oral school at age 3, staying for 5 years at which point the parents insisted on regular school placement. Psychology tests showed better than average organic integrity, a verbal WAIS IQ of 85 and a performance WAIS IQ of 119. She communicates with her family orally, but with all others she can only communicate by writing. The best sentence she produced, when asked what she would like to do in life, was "I really exciting go skiing or get married." She was placed in a manual college program in order to learn skills requisite to taking employment. Her DMQ is also shown in Figure 8.7.

Figure 8.8 shows another 21-year-old's audiogram, for whom a hearing aid was fitted at 2½ years of age, and who also went through an oral program. Psychologic testing showed no perceptual problems, a WAIS verbal IQ of 87,

Table 8.2. Suggested Scale for Direction of Deafness Management Quotient (DMQ)—Total: 100 Points

Residual hearing: 30 points possible
0 = no true hearing
10 = 250-500 < 100 dB   Add 10 points for conductive
20 = 250-500-1000 < 100 dB   element to hearing loss
30 = 2000 < 100 dB
Central intactness: 30 points possible
0 = diagnosis of brain damage
10 = known history of events conducive to birth defects
20 = perceptual dysfunction
30 = intact central processing
Intellectual Factors: 20 points possible
0 = MR < 85 IQ
10 = average → 85-100 IQ
20 = above average: > 100 IQ
Family constellation: 10 points possible
0 = no support
10 = completely supportive and understanding
Socioeconomic: 10 points possible
0 = substandard
10 = completely adequate
Auditory program leading to oral: 81-100 points
Total communicative program: 0-80 points

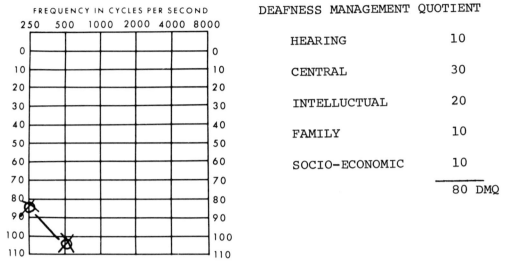

Fig. 8.7. Deafness management quotient of a 21-year-old deaf girl.

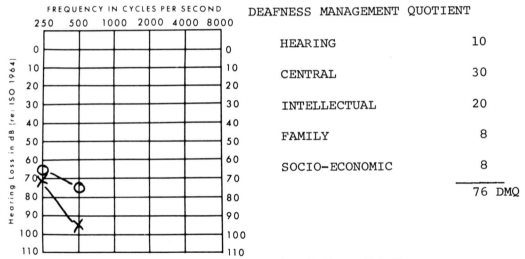

Fig. 8.8. Deafness management quotient of a 21-year-old deaf boy.

and a performance IQ of 113. His communication was limited. The psychologist's comment was: "The usual pidgin English of the deaf." He was directed to a manual college program in order to learn computer programming, which was his vocational choice. His DMQ is also shown in Figure 8.8.

These two children had everything going for them—yet at 21 years they had no place to go. They could not make it in a hearing society nor a deaf group. Twenty years late, they were started on a manual program that hopefully

would give them a place in the sun. These young adults are now difficult problems for vocational rehabilitation counselors.

This suggested scale is meant to be a challenge for professionals to combine their expertise to see whether such a quotient will be effective. If changes should be made in the scales, then they should be made. Perhaps not enough weight has been given the intellectual and central factors. Or possibly the score of 81 as the borderline for an auditory program is too high. Only reference to retrospective studies will reveal the adequacy of the scale. In our experience with adult hearing-impaired individuals, both oral and manual, the scale has been effective in telling us what should have been done when the individual was an infant. Now we are hopeful that it will begin to tell us what should be done *now* for the hearing-impaired infant. If such prediction for management can be achieved, it will mean that we have come a long way on the road toward giving the deaf their birthright: an adequate language system for modern day communication.

Whether such a weighted scale can be developed to be universally useful depends on input from people with a great variety of expertise. Such a scale may be of benefit to the audiologists who elect to look at the ultimate welfare of the child. Another need is to have available in every community a variety of programs from which a selection can be made for each individual child: auditory, oral, or total communication. In this way, the program can be fitted to the child rather than the child to the program. Audiologists must better acquaint themselves with deaf education techniques, not only oral but also manual, and learn what is meant by the concept of total communication. We need to give the infant who requires it, a total program with the complete language forms that will tap his biological language system at the critical age. When these priorities are met, audiologists can assume their places as advocates for the deaf child's maximal welfare.

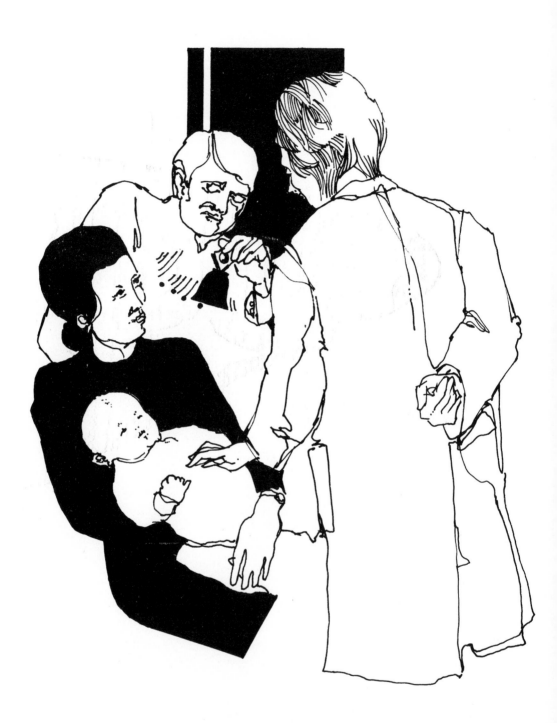

9 CLASSIFICATION OF HEREDITARY DEAFNESS AND AN INDEX OF AUDIOLOGIC DISORDERS

The evaluation of audiologic disorders in children is not an easy task. The clinician must be able to assimilate pieces of information, reach a cohesive and accurate description of the child's hearing status, and make decisions accurately and quickly. It is therefore important to recognize congenital malformations which will alert the clinician to the possibility of an unsuspected hearing loss (Stewart and Bergstrom, 1971).

Many clues may be obtained in your initial observation of the child. As an example, skeletal or facial malformations can alert the clinician to the possible presence of hearing loss; skin disorders may be related to inner ear problems; many chromosome abnormalities have associated hearing loss. Knowledge about the relationship of hearing loss to various types of observable disorders may direct the clinician's attention to specific procedures which will identify the nature of the hearing loss.

The alert clinician is soon aware that malformations and anomalies often "run together." Congenital defects are often caused by prenatal misfortunes which may influence the development of specific body systems or create generalized malformations of all the structures undergoing growth at that time. On the other hand, when multiple congenital malformations appear together frequently, the patient can be described in terms of a "syndrome." The term syndrome is often over-used and misapplied. The difficulties of syndrome classification lie in terminology problems, broad spectra of signs and symptoms, and differences in the basis of diagnosis depending on whether the diagnosis is anatomic, histologic, or hematologic. Often experts disagree on the diagnosis of a syndrome, or the youngster may present such a variety of symptomatic signs that clear-cut diagnosis is not possible. The definition of a syndrome depends on the level of acuity of observation, and becomes easier the more pronounced the accompanying features are demonstrated.

Just because hearing loss may be commonly associated with these disorders, don't be too quick to jump to a conclusion. Many children may likely be candidates for ultimate syndrome diagnosis, but hearing loss will not always be present. In addition, be aware that some of these disorders may manifest progressive-type hearing loss; so that although normal hearing is noted on the initial visit, these children deserve regular reevaluation. The verification of hearing loss is the realm of the audiologist who can substantiate accurately hearing levels in such children with appropriate testing techniques.

A synopsis of various syndromes is presented in an "Index of Birth Defect Syndromes." The material is a summary of information we feel is pertinent to the clinician. The information is by no means intended to be exhaustive or even complete; our intent is to provide a concise, clear, and informative reference regarding special patients who have an inordinately high risk for impairment of their hearing. We recognize that children with symptoms that are variants from our generalized information about each disorder will be seen, and that readers will immediately wish to revise our summary. So be it; our intent is only to provide an orientation, or a guide, to clinicians who might come into contact with children who demonstrate these disorders and to instill a desire to learn more about the disease.

There are many ways of classifying hereditary deafness. Martensson (1960) suggests a classification system that utilizes the genetic mode of transmission, listing various diseases associated with deafness by their mode of inheritance pattern such as dominant, recessive, sex-linked, etc. Kinney (1950) suggests grouping of deafness disorders by clinical manifestations, while Omerod (1960) classifies inherited deafness by the pathology of the auditory

273

system. Proctor and Proctor (1967) provide a classification that combines the genetic and clinical method of grouping under etiologic factors. The recent reference, *Congenital Deafness,* by Black et al. (1971a), presents an excellent summary of hereditary deafness as classified by each of the above mentioned systems. Konigsmark (1969) reports that over 60 types of hereditary deafness can be separated from one another by considering factors such as type of hearing loss, age of onset, severity of hearing loss, mode of genetic transmission, and abnormalities caused in other systems by the abnormal gene or pair of genes. Our choice of classification system (Bergstrom et al., 1971) is ordered around types of hearing loss and body systems as shown in the following section.

CLASSIFICATION OF HEREDITARY DEAFNESS

CONGENITAL SENSORINEURAL HEARING LOSS DISORDERS

Craniofacial and Skeletal Disorders
Absence of tibia
Cleidocranial dysostosis
Diastrophic dwarfism
Hand-hearing syndrome
Klippel-Feil
Saddle nose and myopia
Split-hand and foot
Integumentary and Pigmentary Disorders
Albinism with blue irides
Congenital atopic dermatitis
Ectodermal dysplasia
Keratopachyderma
Lentigines
Onychodystrophy
Partial albinism
Piebaldness
Pili torti
Waardenburg's syndrome
Eye Disorders
Hallgren's
Laurence-Moon-Biedl-Bardet
Nervous System Disorders
Cerebral palsy
Muscular dystrophy
Myoclonic epilepsy
Opticocochleodentate degeneration
Richards-Rundel
Cardiovascular System Disorders
Jervell and Lange-Nielsen
Endocrine and Metabolic Disorders
Goiter
Hyperprolinemia I
Iminoglycinuria
Pendred's

Miscellaneous Somatic Disorders
Trisomy 13-15
Trisomy 18

CONGENITAL CONDUCTIVE HEARING LOSS DISORDERS

Craniofacial and Skeletal Disorders
Apert's syndrome
Fanconi anemia syndrome
Goldenhar's syndrome
Madelung's deformity
Malformed, low set ears
Mohr syndrome
Otopalatodigital
Preauricular appendages
Proximal symphalangism
Thickened ears
Treacher Collins
Integumentary and Pigmentary Disorders
Forney's syndrome
Eye Disorders
Cryptophthalmos
Duane's syndrome
Renal Disorders
Nephrosis, urinary tract malformations
Renal-genital syndrome
Taylor's syndrome

DISORDERS OF CONGENITAL SENSORINEURAL AND/OR CONDUCTIVE HEARING LOSS

Craniofacial and Skeletal Disorders
Achondroplasia
Crouzon's syndrome
Marfan's syndrome
Pierre Robin
Pyle's disease

Integumentary and Pigmentary Disorders
  Knuckle pads and leukonychia
Eye Disorders
  Moebius syndrome
Miscellaneous Somatic Disorders
  Turner's syndrome

PROGRESSIVE HEARING LOSS DISORDERS

**Sensorineural Progressive Hearing
Loss of Later Onset**
  Craniofacial and Skeletal Disorders
    Roaf's syndrome
    Van Buchem's syndrome
  Eye Disorders
    Alstrom's syndrome
    Cockayne's syndrome
    Fehr's corneal dystrophy
    Flynn-Aird
    Norrie's syndrome
    Optic atrophy and diabetes mellitus
    Refsum's syndrome
  Nervous System Disorders
    Acoustic neuromas
    Friedreich's ataxia
    Herrmann's syndrome
    Myoclonic seizures
    Sensory radicular neuropathy
    Severe infantile muscular dystrophy
  Endocrine and Metabolic Disorders
    Alport's syndrome
    Amyloidosis, nephritis, and urticaria
    Hyperprolinemia II
    Hyperuricemia
    Primary testicular insufficiency
**Sensorineural or Conductive Progressive
Hearing Loss**
  Craniofacial and Skeletal Disorders
    Albers-Schönberg disease
    Englemann's syndrome
    Osteogenesis imperfecta
    Paget's disease
  Endocrine and Metabolic Disorders
    Hunter's syndrome
    Hurler's syndrome
**Progressive Conductive or Mixed
Hearing Loss**
  Otosclerosis

Childhood deafness associated with other defects has been observed for hundreds of years

and cited in journal articles too numerous to count. Konigsmark (1969) indicates that about 70 types of hereditary deafness have been identified in man. Only recently, since the mid-1960's, have data been available regarding the relative frequency of various syndrome complexes which include deafness (Fraser et al., 1964; Brown and Chung, 1964; Bergsma, 1973). Most reports and syndrome descriptions are case studies, and the existence of hearing loss may not have been evaluated or was not of significant interest to the author to be included in his report. Confusion between mental retardation and deafness complicates the issue further. In multiple reports of some syndromes by different investigators, the description of the syndromes may be so variable as to raise the question of whether the same or different syndromes are being discussed. Most hereditary deafness is not associated with a syndrome, per se, yet the incidence of children with syndromes in medical settings is sufficient to warrant knowledge by the clinician in relating deafness to common physical anomalies.

Some students may wish to consult more general reference sources for detailed accounts of syndromes included in this section of the book, or to pursue information on syndromes not included in this Index. Such general references cover much more than individual articles, and may touch on many aspects of the disorders not covered in our necessarily scant summaries. Accordingly, such a list is given below which we have found immeasurably useful in our review of birth defects associated with hearing loss.

GENERAL REFERENCES

Bergsma, D. (Ed.): Birth Defects: Atlas and Compendium. Baltimore, The Williams & Wilkins Co., 1973.
Black, F. O., Bergstrom, L., Downs, M., and Hemenway, W. G.: Congenital Deafness. A New Approach to Early Detection Through a High Risk Register. Boulder, University of Colorado Associated Press, 1971.
Ford, F. R.: Diseases of the Nervous System in Infancy, Childhood, and Adolescence, 5th Ed. Springfield, Ill., Charles C Thomas,

Publisher, 1966.

Gellis, S. S., and Feingold, M.: Atlas of Mental Retardation Syndromes. Washington, D. C., U.S. Dept. of HEW, 1968.

Gorlin, R. J., and Pindborg, J. J.: Syndromes of Head and Neck. New York, McGraw-Hill, 1964.

Hemenway, W. G., and Bergstrom, L. (Eds.): Symposium on Congenital Deafness. Otolar-yngol. Clin. North Am. 4: 1971.

Lindsay, J. R.: Profound childhood deafness. Ann. Otol. Rhinol. Laryngol. (Suppl. 5), 82, 1973.

Smith, D. W.: Recognizable Patterns of Human Malformation. Philadelphia, W. B. Saunders Co., 1970.

Warkany, J.: Congenital Malformations. Chicago, Year Book Medical Publishers, 1971.

BIRTH DEFECTS WITH ASSOCIATED HEARING LOSS

Absence of the Tibia. Recessive trait marked by obvious shortened lower legs (Konigsmark, 1969). Skeletal disorder; sensorineural hearing loss.

Achondroplasia. See below in "Index of Birth Defect Syndromes."

Acoustic Neuromas. Dominant. Progressive, bilateral sensorineural hearing loss beginning in the second or third decade of life. Ataxia, visual loss, and involvement of cranial nerves V-X may be seen. Neurofibromas or cafe-au-lait spots are seldom seen. Nervous system disorder; sensorineural progressive hearing loss.

Albers-Schönberg Disease of Osteopetrosis. Recessive. Onset of recurrent cranial nerve palsies, especially facial; may occur in childhood. Brittle but, paradoxically, sclerotic thickened bones. Malignant type leads to obliteration of bone marrow, severe anemia, and rapid demise. Benign type associated with large skull and mandible, excessive height, and leonine facies by teen years. Occasional increased intracranial pressure. Craniofacial and skeletal disorder; progressive sensorineural or conductive hearing loss.

Albinism with Blue Irides. Dominant. Scalp hair white, fine, and silky, sometimes with patches of pigmentation. Few show heterochromia of iris. Fair skin. Integumentary and pigmentary disorder with sensorineural hearing loss.

Alport's Syndrome. See below in "Index of Birth Defect Syndromes."

Alstrom's Syndrome. Recessive. Onset of nystagmus and sensitivity to light; visual loss due to retinal degeneration about age 1. Hearing loss beginning about age 10 and diabetes mellitus in adolescence. Obesity since infancy. Eye disorder with progressive sensorineural hearing loss of late onset.

Apert's Syndrome of Acrocephalosyndactyly. See below in "Index of Birth Defect Syndromes."

Amyloidosis, Nephritis, and Urticaria. Dominant. Onset in teens of recurrent urticaria (vascular reaction of skin with elevated patches and itching) with malaise and chills. Amyloidosis (starchy-like substance in the blood) precedes nephropathy and renal failure. Progression of hearing loss parallels progression of renal failure. Endocrine and metabolic disorder with sensorineural hearing loss of late onset.

Cerebral Palsy. Recessive or sporadic trait. Paralysis due to a lesion of the brain, usually suffered at birth, and characterized by uncontrollable motor spasms.

Cerebral palsy involves paralysis, weakness, incoordination, or other abnormality of motor function due to pathology of the motor control centers of the brain. Damage to the brain may occur during embryonic, fetal, or early infantile life. Essentially nonprogressive, clinical symptoms of the disorder include spasticity (40%), athetosis (40%), ataxia (10%), or combinations of these basic motor dysfunctions. Mental deficiency and convulsive disorders are also common. Feeding problems, retarded growth, eye difficulties such as strabismus and nystagmus, developmental delay, orthopedic problems, communication disorders, and educational problems often are evidenced in varying degrees.

Damage to the brain may occur during embryonic, fetal, or early infantile life and may result from an antecedent disorder such as trauma, metabolic disorder or infection, destructive intercranial cerebral processes, and/or developmental defects of the brain. Location of the lesion may be in cerebral cortex, basal ganglia, or other sites in the pyramidal system or extrapyramidal system; coexistent involvement in both systems is observed. Less frequently, cerebellar damage may be evident. Patients may have mild to moderate sensorineural hearing loss, typically more severe in high frequencies.

Cleidocranial Dysostosis. Dominant inheritance. See below in "Index of Birth Defect Syndromes."

Cockayne's Syndrome. Recessive. Dwarfism, mental retardation, retinal atrophy, and motor disturbances. Progressive disorder. Appearance normal at birth. Growth and development normal through first year. During second year growth falls below normal range and mental-motor development becomes abnormal. Minimal diagnostic characteristics include dwarfism, retinal degeneration, microcephaly, cataracts, neurologic impairment including progressive mental retardation, sun-sensitive skin, thickening of the skull bones, disproportionately long extremities with large hands and feet, eye disorder, and progressive sensorineural hearing loss of later onset.

Congenital Atopic Dermatitis. Recessive. Congenital moderate hearing loss which may not be detected until school years. About age 10, affected persons develop lichenified, skin eruptions especially on forearms, hands, elbows, and sometimes the waist. Integumentary and pigmentary disorder with congenital sensorineural hearing loss.

Crouzon's Syndrome of Craniofacial Dysostosis. See below in "Index of Birth Defect Syndromes."

Cryptophthalmus. Recessive. Adherent eyelids which hide the eyes, often accompanied by external ear malformations. In its most severe form, it is bilateral without recognizable differentiation of the lids and its associated structures of lashes and brows; in less severe form, the upper or lower lid may be absent. Eye disorder which may be accompanied by congenital conductive hearing loss.

Diastrophic Dwarfism. Recessive trait. Marked shortness of stature, characteristic hand deformity with short fingers, and severe bilateral clubfoot. The auricles show cystic swellings in infancy which later develop into cauliflower-like deformities which may calcify. There is a 25% incidence of cleft palate (Hall, 1969). Craniofacial disorder; congenital sensorineural hearing loss.

Duane's Syndrome. Recessive. Congenital paralysis of the sixth nerve manifested by a partial or complete failure to abduct eyes, retraction of globe in adduction. Usually unilateral, and may be accompanied by external ear malformation. Eye disorder with congenital conductive hearing loss.

Ectodermal Dysplasia. Sparce, thin, fragile hair on head, eyebrows, and body with reduced tensile strength. Thick nails with subungual infections. Thick rough skin of palms and soles with brownish pigmentation. Normal sweat glands and teeth. Integumentary and pigmentary disorder with congenital sensorineural hearing loss.

Engelmann's Syndrome or Diaphysial Dysplasia. Dominant. Onset in first and second decades of life of progressive cortical thickening of diaphysial regions of long bones and of skull. Cranial nerve symptoms may be seen. Craniofacial disorder; sensorineural or conductive progressive hearing loss.

Fanconi Anemia Syndrome. Recessive. Includes absence or deformity of thumbs; other skeletal, heart, and kidney malformations; skin pigmentation; and mental retardation (McDonough, 1970). Craniofacial-skeletal disorder; congenital conductive hearing loss.

Fehr's Corneal Dystrophy. Recessive. Progressive visual loss to blindness by about age 40. Eye disorder; progressive sensorineural hearing loss of later onset.

Forney's Syndrome. Dominant. Lentigines,

mitral valve insufficiency and skeletal malformations. Integumentary-pigmentary disorder; congenital conductive hearing loss.

Flynn-Aird. Dominant. Progressive myopia, cataracts, retinitis pigmentosa, and hearing loss beginning in first decade of life. Ataxia, shooting pains, and joint symptoms beginning in second decade. Eye disorder; sensorineural progressive hearing loss of later onset.

Friedreich's Ataxia. Recessive. Childhood onset of nystagmus, ataxia, optic atrophy, hyperreflexia, and hearing loss. Nervous system disorder; progressive sensorineural hearing loss of later onset.

Goiter, Stippled Epiphysis and High Protein-Bound Iodine (PBI). Congenital metabolic defect associated with thyroid over-activity, congenital profound sensorineural deafness, bird-like facies, pigeon breast, and winged scapulae. Goiter appears in early infancy. Endocrine-metabolic disorder; congenital sensorineural hearing loss.

Goldenhar's Syndrome or Oculoauriculovertebral Dysplasia. Recessive. See below in "Index of Birth Defect Syndromes."

Hallgren's Syndrome. Recessive trait. Described by Hallgren in 1959. Retinitis pigmentosa, progressive ataxia, and mental retardation in 25% of cases. Of such patients 90% have profound deafness and 90% have a gait disturbance. Eye disorder; congenital sensorineural hearing loss.

Hand-Hearing Syndrome. Dominant inheritance, recently described by Stewart and Bergstrom (1971). This disorder has typical congenital hand malformations with flexion contractures and muscular atrophy. Craniofacial-skeletal disorder; congenital sensorineural hearing loss.

Herrmann's Syndrome. Dominant. Late childhood or adolescent onset of photomyoclonus and hearing loss followed by diabetes mellitus, progressive dementia, pyelonephritis, and glomerulonephritis. Nervous system disorder; sensorineural progressive hearing loss of later onset.

Hurler's Syndrome (Recessive) and Hunter's Syndrome (X-linked). See below in "Index of Birth Defect Syndromes."

Hyperprolinemia I. Dominant. No proven association with clinical disease, although identified frequently in pedigrees with renal disease or convulsive disorders. May demonstrate seizures, growth retardation, and microscopic hematuria. Endocrine-metabolic disorder; congenital sensorineural hearing loss.

Hyperprolinemia II. Dominant. Ichthyosis, renal disease manifested by hematuria, calculi, renal cysts, and renal failure. Endocrine-metabolic disorder; sensorineural progressive hearing loss of later onset.

Hyperuricemia. Dominant. Early pubescent onset of hyperuricemia, followed by progressive sensorineural hearing loss, ataxia, and renal failure. Cardiopathy, myopathy, and gout have been seen in some patients. Endocrine-metabolic disorder; sensorineural progressive hearing loss of later onset.

Iminoglycinuria. Dominant trait. Selective impairment of cellular transport of the iminoglycine group of amino acids. No specific physical findings. Endocrine-metabolic disorder; congenital sensorineural hearing loss.

Jervell and Lange-Nielsen Syndrome. Recessive trait. Described by Jervell and Lange-Nielsen in 1957 as congenital total deafness and functional heart disease, with possible sudden death. Afflicted individuals usually die in childhood, but postmortem examination shows no organic heart defect. Cardiovascular system disorder; congenital sensorineural hearing loss.

Keratopachyderma, Digital Constrictions. Dominant trait. Hyperkeratosis of palms, soles, elbows, and knees. Digital band-like constrictions of finger creases develop about age 4 or 5. Patients show congenital high frequency sensorineural hearing loss. Integumentary-pigmentary disorder; congenital sensorineural hearing loss.

Klippel-Feil Syndrome. See below in "Index of Birth Defect Syndromes."

Knuckle Pads and Leukonychia. Dominant. Callous-like thickening over dorsal aspects of interphalangeal joints of fingers and toes first observed in infancy and early childhood. Progressive whitening of finger and toe nails. Integumentary-pigmentary disorder; congenital sensorineural or conductive hearing loss.

Laurence-Moon-Biedl-Bardet Syndrome. Recessive inheritance. Recognized in 1866 as

dwarfism accompained by obesity, hypo-
gonadism, retinitis pigmentosa, night blindness, and mental retardation. Eye disorder;
congenital sensorineural hearing loss.

Lentigines. Dominant trait. Freckly eruption of
brown spots on the skin, appearing about age
2 years. Electrocardiographic anomalies, retardation of growth, abnormalities of the
genitalia, and ocular hypertelorism. Integumentary-pigmentary disorder; congenital
sensorineural hearing loss.

Madelung's Deformity. Dominant. Mild dwarfism with thickening of the long bones,
limitation of motion at elbow and wrist, club
foot, spina bifida occulata, accompanied by
pain during periods of skeletal growth (Nassif
and Harboyan, 1970). Facioskeletal disorder
with congenital conductive hearing loss.

Malformed, Low Set Ears. Recessive. Mild to
moderate hearing loss, always conductive,
and usually worse in the most affected
external ear. Mental retardation in 50% of
cases. Craniofacial disorder; congenital conductive hearing loss.

Marfan's Syndrome. Dominant inheritance.
May also show progressive-type hearing loss.
Individual appears thin and elongated, with
long, spidery fingers, pigeon breast, hammer
toes, lateral deviation of the spine, and a long
head. Craniofacial-skeletal disorder; congenital sensorineural and/or conductive hearing
loss.

Moebius Syndrome. Recessive. Bilateral congenital facial paralysis, severe but incomplete, with varying degrees of ophthal-
moplegia, external ear malformations,
micrognathia. Hands, feet, or digits may be
missing; tongue paralysis and mental retardation may be present. Middle ear anomalies
may be associated, as well as aberrant facial
nerve. Eye disorder; congenital sensorineural
and/or conductive hearing loss.

Mohr Syndrome or Oral-Facial-Digital II. Recessive trait. Involves oral, facial, and digital
abnormalities including nodular tongue, midline cleft lip, small mandible, polydactyly,
syndactyly, bifid tip of nose, thick lingual
frenum, and widely spaced medial canthi of
eyes. No effect on intelligence, but conductive loss may interfere with learning, and oral

deformities may cause speech dysfluencies.
Craniofacial-skeletal disorder; congenital conductive hearing loss.

Muscular Dystrophy. Recessive trait. Muscle
wasting with possible later retinal detachment. Nervous system disorder; congenital
sensorineural hearing loss.

Myoclonic Epilepsy. Recessive. A seizure disorder characterized by "absence" attacks and
myoclonic jerks usually involving the muscles
of the face and arms in a symmetric fashion.
Nervous system disorder; congenital sensorineural hearing loss.

Myoclonic Seizures. Also includes cerebellar
ataxia and hearing loss. Nervous system
disorder; progressive sensorineural hearing
loss of later onset.

Myopia and Mental Retardation. Recessive
genetic trait. Congenital severe myopia and
mild retardation. Eye disorder; congenital
sensorineural hearing loss.

Nephrosis, Urinary Tract Malformations. Sex-
linked or recessive. Bifid uvula and shorten-
ing or broadening of the distal parts of
fingers and toes. Renal disorder; congenital
conductive hearing loss.

Norrie's Syndrome. Recessive. Congenital blindness due to pseudotumor retini. Hearing loss
in 25% to 30% of patients. Eye disorder;
progressive sensorineural hearing loss.

Onychodystrophy. Recessive. Characterized by
soft, brown, pitted teeth; short, small finger
and toe nails; diminished sweat gland response; rough, dry skin; and scalp dermatitis
(Feinmesser and Zelig, 1961). Integumentary-pigmentary disorder; congenital sensorineural hearing loss.

Optic Atrophy and Diabetes Mellitus. Recessive. Progressive visual and hearing losses first
decade of life. Onset of mild diabetes first or
second decade. Eye disorder; congenital
progressive sensorineural hearing loss of later
onset.

Optic Atrophy and Polyneuropathy. Recessive
or sex-linked. Progressive congenital hearing
loss, with progressive peripheral neuropathy
and optic atrophy. Eye disorder; congenital
sensorineural hearing loss.

Opticocochleodentate Degeneration. Recessive
trait. Characterized by blindness, optic atrophy, and motor spasticity. Nervous system

disorder; congenital sensorineural hearing loss.

Osteogenesis Imperfecta. See below in "Index of Birth Defect Syndromes."

Otopalatodigital Syndrome. Recessive. Cleft palate, stubby clubbed fingers and toes, wide-spaced nasal bridge giving pugilistic facies, low set and small ears, winged scapulae, downward obliquity of the eyes, and down-turned mouth. Craniofacial-skeletal disorder; congenital conductive hearing loss.

Partial Albinism. Sex-linked or recessive inheritance. May have absence of pigment in iris, sclera, fundus with associated ophthalmologic disorders. May demonstrate total deafness. Integumentary-pigmentary disorder; congenital sensorineural hearing loss.

Paget's Disease or Osteitis Deformans. Dominant. Onset in middle age of long bone and cranial deformities and cranial nerve palsies. Craniofacial-skeletal disorder; sensorineural or conductive progressive hearing loss.

Pendred's Syndrome. Recessive trait. Described in 1896 by Pendred as nonendemic goiter and total deafness. In 1927 Brian concluded that the deafness and goiter were independent manifestations of the same recessive genetic defect. A very common disorder, it is estimated that 10% of recessive deafness is due to this syndrome. The etiology involves abnormal metabolism of iodine. The goiter, or thyroid enlargement, appears during childhood, and the gland becomes nodular during adult life. Deafness is sensorineural and most severe in high frequencies. Endocrine and metabolic disorder; congenital sensorineural hearing loss.

Piebaldness. Sex-linked or recessive. Absence of skin pigmentation primarily on the ventral surfaces of the body, with normal pigmentation on the occiput, back of the neck and mid-dorsal surface of the trunk. Heterochromia is occasionally present, or blue irides. Integumentary-pigmentary disorder; congenital sensorineural hearing loss.

Pierre Robin Syndrome. Dominant. Oral findings include cleft palate, smallness of the jaw and chin, and downward displacement or retraction of the tongue. Ears may be low set. About 20% of cases associated with mental retardation. Craniofacial-skeletal disorder; congenital sensorineural and/or conductive hearing loss.

Pili Torti. Recessive. Dry, brittle, twisted hair. Integumentary-pigmentary disorder; congenital sensorineural hearing loss.

Preauricular Appendages. Dominant. May be seen in patients with normal pinnae, deformed or low set ears. Includes preauricular pits which frequently become infected, and external auditory atresia. Craniofacial-skeletal disorder; congenital conductive hearing loss.

Primary Testicular Insufficiency. X-linked, recessive, or sex-limited dominant. Early onset of blindness; onset by school years of "partial" hearing loss; normal virilization, small testes, and hyperuricemia (Weinstein, et al., 1969).Endocrine-metabolic disorder; sensorineural progressive hearing loss of later onset.

Proximal Symphalangism. Dominant. Stiff fingers and toes due to bony ankylosis of the proximal interphalangeal joints. Conductive loss due to stapes fixation. Skeletal disorder; congenital conductive hearing loss.

Pyle's Disease of Craniometaphysial Dysplasia. Dominant. Hearing loss may also be progressive and is usually of the mixed type. Patient characterized by splayed appearance of the long bones. Craniofacial-skeletal disorder; congenital sensorineural and/or conductive hearing loss.

Refsum's Syndrom. Recessive. Onset in second decade with visual loss and night blindness due to retinitis pigmentosa, progressive ataxia, muscle wasting, and peripheral sensory loss. Ichthyosis. Biochemical defects. Eye disorder; sensorineural progressive hearing loss of late onset.

Renal-Genital Syndrome. Recessive. Low set ears; stenotic external canals may be present; vaginal atresia. Renal disorder; congenital conductive hearing loss.

Richards-Rundel. Recessive. Congenital, severe, progressive hearing loss. Ataxia, muscle wasting in early childhood. Nystagmus, absent deep tendon reflexes, mental retardation, and failure to develop secondary sexual characteristics. Nervous system disorder; congenital sensorineural hearing loss.

Roaf's Syndrome. Not hereditary. Congenital or early retinal detachment, cataracts, myopia, shortened long bones, and mental retardation. Craniofacial-skeletal disorder; sensorineural progressive hearing loss of later onset.

Saddle Nose and Myopia. Dominant trait, characterized by severe myopia, cataracts and congenital saddle nose deformity (Ruppert et al., 1970). Craniofacial-skeletal disorder; congenital sensorineural hearing loss.

Sensory Radicular Neuropathy. Dominant. Onset in late teens or early adulthood of painless ulcerations of feet and progressive sensorineural hearing loss. Nervous system disorder; sensorineural progressive hearing loss of later onset.

Severe Infantile Muscular Dystrophy. Recessive. Congenital facial weakness with resultant difficulty in hearing, followed by abnormal gait, weakness of proximal and distal musculature. Nervous system disorder; sensorineural progressive hearing loss of later onset.

Split-Hand and Foot. Recessive inheritance. Hands show partial syndactyly and absence of some fingers. Diminished vestibular response (Konigsmark, 1969). Skeletal disorder; congenital sensorineural hearing loss.

Taylor's Syndrome. Recessive trait. Unilateral microtia or anotia (congenital absence of the external ears), with unilateral facial bone hypoplasia. Renal disorder; congenital conductive hearing loss.

Thickened Ears. Dominant. Craniofacial disorder; congenital conductive hearing loss.

Trisomy 13-15. See below in "Index of Birth Defect Syndromes."

Trisomy 18. See below in "Index of Birth Defect Syndromes."

Treacher Collins Syndrome or Mandibular Dysostosis. See below in "Index of Birth Defect Syndromes."

Turner's Syndrome. Chromosome defect, not inherited. Low hairline, webbing of neck, widely spaced nipples, shield-like chest, webbing of digits. Chromosomal abnormality recognizable at birth by webbing or loose folds of skin of short neck, swelling of dorsa of hands and feet, deep creases on thickened palms and soles, hypertelorism, epicanthic folds, ptosis of upper lids, elongated "gothic" ears, high arched palate, micrognathia, pinpoint nipples, and enlarged clitoris. Fingernails are hypoplastic and appear small. Later manifestations include shortness of stature, ocular manifestations, hearing impairment, impairment of taste, congenital cardiovascular disease, anomalies of kidneys, and sexual infantilism. It occurs only in females. Mentality may be normal. Mild sensorineural and conductive hearing loss has been reported. Anderson et al. (1969) reported audiometric findings from 79 patients with Turner's syndrome. Of the 79 patients, 64% had sensorineural hearing loss with a bilaterally symmetrical dip in the mid-frequency range. An additional 22% showed a conductive or mixed hearing loss. Conductive hearing loss has been attributed to frequent middle ear infections in infancy and early childhood, but congenital hearing loss has also been observed.

Usher's Syndrome. Recessive. This syndrome of familial retinitis pigmentosa and deafness was first described by Von Graefe in 1858 and later by Usher (1914). Clinical symptoms include increasing contraction of the visual field, causing night blindness and possible cataracts. The hearing loss is bilateral, cochlear, and usually develops late after the patient's visual fields have narrowed. A chronic progressive degenerative disease of the inner layer of the retina. Eye disorder; congenital sensorineural hearing loss.

Van Buchem's Syndrome or Generalized Cortical Hyperostosis. Recessive. Onset during puberty. Lion-like facial expression, square jaw, optic atrophy. Craniofacial-skeletal disorder; sensorineural hearing loss of later onset.

Waardenburg's Syndrome. See below in "Index of Birth Defect Syndromes."

Wildervanck's Syndrome or Otofaciocervical Dysmorphia. Dominant. Depressed nasal root, protruding narrow nose, narrow elongated face, flattened maxilla and zygoma, prominent ears, preauricular fistulas, poorly developed neck muscles. Combines the Klippel-Feil characteristics with retraction of the eyeball, sixth nerve paralysis, and total deafness. Integumentary and pigmentary disorder; congenital sensorineural hearing loss.

AN INDEX
OF SELECTED
BIRTH DEFECT SYNDROMES

ACHONDROPLASIA
(Chondrodystrophia Fetalis)

(Figs. 9.1, 9.2)

MAJOR DIAGNOSTIC FEATURES

A congenital skeletal anomaly characterized by slow growth of cartilage, retarded endochondrial ossification, and almost normal periosteal bone formation. As a result those affected are very ᐧshort in stature with disproportionately short limbs, large heads with prominent foreheads, depressed nasal bridge, and "button" nose. Mentality is usually normal but retardation may appear secondary to hydrocephalus and increased cranial pressure. Deafness may be present. Respiratory, pulmonary, and other complications increase with age. Diagnosis may be suspected by clinical examination, but is confirmed by radiographic evaluation.

ETIOLOGY

Hereditary dominant disorder. However, over 80% of cases are due to fresh mutation, both parents being normal. Incidence increases with increasing parental age.

RELATED AUDITORY PROBLEMS

Both conductive and/or sensorineural loss

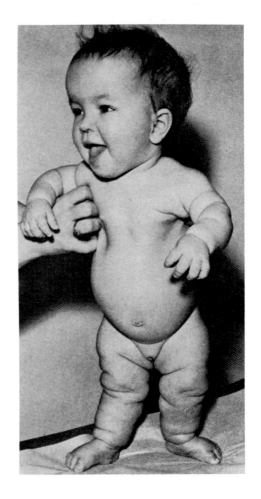

Fig. 9.1. Achondroplasia. Note short stature, disproportionate length legs, and large head. (With permission from T. H. Shepard and B. Graham: The congenitally malformed: achondroplastic dwarfism; diagnosis and management. Northwest Med. 66: 451-456, 1967.)

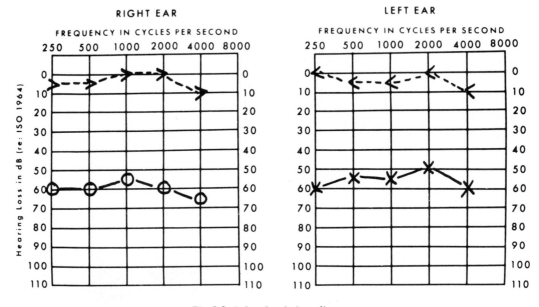

Fig. 9.2. Achondroplasia audiogram.

may be present. Middle ear anomalies include fusion of ossicles to surrounding bony structures as well as dense thick trabeculae without islands of cartilage in the endochondrial and periosteal bone. Associated anomalies of the inner ear include deformed cochlea and thickened intercochlear partitions. Incidence of serous otitis high.

GENERAL TREATMENT

Genetic counseling, surgical treatment as indicated.

REFERENCES

Cohen, M. E., et al.: Neurological abnormalities in achondroplastic children. J. Pediatr. 71: 367, 1967.

Langer, L. O., Jr.: Achondroplasia: Clinical radiologic features with comment on genetic implications. Clin. Pediatr. (Philadelphia) 7: 474–478, 1968.

Langer, L. O., Jr., et al.: Achondroplasia. Am. J. Roentgenol. 100: 12–15, 1967.

Shepard, T. H., and Graham, B.: The congenitally malformed: Achondroplastic dwarfism; diagnosis and management. Northwest Med. 66: 4, 451–456, 1967.

Yarington, C. T., and Sprinkle, P.: Hearing problems in certain forms of osteodystrophy: The chondrodystrophies. EENT Monthly 46: 1136–1138, 1967.

ALPORT'S SYNDROME
(Hereditary Nephritis and Nerve Deafness)

(Fig. 9.3)

MAJOR DIAGNOSTIC FEATURES

Renal disorder associated with deafness and ocular anomalies. More common in males than females. Few symptoms present at birth. Progressive characteristics include urinary hematuria and proteinuria, hypertension, deafness, cataracts, spherophakia, and anterior lenticonus.

ETIOLOGY

Autosomal dominant, transmitted by females but more common in males.

RELATED AUDITORY PROBLEMS

Bilateral progressive sensorineural hearing loss present in about 50% of cases. Audiograms generally show high frequency sensorineural loss in children after age 8, sloping sensorineural loss in early adult life, and possible complete loss of hearing in those most severely affected. Hearing loss at 4000 Hz has also been reported. Loudness recruitment, high SISI scores, absent tone decay, Type II Bekesy tracings are typical.

GENERAL TREATMENT

As indicated, generally results in death during third decade of life. Males have poorest outlook with death from uremia likely in teens or before third decade. Female survival is more variable, but they may also die of uremia.

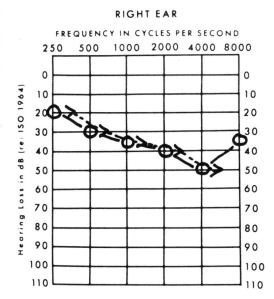

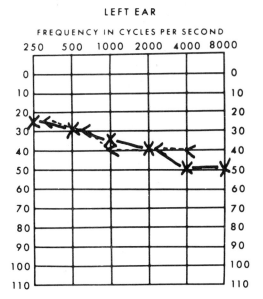

Fig. 9.3. Alport's syndrome audiogram. (With permission from W. T. Johnson and P. J. Hagen: Hereditary nephropathy and loss of hearing. Arch. Otolaryngol. 82: 166-172, 1965.)

REFERENCES

Bergstrom, L., Jenkins, P., Sando, I., and English, G. M.: Hearing loss in renal disease: Clinical and pathological studies. Ann. Otol. Rhinol. Laryngol. 82: 555–577, 1973.

Cohen, M. M., Cassady, G., and Hanna, B. L.: A genetic study of hereditary renal dysfunction with associated nerve deafness. Am. J. Hum. Genet. 13: 379, 1961.

Ferguson, A., and Rance, P.: Hereditary nephropathy with nerve deafness

(Alport's syndrome). Am. J. Dis. Child. 124: 84–88, 1972.

Goldbloom, R. B., Fraser, F. C., Waugh, D., Aronovitch, M., and Wiglesworth, F. W.: Hereditary renal disease associated with nerve deafness and ocular lesions. Pediatrics 20: 241, 1957.

Johnson, W. T., and Hagan, P. J.: Hereditary nephropathy and loss in hearing. Arch. Otolaryngol. 82: 166–172, 1965.

Perkoff, G. T.: The hereditary renal diseases. N. Engl. J. Med. 277: 79–85, 129–138, 1967.

APERT'S SYNDROME
(Acrocephalosyndactyly)

(Figs. 9.4–9.6)

MAJOR DIAGNOSTIC FEATURES

Skeletal and associated skull malformations which include craniofacial dysostosis, syndactyly, brachiocephaly, hypertelorism, bilateral proptosis, saddle nose, high arched palate, ankylosis of joints, and spinal bifida. Syndactyly (fusion of fingers and toes) is complete on both hands and feet. Hearing loss common. Characteristic "tower skull." Detectable at birth.

ETIOLOGY

Most reported cases appear sporadic. When reproduction is possible, the disorder is apparently of autosomal dominant transmission. There also appears to be a high mutation rate related to increasing parent age. Manifestation present at birth.

RELATED AUDITORY PROBLEMS

Audiometric findings usually indicate flat conductive loss. However, a sensorineural component is suspected in some cases. Surgical explorations have revealed congenital stapedial footplate fixation, abnormal patency of cochlear aqueduct, and enlarged internal auditory meati. Impedance audiometry shows manifestations of conductive hearing loss with low compliance and absent acoustic reflexes.

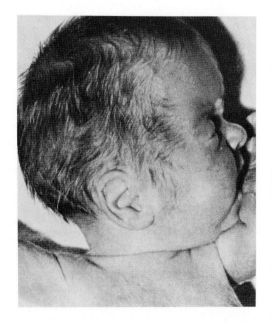

Fig. 9.4. Apert's syndrome with typical broad, flat skull, protrusion of the eyes, and flat maxillae. (With permission from F. O. Black, L. Bergstrom, W. G. Hemenway, and M. P. Downs: A high risk registry to find congenital deafness. Otolaryngol. Clin. North Am. 4: 369-399, 1971.)

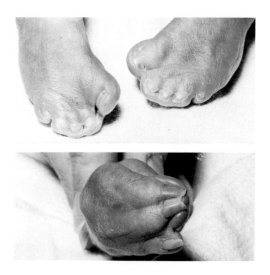

Fig. 9.5. Apert's syndrome with syndactyly of the hands and feet.

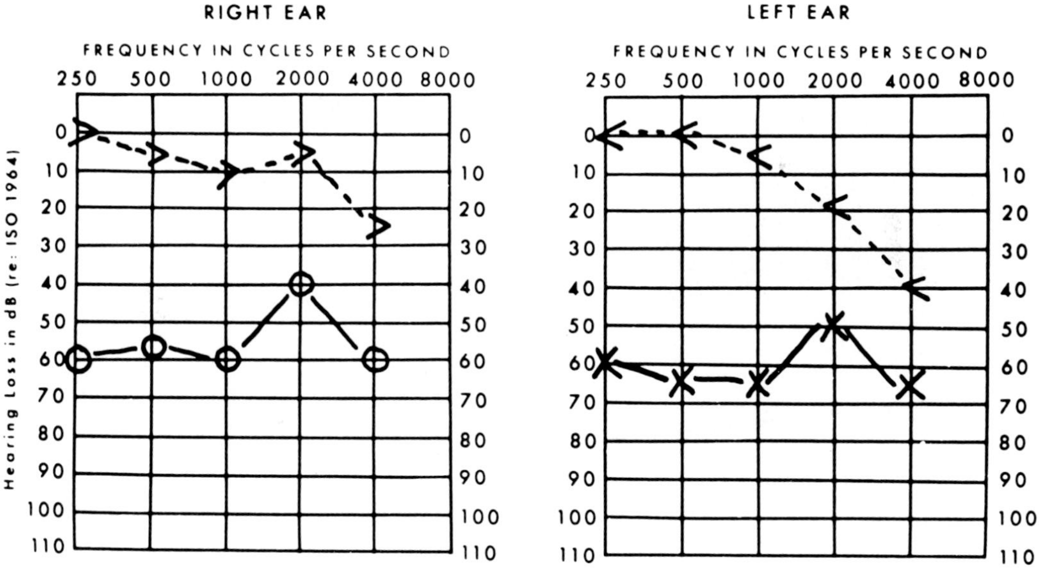

RIGHT EAR

FREQUENCY IN CYCLES PER SECOND

LEFT EAR

FREQUENCY IN CYCLES PER SECOND

Fig. 9.6. Apert's syndrome audiogram.

GENERAL TREATMENT

Surgical correction of skull and digital malformations if possible. Genetic counseling. Stapedectomy or hearing aid.

REFERENCES

Bergstrom, L., and Neblett, L. M.: Otologic manifestations of acrocephalosyndactylie. Arch. Otolaryngol. 96: 117-123, 1972.

Blank, C. E.: Apert's syndrome (a type of acrocephalosyndactyly): Observations on a British series of forty-nine cases. Ann. Hum. Genet. 24: 151-164, 1960.

Park, E. A., and Powers, G. F.: Acrocephaly and scaphocephaly with symmetrically distributed malformations of extremities: A study of so-called "acrocephalosyndactylism." Am. J. Dis. Child. 20: 235, 1920.

CLEIDOCRANIAL DYSOSTOSIS
(Cleidocranial Dysplasia; Osteodental Dysplasia)

(Figs. 9.7, 9.8)

MAJOR DIAGNOSTIC FEATURES

A general disorder of skeleton due to retarded ossification of membranous and cartilaginous precursors of bone characterized by congenital absence of clavicles, softness of skull, and irregular ossification of bones. In addition shortness of stature, narrow drooping shoulders, widely spaced eyes, irregular or absent teeth, and high arched palate or submucous cleft have been noted. Mental development is usually normal. Chromosome analyses show normal karyotypes.

ETIOLOGY

Autosomal dominant with high penetrance and wide variability in expression. About one-third of the cases appear to be sporadic.

RELATED AUDITORY PROBLEMS

Occasional deafness is reported. May be conductive or sensorineural due to retarded bone ossification.

GENERAL TREATMENT

Generally, treatment is limited as no serious

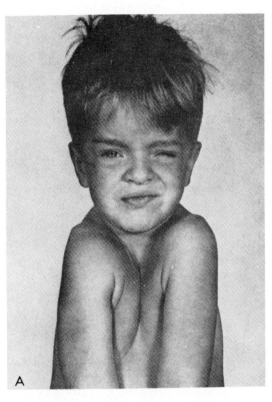
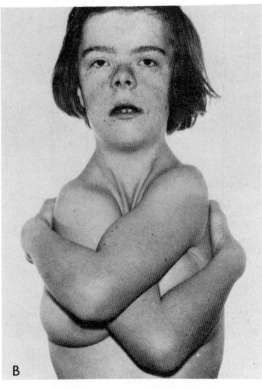

A

B

Fig. 9.7. Children with cleidocranial dysostosis. (Figures reproduced with permission. Boy (A) from I. S. Jaffee: Congenital shoulder-neck-auditory anomalies. Laryngoscope 58: 2119-2139, 1968; girl (B) from J. Fons: Ear malformations in cleidocranial dysostosis. Acta Otolaryngol. 67: 483-489, 1969.)

RIGHT EAR

LEFT EAR

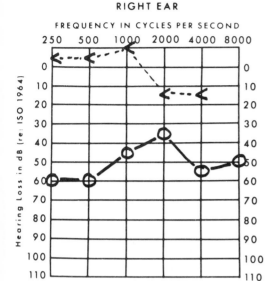

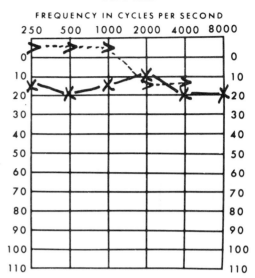

Fig. 9.8. Cleidocranial dysostosis audiogram. (With permission from J. Fons: Ear malformations in cleidocranial dysostosis. Acta Otolaryngol. 67: 483-489, 1969.)

handicap is evidenced. Dental and orthodontic treatment may be indicated. Genetic counseling is recommended.

REFERENCES

Fons, J.: Ear malformations in cleidocranial dysostosis. Acta Otolaryngol. (Stockh) 67: 483–489, 1969.

Forland, M.: Cleidocranial dysostosis: A review of the syndrome and report of a sporadic case with hereditary transmission. Am. J. Med. 33: 792, 1962.

Herndon, C. N.: Cleidocranial dysostosis. Am. J. Hum. Genet. 3: 314, 1951.

Jaffee, B. S.: Congenital shoulder-neck-auditory anomalies. Laryngoscope 58: 10, 2119–2139, 1968.

CROUZON'S SYNDROME
(Craniofacial Dysostosis)

(Figs. 9.9, 9.10)

MAJOR DIAGNOSTIC FEATURES

Abnormally shaped head characterized by a central prominence in the frontal region, a peculiar nose resembling a beak, and marked bilateral exophthalmos caused by premature closure of cranial sutures. Mentality may be low but usually is not unless there is brain damage secondary to increased intracranial pressure. Hearing loss. Bifid uvula and cleft palate may be present.

ETIOLOGY

Autosomal dominant with variable expression. Approximately one-fourth of reported cases arise as fresh mutations. Detected at birth or during first year.

RELATED AUDITORY PROBLEMS

Ears may be low set. Occasional deafness is reported, generally nonprogressive and conductive. Middle ear manifestations include deformed stapes with bony fusion of promontory, ankylosis of malleus to outer wall of the epitympanum, distortion and narrowing of middle ear space, and absence of the tympanic membrane. Stenosis or atresia of external canal common. Impedance audiometry may confirm presence of conductive hearing loss.

GENERAL TREATMENT

Early surgical intervention is usually recommended to prevent damage to the brain and eyes. Genetic counseling is recommended.

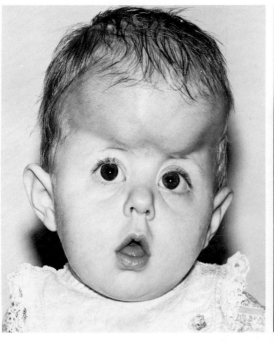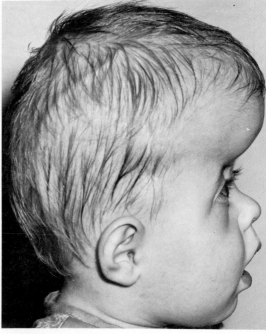

Fig. 9.9. Crouzon's syndrome. Deformity may vary with specific cranial sutures involved.

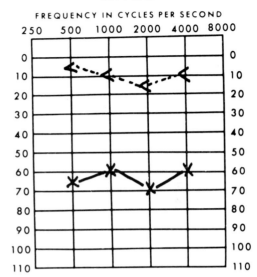

Fig. 9.10. Crouzon's syndrome audiogram. (With permission from F. O. Black, L. Bergstrom, M. P. Downs, and W. G. Hemenway: Congenital Deafness. Boulder, Colorado Associated Univ. Press, 1971.)

REFERENCES

Baldwin, J. L.: Dysostosis craniofacialis of Crouzon. Laryngoscope 78: 10, 1660–1675, 1968.
Dodge, H. W., Jr., Wood, M. W., and Kennedy, R. L. J.: Craniofacial dysostosis: Crouzon's disease. Pediatrics 23: 98, 1959.
Parks, M. M., and Castenbader, F. D.: Craniofacial dysostosis (Crouzon's disease). Am. J. Ophthalmol. 33: 77, 1950.
Schiller, J. G.: Craniofacial dysostosis of Crouzon: A case report and pedigree with emphasis on heredity. Pediatrics 23: 67, 1959.
Vulliamy, D. G., and Normandale, P. A.: Craniofacial dysostosis in a Dorset family. Arch. Dis. Child. 41: 375, 1966.

DOWN'S SYNDROME

(Figs. 9.11–9.13)

MAJOR DIAGNOSTIC FEATURES

Most common characteristics are facial appearance including epicanthal folds, oblique palpebral fissures, broad bridge of the nose, protruding tongue, open mouth, square-shaped ears, and flattened facial profile; mental retardation; muscular hypotonia; and congenital heart disease. Hands are also notably short and broad with simian line, abnormal dermatoglyphics.

ETIOLOGY

Majority are trisomic for chromosome 21 due to nondisjunction. Risk of trisomy 21 increases as maternal age increases. Translocation and mosaic types occur less frequently but can be carried by normal-appearing parent or sibling.

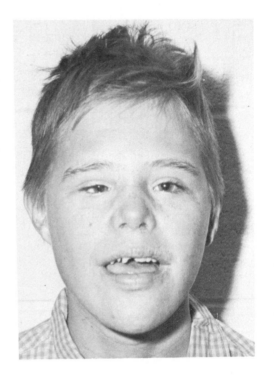

Fig. 9.11. Down's syndrome.

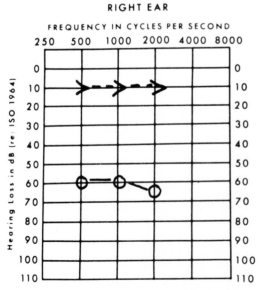
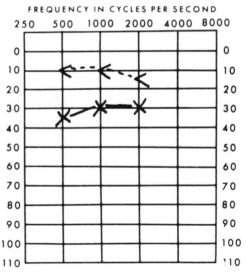

Fig. 9.12. Down's syndrome audiogram.

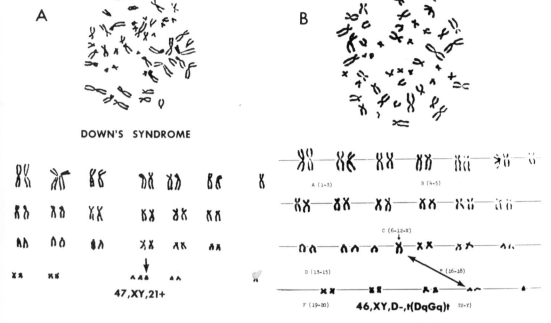

Fig. 9.13. Karyotypes of Down's syndrome. Note extra 21st chromosome (A) and translocation (B). Clinical manifestations of syndrome are indistinguishable in either pattern. (Courtesy A. Robinson, M.D., Cytogenetics Laboratory, University of Colorado Medical Center, Denver.)

RELATED AUDITORY PROBLEMS

Although hearing loss is not a typical feature of Down's syndrome, a higher incidence of hearing loss is found among a Down's syndrome population than among a normal population. Surveys have shown that over half of a Down's population suffer from conductive or mixed hearing loss as a result of middle ear infections or disease. A higher susceptibility to upper respiratory infections, as well as infections of sinuses and middle ears due to abnormal skull development has been postulated. Sensorineural loss has also been found. Impedance audiometry may clarify presence of conductive element to the hearing loss.

GENERAL TREATMENT

Special educational programming. Correction of congenital malformations as need arises.

REFERENCES

Federman, D. D.: Down's syndrome. Clin. Pediatr. (Phila.) 4: 331, 1965.
Fulton, R. T., and Lloyd, L. L.: Hearing impairment in a population of children with Down's syndrome. Am. J. Ment. Defic. 73: 298, 1968.
Glovsky, L.: Audiological assessment of a Mongoloid population. Trans. Sch. Bull. 63: 27–36, 1966.
Hall, B.: Mongolism in newborn infants. Clin. Pediatr. (Phila.) 5: 4, 1966.
Yannet, H.: Mental Retardation. In Textbook of Pediatrics, 8th Ed., edited by W. Nelson, pp. 1232–1243, Philadelphia, W. B. Saunders Co., 1964.

GOLDENHAR'S SYNDROME

(Figs. 9.14, 9.15)

MAJOR DIAGNOSTIC FEATURES

Eye abnormalities include cleft of upper lid, epibulbar dermoids, extraocular muscle defects, and antimongoloid obliquity. Auricular abnormalities include auricular appendices, unilateral posteriorly placed ear, unilateral microtia, atresia of external auditory meatus, and blind-ended fistulas. Oral abnormalities include unilateral facial hypoplasia of ramus and condyle, high arched palate, and open bite. Musculoskeletal abnormalities such as hemivertebrae and club foot. Congenital heart disease. Mental retardation not common.

ETIOLOGY

Unknown. Most cases are sporadic. Possibly secondary to vascular abnormality during embryologic development of first and second arches.

RELATED AUDITORY PROBLEMS

Conductive loss present in 40% to 50% of reported cases due to atresia of external auditory canals.

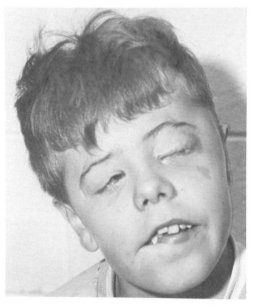

Fig. 9.14. Goldenhar's syndrome. Eye, ear, and oral anomalies.

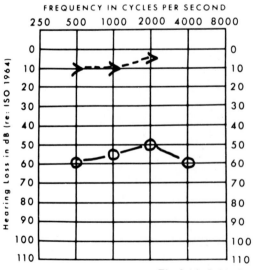

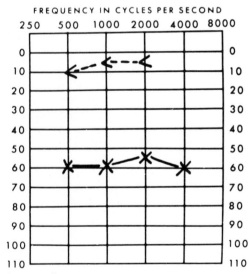

Fig. 9.15. Goldenhar's syndrome audiogram.

GENERAL TREATMENT

Surgical correction of ocular and dental abnormalities; plastic surgery; other as indicated.

REFERENCES

Dumars, K., and Charles, M. A.: Oculo-auriculo-vertebral dysplasia: Goldenhar's syndrome. Rocky Mt. Med. J. 65: 44, 1968.
Mahneke, A.: Epibulbar dermoids: Preauricular appendices combined with unilateral malformation of the face. Acta Ophthalmol. (Kbh.) 34: 412–420, 1956.

HUNTER'S-HURLER'S SYNDROME

(Figs. 9.16–9.18)

MAJOR DIAGNOSTIC FEATURES

Normal appearance at birth but during early months of life onset of progressive abnormal traits. Disorder has been described as "inborn error of metabolism." Diagnostic features include coarse facial features, depressed nasal bridge, corneal clouding, hepatosplenomegaly, joint stiffness, and thoracolumbar kyphosis. As children grow older other features may develop including abundance of fine body hair, enlarged head, prominent eyebrows, thick lips, prominent abdomen, limitation of joint mobility, decline in mental development, cardiac anomalies, deafness, blindness. Diagnosis is based on presence of mucopolysaccharides in urine and tissues. Hunter's and Hurler's are identical clinically. Hunter's is generally less severe and

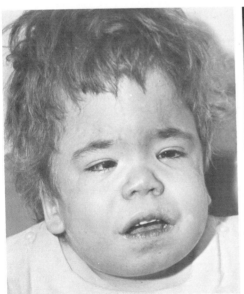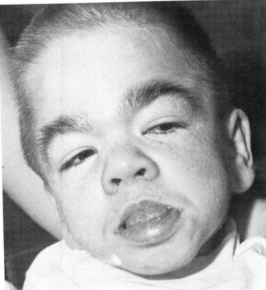

Fig. 9.16. Hunter's-Hurler's syndrome.

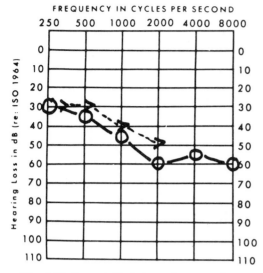
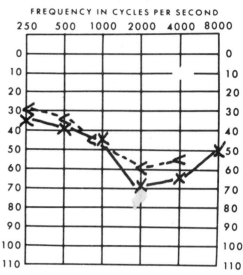

RIGHT EAR

FREQUENCY IN CYCLES PER SECOND

LEFT EAR

FREQUENCY IN CYCLES PER SECOND

Fig. 9.17. Hunter's-Hurler's syndrome audiogram. (With permission from F. O. Black, L. Bergstrom, M. P. Downs, and W. G. Hemenway: Congenital Deafness. Boulder, Colorado Associated Univ. Press, 1971.)

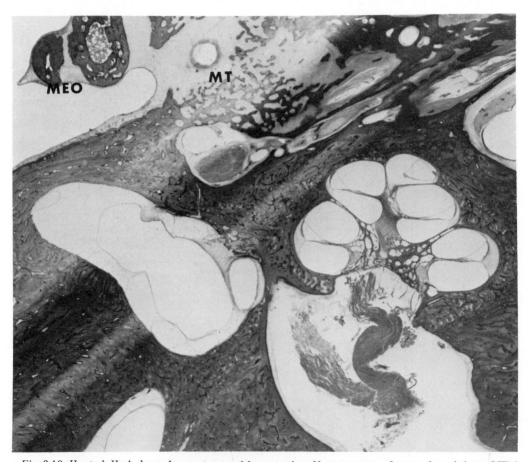

Fig. 9.18. Hunter's-Hurler's syndrome, temporal bone section. Note presence of mesenchymal tissue (MT) in the epitympanum area anterior to the middle ear ossicles (MEO). The inner ear in this case appears to be normal. (Courtesy of George Singleton, M.D., University of Florida, Gainesville.)

affects only males. Hurler's can affect both sexes.

ETIOLOGY

Hurler's felt to be familial, autosomal recessive. Hunter's is x-linked. Features develop because of progressive deposition of acid mucopolysaccharide in various tissues.

RELATED AUDITORY PROBLEMS

Hearing loss may be sensorineural or conductive, the latter usually due to refractory mucoid otitis media. Hearing loss has been seen in 5.2% of reported Hurler's and 43% of Hunter's. Temporal bone findings include absence of incudomalleolar joint, fibrous tissue invasion into otic capsule with presence of "gargoyle cells," multiple bony outgrowths into the middle ear, obliteration of the oval window and round window areas with mesenchymal tissue, a small middle ear space filled with mesenchymal tissue, a small mastoid antrum, poor development of the mastoid, and hypertrophy of the mucosa. Impedance audiometry may be the most suitable means of testing these patients.

GENERAL TREATMENT

No curative therapy. Surgery for cosmetic and functional improvement, physical therapy, genetic counseling.

REFERENCES

Kelemen, G.: Hurler's syndrome and the hearing organ. J. Laryngol. Otol. 80: 791, 1966.

Leroy, J. G., and Crocker, A. C.: Clinical definition of Hurler-Hunter phenotypes. Am. J. Dis. Child. 112: 518, 1966.

Maroteaux, P., and Lamy, M.: Hurler's disease, Morquio's disease, and related mucopolysaccharidoses. J. Pediatr. 67: 312, 1965.

Singleton, G. T.: The Alterations in Hearing and Histopathologic Changes in Hurler's Syndrome. Symposium on Hearing Disorders in Children, University of Oklahoma, January 18–19, 1968.

Wolff, D.: Microscopic study of temporal bones in dysostosis multiplex (gargoylism). Laryngoscope 52: 218, 1942.

KLIPPEL-FEIL SYNDROME
(Wildervanck's Syndrome; Brevicollis; Cervico-oculoacoustic)

(Figs. 9.19, 9.20)

MAJOR DIAGNOSTIC FEATURES

Involves fusion of some or all cervical vertebrae and is characterized by a short neck with limited mobility which gives the impression that the head sits on the shoulders. Other malformations may occur such as club-foot and cleft palate. Associated neurologic disturbances; mirror movements.

ETIOLOGY

Debated. If familial, autosomal dominance with poor penetrance and variable expression. Faulty segmentation of mesodermal somites in utero, defects in maternal intestinal tract, environmental factors have been suggested. Various chromosomal abnormalities have been reported on occasion.

RELATED AUDITORY PROBLEMS

May range from mild conductive to profound sensorineural. Temporal bone and roentgenogram findings include narrow to absent external auditory meatus and/or middle ear space, deformed ossicles, narrow oval window niche, underdevelopment of cochlea and vestibular structures, absence of semicircular canals, absence of eighth cranial nerve. Central nervous system involvement is also frequently described and may contribute to audiologic findings. Impedance audiometry may show conductive element accompanying profound sensorineural hearing loss.

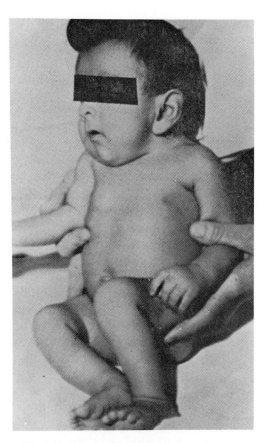

Fig. 9.19. Infant with Klippel-Feil syndrome. Note short neck which gives the appearance of the head sitting on the shoulders. (With permission from F. O. Black, L. Bergstrom, M. P. Downs, and W. G. Hemenway: Congenital Deafness. Boulder, Colorado Associated Univ. Press, 1971.)

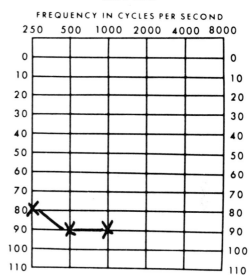

Fig. 9.20. Klippel-Feil syndrome audiogram. (With permission from F. O. Black, L. Bergstrom, M. P. Downs, and W. G. Hemenway: Congenital Deafness. Boulder, Colorado Associated Univ. Press, 1971.)

REFERENCES

Erskine, C. A.: An analysis of the Klippel-Feil syndrome. AMA Arch. Pathol. 41: 269–281, 1946.

Forney, W. R., Robinson, S. J., and Pascoe, D. J.: Congenital heart disease, deafness, and skeletal malformations: A new syndrome. J. Pediatr. 68: 14, 1966.

Palant, D. I., and Carter, B. L.: Klippel-Feil syndrome and deafness. A study with polytomography. Am. J. Dis. Child. 123: 3, 218–220, 1972.

Stark, E., and Borton, T. E.: Hearing loss and the Klippel-Feil syndrome: Case report. Am. J. Dis. Child. 123: 3, 233–235, 1972.

Thomson, J. A.: Case of the Klippel-Feil syndrome. Arch. Dis. Child. 12: 127–131, 1937.

McLay, K., and Maran, A. G. D.: Deafness and the Klippel-Feil syndrome. J. Laryngol. Otol. 83: 175–184, 1969.

LONG ARM 18 DELETION SYNDROME

(Figs. 9.21–9.23)

MAJOR DIAGNOSTIC FEATURES

Abnormalities include mental retardation, microcephaly, short stature, hearing impairment with malformations of auricles and external auditory canals, retinal changes, facial peculiarities, and a high count of whorls on the fingers. Congenital heart disease, horseshoe kidney, cryptorchidism, spinal defects, and foot abnormalities have also been described.

ETIOLOGY

Genetic imbalance syndrome involving partial deletion of the long arm of the 18th chromosome. If translocation is responsible for deletion, transmission to children is possible.

RELATED AUDITORY PROBLEMS

Conductive hearing loss associated with external and middle ear anomalies most frequently reported. Temporal bone study has shown collapsed Reissner's membrane in all turns of the cochlea; rolled and retracted tectorial membrane, hypoplastic cochlear aqueduct.

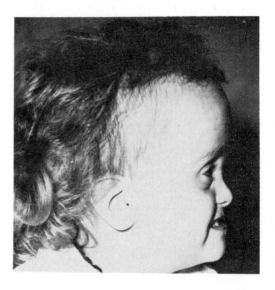

Fig. 9.21. Long arm 18 deletion syndrome. Note altered pinna, prominent forehead and nasolabial fold. [With permission from D. Bergsma: Birth Defects: Atlas and Compendium. Baltimore, National Foundation–March of Dimes (Williams & Wilkins Co.), 1973.]

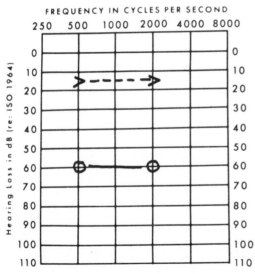

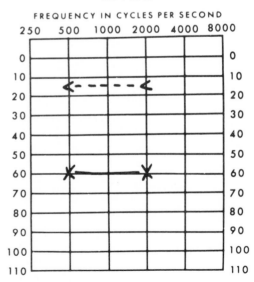

Fig. 9.22. Long arm 18 deletion syndrome audiogram.

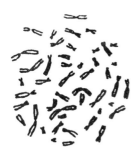

PARTIAL DELETION OF 18 LONG ARM

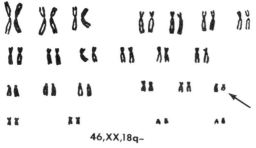

46,XX,18q–

Fig. 9.23. Karyotype of partial deletion of long arm 18. (Courtesy A. Robinson, M.D., Cytogenetics Laboratory, University of Colorado Medical Center, Denver.)

GENERAL TREATMENT

Surgical repair of correctable defects. Attention to learning and hearing problems.

REFERENCES

Bergstrom, L., Hemenway, W. G., and Sando, I.: Pathological changes in congenital deafness. Laryngoscope 82: 1777–1792, 1972.

Insley, J.: Syndrome associated with a deficiency of part of the long arm of chromosome. Arch. Dis. Child. 42: 140, 1967.

Wertelecki, W., Schindler, A. M., and Gerald, P. S.: Partial deletion of chromosome 18: A syndrome. Lancet 2: 641, 1966.

OSTEOGENESIS IMPERFECTA
(Van Der Hoeve's Disease)

(Figs. 9.24, 9.25)

MAJOR DIAGNOSTIC FEATURES

High percentage of infant death, multiple fractures may be present at birth, weak joints, blue sclera, thin and translucent skin, yellowish-brown and easily broken teeth, deafness. Deformities such as kyphoscoliosis and pectus excavation, internal hydrocephalus, nerve root compression, cardiovascular lesions, and thin atrophic skin may also occur.

ETIOLOGY

Hereditary autosomal dominant, present at birth. Majority of severe cases are sporadic.

RELATED HEARING PROBLEMS

Of reported cases, 60% have conductive hearing loss reportedly due to otosclerotic changes, the footplate of the stapes, and the posterior semicircular canal. Temporal bone

RIGHT EAR

LEFT EAR

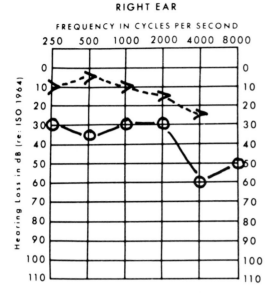

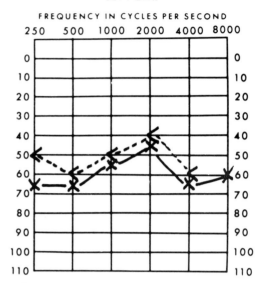

Fig. 9.24. Osteogenesis imperfecta audiogram.

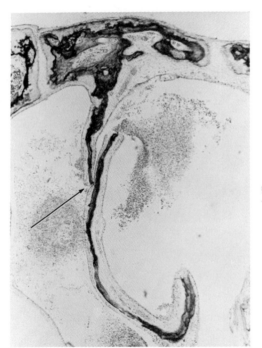

Fig. 9.25. Healed fracture (arrow) of extremely delicate posterior stapedial crus in a case of osteogenesis imperfecta. (With permission from L. Bergstrom, W. G. Hemenway, and I. Sando: Pathological changes in congenital deafness. Laryngoscope 82: 1777-1792, 1972.)

findings show diminished or immature bone formation in otic capsule and ossicles. Degeneration of stapes crura so no contact is possible between crura and footplate. Sensorineural hearing loss has also been demonstrated in high frequencies.

GENERAL TREATMENT

Genetic counseling, magnesium therapy, orthopedic correction.

REFERENCES

Altman, F.: The temporal bone in osteogenesis imperfecta congenita. Arch. Otolaryngol. 75: 486–497, 1959.
Hall, J. G., and Rohrt, T.: The stapes in osteogenesis imperfecta. Acta Otolaryngol. (Stockh.) 65: 345–348, 1968.
Herndon, C. N.: Osteogenesis imperfecta: Some clinical and genetic considerations. Clin. Orthop. 8: 132, 1956.
Opheim, O.: Loss of hearing following the syndrome of Van Der Hoeve—de Kleyn. Acta Otolaryngol. (Stockh.) 65: 337–344, 1967.

RUBELLA, CONGENITAL

(Figs. 9.26–9.29)

MAJOR DIAGNOSTIC FEATURES

Fetal infection with rubella virus may result in spontaneous abortion, stillbirth, or a variety of birth defects occurring singularly or in combination. Transient neonatal manifestations include low birth weight, hepatosplenomegaly, purpura, bulging anterior suture, corneal clouding, and jaundice. Anemia, pneumonia, meningitis, encephalitis, and intermittent rash may develop. Permanent stigmata include deafness, visual defects, microcephaly, mental retardation, cardiac defects, behavioral problems.

ETIOLOGY

Rubella virus infection.

RELATED AUDITORY PROBLEMS

Sensorineural, severe to profound, sometimes complicated by a conductive element. Patho-logic findings have included abnormalities in stria vascularis, tectorial membrane, hair cells in Corti's organ and sacculus, and cochleosaccular degeneration of Scheibe. Additional pathologic findings have included: specific distribution of severely degenerated hair cells in the cochlea, eosinophilic material in perilymphatic space most likely coming from vessels in the scala tympani, slight distortion of cochlear second turn and Rosenthal's canal, and stapes anomalies. Audiograms are variable.

Evidence of central deafness as a result of central nervous system lesion has been reported.

GENERAL TREATMENT

Treatment for specific defects. Surgery for cataracts or glaucoma when indicated. Amplifi-

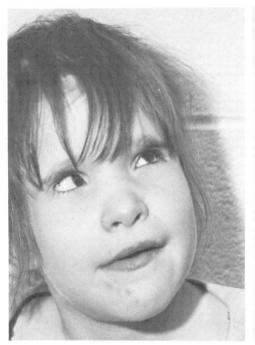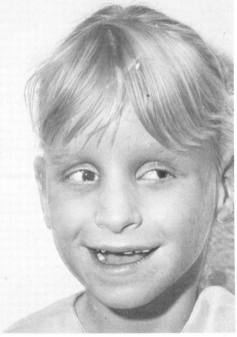

Fig. 9.26. Children with many problems associated with maternal rubella.

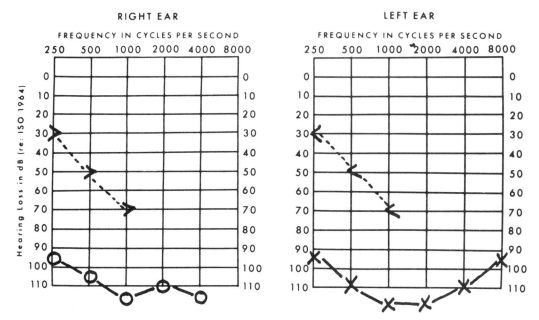

Fig. 9.27. Rubella audiogram. (With permission from F. O. Black, L. Bergstrom, M. P. Downs, and W. G. Hemenway: Congenital Deafness. Boulder, Colorado Associated Univ. Press, 1971.)

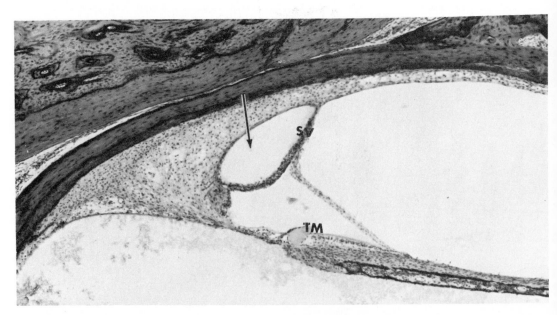

Fig. 9.28. Cystic structure (arrow) in the stria vascularis (SV) of the basal cochlear turn, and rolled-up tectorial membrane (TM) in the inner sulcus. Tectorial membrane is covered by a single layer of cells. (With permission from W. G. Hemenway, I. Sando, and D. McChesney: Temporal bone pathology following maternal rubella. Arch. Klin. Exp. Ohren. Nasen. Kehlkopfheilkd. 193: 287, 1969.)

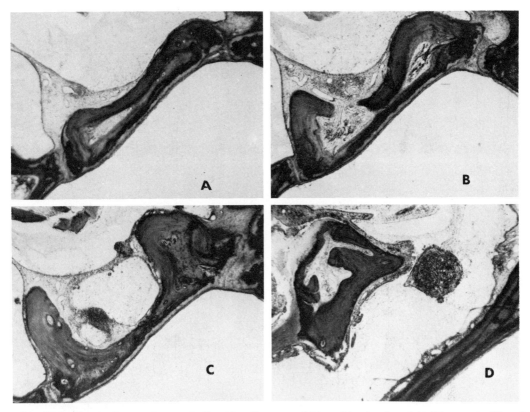

Fig. 9.29. Abnormal stapes due to rubella with rudimentary thickened head and neck in (D), crura in (C), and footplate in (A) and (B).

cation and auditory training when significant hearing loss is determined.

REFERENCES

Bordley, J. E., Brookhouser, P. E., and Worthington, E. L.: Viral infections and hearing. A critical review of the literature. 1969–1970. Laryngoscope 82: 4, 557–577, 1972.

Borton, T. E., and Stark, E. W.: Audiological findings in hearing loss secondary to maternal rubella. Pediatrics 45: 225, 1970.

Browder, J. A.: Hearing loss caused by prenatal rubella. Rocky Mt. Med. J. 68: 12, 43–46, 1971.

Hemenway, W. G., Sando, I., and McChesney, D.: Temporal bone pathology following maternal rubella. Arch. Klin. Exp. Ohren. Nasen. Kehlkopfheilkd. 193: 287, 1969.

Peck, J. E.: Hearing deficit following maternal rubella. J. Pediatr. 81: 12, 414–415, 1972.

TREACHER-COLLINS SYNDROME
(Mandibulofacial Dysostosis; First Arch Syndrome)

(Figs. 9.30–9.33)

MAJOR DIAGNOSTIC FEATURES

Facial bone abnormalities of structures formed from the first branchial arch including downward sloping palpebral fissures, depressed cheek bones, deformed pinna, receding chin, and large fish-like mouth with frequent dental abnormalities. Atresia of auditory canal, defects of auditory canal and ossicles, and cleft palate are most common. Mental deficiency reported in about 5% of cases.

ETIOLOGY

Genetic defect leading to multiple congenital anomalies. Autosomal dominant with high penetrance and variable expression. More than half of cases reported are fresh mutations.

RELATED AUDITORY PROBLEMS

The external ears may be small, displaced, or simply nubbins. Atresia of external auditory canal is common. The middle ear is often poorly developed, the tympanic ossicles being absent or deformed. Hypoplasia of the horizontal semicircular canal and of the cochlea has been observed, as have branching of nerve to horizontal canal cristae bilaterally and abnormalities of bony and membranous vestibular labyrinth. Deafness generally complete conductive, but may be sensorineural.

GENERAL TREATMENT

Genetic counseling, surgical repair of ear anomalies, hearing aid if recommended, orthodontic treatment, and speech therapy if indicated.

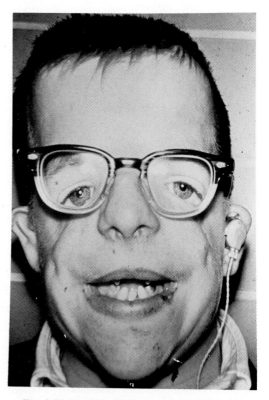

Fig. 9.30. Treacher-Collins syndrome. Note low set ears, eye slant, and flattening of the zygoma.

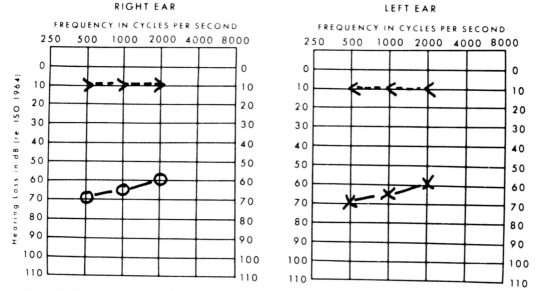

Fig. 9.31. Treacher-Collins syndrome audiogram. (With permission from F. O. Black, L. Bergstrom, M. P. Downs, and W. G. Hemenway: Congenital Deafness. Boulder, Colorado Associated Univ. Press, 1971.)

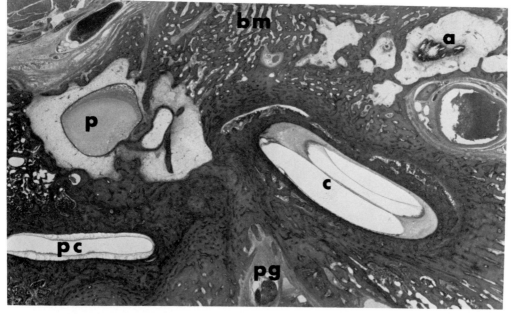

Fig. 9.32. Histopathologic section from a Treacher-Collins patient. The middle ear cavity has inadequate space for ossicles, and a mass of bone (bm) attached to the promontory divides the hypotympanum into a posterior (p) and anterior (a) space. The cochlea (c) is essentially normal; the jugular ganglion (pg) is anterior to the posterior semicircular canal (pc). Another section from this case is shown in Figure 1.1 showing a columellar-type stapes. (With permission from I. Sando, W. G. Hemenway, and W. R. Morgan: Histopathology of temporal bones in mandibulofacial dysostosis. Trans. Am. Acad. Ophthalmol. Otolaryngol. 72: 913-924, 1968.)

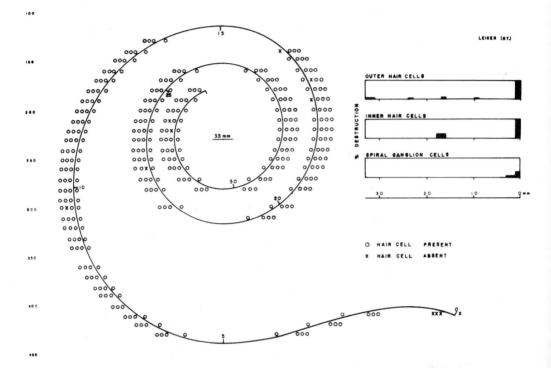

Fig. 9.33. Cochleogram of Treacher-Collins case, right ear. The cochlea has 2.5 turns and is 33 mm long (within normal limits). Some loss of inner and outer hair cells and spiral ganglion cells may be noted in extreme basal end of cochlea. (With permission from I. Sando, W. G. Hemenway, and W. P. Morgan: Histopathology of temporal bones in mandibulofacial dysostosis. Trans. Am. Acad. Ophthalmol. Otolaryngol. 72: 913-924, 1968.)

REFERENCES

Fernandez, A. O., and Ronis, M. L.: The Treacher-Collins syndrome. Arch. Otolaryngol. 80: 505, 1964.
Frazen, L. E., et al.: Mandibulofacial dysostosis. Am. J. Dis. Child. 113: 405, 1967.
Herbets, G.: Otological observations on the Treacher-Collins syndrome.

Acta Otolaryngol. 54: 457, 1962.
Lindsay, J. R.: Inner ear pathology in congenital deafness. Otolaryngol. Clin. North Am. 4: 249, 1971.
Sando, I., Hemenway, W. G., and Morgan, W. R.: Histopathology of temporal bones in mandibulofacial dysostosis. Trans. Am. Acad. Ophthalmol. Otolaryngol. 72: 913-924, 1968.

TRISOMY 13–15

(Figs. 9.34–9.36)

MAJOR DIAGNOSTIC FEATURES

Chromosomal aberration resulting in minimal characteristics of microphthalmia, cleft lip and palate, and polydactyly. A host of other abnormalities may be present including mental retardation; deafness; broad nose; hypotelorism; microcephaly; heart and/or skin defects; retroflexed thumbs; "rocker-bottom" feet; seizures; renal, abdominal, and genitalia abnormalities. Those affected frequently suffer with feeding problems, failure to thrive, jitteryness, apneic spells, hypotonia, and jaundice.

ETIOLOGY

Meiotic nondisjunction appears to be the cause of the extra chromosome in 13-15 group. Trisomy 13 syndrome with 47 chromosomes frequently associated with increased maternal age.

RELATED AUDITORY PROBLEMS

External ears are low set. Middle ear findings have included deformed stapes, distorted incudostapedial joint posteriorly, and absence of stapedial muscle and tendon. Inner ear abnormalities have included distorted and shortened cochlea, shortened endolymphatic valve, abnormal branch of nerve to posterior semicircular canal crista from posterior cranial fossa, degeneration of organ of Corti, tectorial membrane, stria vascularis, and saccule. Other studies have been normal.

GENERAL TREATMENT

Genetic counseling, other as may be indicated. Prognosis is poor; 95% die by 3 years.

REFERENCES

Black, F. O., Sando, I., Wagner, J. A., and Hemenway, W. G.: Middle and inner ear abnormalities. Arch. Otolaryngol. 93: 615–619, 1971.
Cohen, P. E.: The "D" syndrome. Am. J. Dis. Child. 111: 235, 1966.
Kos, A. O., Schuknecht, H. F., and Singer, J. D.: Temporal bone studies in 13-15 and 18 trisomy syndrome. Arch. Otolaryngol. 83: 439–445, 1966.
Maniglia, J. M., Wolff, D., and Herques, A. S.: Congenital deafness in 13-15 syndrome. Arch. Otolaryngol. 92: 181–188, 1970.
Scherz, R. G., Fraga, J. R., and Reichelderfer, T. E.: A typical example of 13-15 trisomy in a Negro boy. Clin. Pediatr. (Phila.) 11: 4, 246–248, 1972.
Taylor, A. I.: Autosomal trisomy syndromes: A detailed study of twenty-seven cases of Edward's syndrome and twenty-seven cases of Patan's syndrome. J. Med. Genet. 5: 227, 1968.

Fig. 9.34. Trisomy 13-15 (D_1) karyotype showing 47 chromosomes with extra chromosome (arrow). (Courtesy of A. Robinson, M.D., Cytogenetics Laboratory, University of Colorado Medical Center, Denver.)

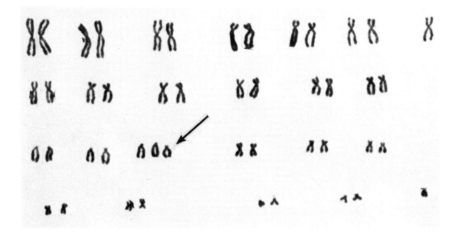

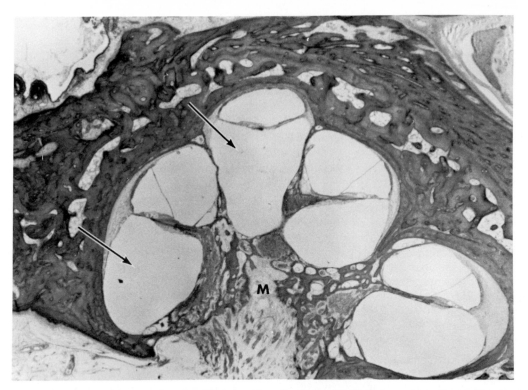

Fig. 9.35. Temporal bone section through the cochlea of a trisomy 13-15 (D₁) case. Note distorted basal and apical cochlear turns (arrows). The modiolus (M) is incompletely developed. (With permission from F. O. Black, I. Sando, J. A. Wagner, and W. G. Hemenway: Middle and inner ear abnormalities, 13-15 (D₁) trisomy. Arch. Otolaryngol. 93: 615-619, 1971.)

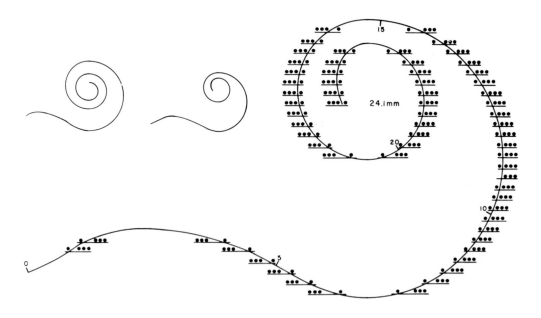

● ●●● HAIR CELLS PRESENT

Fig. 9.36. Cochleogram (left ear) from trisomy 13-15 (D₁) showing incomplete development of cochlea with only 2-1/8 turns and 24.1 mm in length. Note comparative normal and abnormal cochlear coils and length as shown in upper left. Hair cells are present in their anticipated anatomic distribution. (With permission from F. O. Black, I. Sando, J. A. Wagner, and W. G. Hemenway: Middle ear and inner ear abnormalities 13-15 (D₁) trisomy. Arch. Otolaryngol. 93: 615-619, 1971.)

TRISOMY 18

(Figs. 9.37, 9.38)

MAJOR DIAGNOSTIC FEATURES

Due to chromosomal aberration, features present at birth include being underweight with an undernourished appearance, possible limpness at first soon becoming hypertonic. Microcephaly with triangular shape due to occipital prominence and receding chin. Skin is loose. Flexion of hand with overlapping of index finger over third, "rocker-bottom" feet, short sternum, small pelvis, and agenesis of bones of the extremities. Congenital heart disease, renal abnormalities, cleft lip and plate, deformed ears may also be present. Mental retardation usually profound.

ETIOLOGY

Due to nondisjunction of one chromosome in 17-18 group. Advanced maternal age is common. Possibility of recurrence in same family is rare unless translocation is present.

RELATED AUDITORY PROBLEMS

Audiometric testing shows failure to respond to sound. Middle ear anomalies include malformed stapes, deformed incus and malleus, exposed stapedial muscle in the middle ear cavity, absence of stapedial tendon, absence of pyramidal eminence, a split tensor tympanic muscle in separate bony canals, abnormal course of the facial and chorda tympani nerves, and underdevelopment of facial nerve.

Other anomalies reported include atresia of external canals, decreased spiral ganglion cells, anomalies of cochlea, absence of utriculoendolymphatic valve, and absence of semicircular canals and cristae.

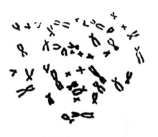

TRISOMY 18

47,XX,18+

Fig. 9.37. Trisomy 18 karyotype. Note extra chromosome (arrow). (Courtesy of A. Robinson, M.D., Cytogenetics Laboratory, University of Colorado Medical Center, Denver.)

GENERAL TREATMENT

Genetic counseling, other treatment as indicated. By 1 year 90% will die.

REFERENCES

Chrysostomidou, D. M., Caslaris, E., Alexion, D., and Bartsocas, C. S . Trisomy 18 in Greece. Acta Paediatr. Scand. 60: 591–593, 1971.

Kelemen, G., Hooft, C., and Kluyskens, P.: The inner ear in autosomal trisomy. Pract. Otorhinolaryngol. (Basel) 30: 251–258, 1968.

Kos, A. O., Schuknecht, H. F., and Singer, J. D.: Temporal bone studies in 13-15 and 18 trisomy syndromes. Arch. Otolaryngol. 83: 439–445, 1966.

Sando, I., Bergstrom, L., Wood, R. P., and Hemenway, W. G.: Temporal bone findings in trisomy 18 syndrome. Arch. Otolaryngol. 91: 552–559, 1969.

Smith, D. W.: The number 18 trisomy syndrome. J. Pediatr. 60: 513, 1962.

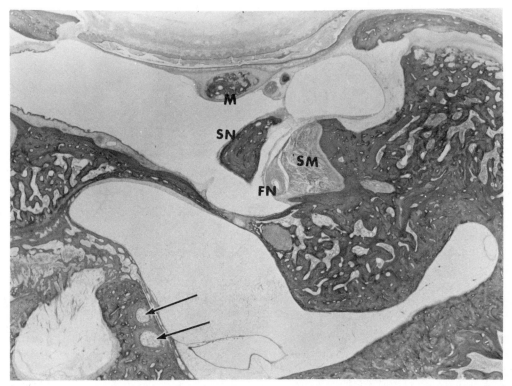

Fig. 9.38. Trisomy 18 temporal bone section with double singular canal (arrows) which contains nerve to posterior semicircular canal crista. Note thickened stapes neck (SN), underdeveloped facial nerve (FN), exposed stapedial muscle (SM), and anomalous malleous (M). (With permission from I. Sando, L. Bergstrom, R. P. Wood, and W. G. Hemenway: Temporal bone findings in trisomy 18 syndrome. Arch Otolaryngol. 91: 552-559, 1969.)

WAARDENBURG'S SYNDROME

(Figs. 9.39, 9.40)

MAJOR DIAGNOSTIC FEATURES

The most obvious characteristics include white forelock, lateral displacement of medial canthi, iris bicolor or blue irides, prominence of root of nose, hyperplasia of medial portion of eyebrows, congenital deafness. Other findings include thin nose with flaring alae nasae, "cupid bow" configuration of lips, prominent mandible, and occasional cleft or high arched palate. All characteristic features are not found in each patient. Mental retardation not typical.

ETIOLOGY

Inherited as autosomal dominant characteristic with variable penetrance.

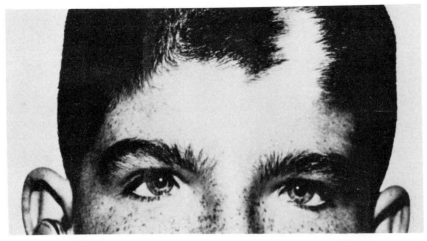

Fig. 9.39. Waardenburg's syndrome. Note white forelock in hair and lateral displacement of median canthi. [With permission from D. Bergsma: Birth Defects: Atlas and Compendium. Baltimore, National Foundation–March of Dimes (Williams & Wilkins Co.), 1971.

RIGHT EAR

FREQUENCY IN CYCLES PER SECOND

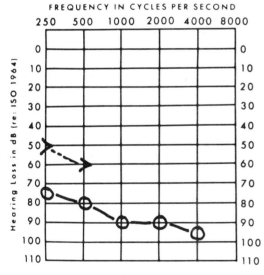

LEFT EAR

FREQUENCY IN CYCLES PER SECOND

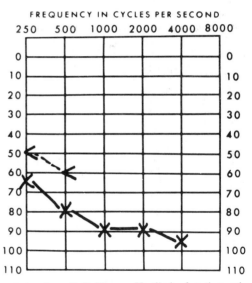

Fig. 9.40. Waardenburg's syndrome audiogram. (With permission from R. E. Marcus: Vestibular function and additional findings in Waardenburg's syndrome. Acta Otolaryngol. (Suppl.) 229, 1968.)

RELATED AUDITORY PROBLEMS

Congenital sensorineural, may be unilateral, may be progressive. Hearing impairment may be evidenced primarily in low and middle frequencies, but profound loss can also be present. Principal histopathologic findings are absence of organ of Corti, atrophy of spiral ganglion with paucity of nerve fibers.

REFERENCES

DiGeorge, A. M., Olmstead, R. W., and Harley, R. D.: Waardenburg's syndrome. J. Pediatr. 57: 649–669, 1960.
Fisch, L.: Deafness as part of an hereditary syndrome. J. Laryngol. Otol. 73: 355–382, 1959.
McKusick, V. A.: Medical genetics. J. Chronic Dis. 12: 129–132, 1960.
Proctor, C. A., and Proctor, B.: Understanding hereditary nerve deafness. Arch. Otolaryngol. 85: 23–40, 1967.
Waardenburg, P. J.: A new syndrome combining developmental anomalies of the eyelids, eyebrows and nose root with pigmentary defects of the iris and head hair with congenital deafness. Am. J. Hum. Genet. 3: 195–253, 1951.

CONCLUSION

The field of preventive medicine gives us an analogue: it has been said that "medicine is unique among the sciences in that it strives incessantly to defeat the object of its own invention." This object, of course, is disease—and there is a parallel in audiology. Since our beginnings in the mid-forties, we have measured, described, researched, catalogued, analyzed, and synthesized the entity of hearing loss exhaustively—and now, having defined it, we must busy ourselves with preventing the devastation of its effects on children. In such terms preventive audiology becomes a viable endeavor—a discipline devoted to preventing the effects of ear disease on the individual who suffers from it. Such prevention can only be accomplished by early detection of the condition and by proper provision for remedial therapy and education.

"We must be patient and await fresh methods and occasions for research. We must be ready, too, to abandon a path which we have followed for a time, if it seems to be leading to no good end."

Sigmund Freud (1948)
Beyond the Pleasure Principle

BIBLIOGRAPHY

Accreditation Council for Facilities for the Mentally Retarded: Standards for Residential Facilities for the Mentally Retarded. Chicago. Joint Commission on Accreditation of Hospitals, 1971.

A Comprehensive Plan for Hearing-Impaired Children in Illinois. Springfield, Illinois. Illinois State Dept. of Public Health, 1968.

Ades, H. W.: Central auditory mechanisms. In Handbook of Physiology, edited by J. Fields, H. W. Magoun, and V. E. Hall, Vol. 1. Washington, D.C., American Physiological Society, 1959.

Alberman, E. D., and Goldstein, H.: The AT RISK register: A statistical evaluation. Br. J. Prev. Soc. Med. 24: 129–135, 1970.

Alberti, P. W. R. M., and Kristensen, R.: The clinical application of impedance audiometry Laryngoscope 80: 735–346, 1970.

Albrite, J. P., Butler, R. A., and Galloway, F. T.: The cochleopalpebral reflex in normal hearing and hard-of-hearing persons. Arch. Otolaryngol. 64: 402–408, 1956.

Aldrich, C. A.: New test for hearing in the newborn: Conditioned reflex. Am. J. Dis. Child. 35: 36–37, 1928.

Alpiner, J.: Personal correspondence. University of Denver, Speech and Hearing Clinic, 1971.

Altman, M. M.: Methods for early detection of hearing loss in infants, final report. Rambam Govt. Hospital, Haifa, Israel, 1968.

Altmann, F.: Histologic picture of inherited nerve deafness in man and animals. Arch. Otolaryngol. 51: 852–890, 1950.

American Speech and Hearing Association. Proceedings of a conference on hearing aid evaluation procedures. ASHA 2: 1967.

American Speech and Hearing Association: A Guide to Clinical Services in Speech Pathology and Audiology. Washington, D.C., 1973.

Ames, M. D., Plotkin, S. A., Winchester, R. A., and Atkins, T. E.: Central auditory imperception: A significant factor in congenital rubella deafness. JAMA, 213: 419–421, 1970.

Amon, C.: Project Parent-Child: A model for prescriptive intervention. Presented at ASHA Convention, San Francisco, 1972.

Anderson, H.: Acoustic Intra-Aural Reflexes in Clinical Diagnosis. Stockholm, Karolinska Sjukhuset, 1969.

Anderson, H., and Barr, B.: Congenital pseudo-mixed deafness. Laryngoscope 77: 1825–1839, 1967.

Anderson, H., Filipsson, R., Fluur, E., Koch, B., Lindsten, J., and Wedenberg, E.: Hearing impairment in Turner's syndrome. Acta Otolaryngol. (Suppl.) 247: 1 26, 1969.

Anderson, H., and Wedenberg, E.: Audiometric identification of normal hearing carriers of genes for deafness. Acta Otolaryngol. (Stockh.) 65: 535–554, 1968.

Anderson, M. S., and Bentinck, B. R.: Intracranial schwannoma in a child. Cancer 29: 231–234, 1972.

Andreev, A. M., Arapova, A. A., and Gersuni, S. V.: On the electrical potentials of the human cochlea. J. Physiol. USSR 26: 205–212, 1941.

Anson, B. J.: An Atlas of Human Anatomy, 2nd Ed. Philadelphia, W. B. Saunders, 1963.

Anson, B. J.: Developmental anatomy of the ear. In Otolaryngology. Vol. I. Basic Sciences and Related Disciplines, edited by M. M. Paparella and D. A. Shumrick. Philadelphia, W. B. Saunders, 1973.

Anson, B. J., and Donaldson, J. A.: The Surgical Anatomy of the Temporal Bone and Ear. Philadelphia. W. B. Saunders. 1967.

Anthony, D. A., et al.: Seeing Essential English. Univ. Northern Colo., Greeley, 1971.

Aran, J. M.: The electrocochleogram: Recent results in children and in some pathological cases. Arch. Klin. Exp. Ohren. Nasen. Kehlkopfheilkd. 198: 128–141, 1971.

Aran, J. M., and LeBert, G.: Les réponses nerveuses cochleaires chez l'homme: Image du fonctionnement de l'oreille et nouveau test d'audiométrie objective. Rev. Laryngoscope (Bordeaux) 89: 361, 1968.

Arey, L. B.: Developmental Anatomy. Philadelphia, W. B. Saunders, 1940.

Auditory Screening for Infants (Hardy and Dougherty): Film from the Division of Maternal and Child Health, Maryland State Dept. of Health, 1959.

Auditory Screening of Infants (M. P. Downs): Film from Nebraska Educ. Television Council for Higher Education, Lincoln, 1971.

Babbidge, H. S.: Education of the Deaf. A Report to the Secretary of Health, Education, and Welfare by his Advisory Committee on the Education of the Deaf. U.S. Govt. Printing Office, 1965, 0-765-119.

Baker, H. J., and Leland, B.: Detroit tests of learning aptitude—oral directions and oral commissions. In Detroit Tests of Learning Aptitude. Detroit, Bobbs-Merrill, 1935.

Ballenger, J. J.: Diseases of the Nose, Throat and Ear, 11th Ed. Philadelphia, Lea & Febiger, 1969.

Barnett, A. B., and Goodwin, R. S.: Averaged evoked electroencephalographic responses to clicks in the human newborn. EEG Clin. Neurophysiol. 18: 441–450, 1965.

Barr, B.: Pure tone audiometry for pre-school children: A preliminary report. Acta Otolaryngol. [suppl.], (Stockh.) 110: 89, 1954.

Barr, B., and Anderson, H.: Congenital pseudo-mixed deafness. Laryngoscope 77: 1825–1839, 1967.

Barr, B., and Wedenberg, E.: Prognosis of perceptive hearing loss in children with respect to genesis and use of hearing aid. Acta Otolaryngol. (Stockh.) 59: 462–472, 1965.

Bartoshuk, A. K.: Response decrement with repeated elicitation of human neonatal cardiac acceleration to sound. J. Comp. Physiol. Psychol. 55: 9–13, 1962a.

Bartoshuk, A. K.: Human neonatal cardiac acceleration to sound: Habituation and dishabituation. Percept. Mot. Skills 15: 15–27, 1962c.

Bartoshuk, A. K.: Human neonatal cardiac responses to sound: A power function. Psychon. Sci. 1: 151–152, 1964.

Bayley, N.: The development of motor abilities during the first three years. Monogr. Soc. Res. Child. Dev. 1: 1–25, 1935.

Beadle, K. R., and Crowell, D. H.: Neonatal electrocardiographic responses to sound: Methodology. J. Speech Hear. Res. 5: 112–123, 1962.

Beagley, H. A., and Knight, J. J.: The evaluation of suspected non-organic hearing loss. J. Laryngol. Otol. 82: 693–705, 1968.

Beal, D. R.: Prevention of otitis media in the Alaskan native. In Otitis Media, edited by A. Glorig and K. Gerwin, pp. 156–162. Springfield, Ill., Charles C Thomas, Publisher, 1972.

Beck, H. L.: Counseling parents of retarded children. Children 6: 225–230, 1959.

Belzile, M., and Markle, D. M.: A clinical comparison of monaural and binaural hearing aids worn by patients with conductive or perceptive deafness. Laryngoscope 69: 1317–1323, 1959.

Bench, R. J.: Sound transmission to the human foetus through the maternal abdominal wall. J. Genet. Psychol. 113: 85 87, 1968.

Bench, R. J.: Infant audiometry. Sound 4: 72–74, 1971.

Bench, R. J., and Boscak, N.: Some applications of signal detection theory to paedo-audiology. Sound 4: 3, 1970.

Bender, R., and Wig, E.: Binaural hearing aids for hearing impaired children in elementary schools. Volta Review, 64: 537–542, 1962.

Bennett, M., Ward, P. H., and Tait, C. A.: Otologic-audiologic study of cleft palate children. Laryngoscope 78: 1011–1019, 1968.

Bennett, S. M.: A group test of hearing for six-year-old children. Br. J. Educ. Psychol. 21: 45–52, 1951.

Bentzen, O., and Courtois, J.: Statistical analysis of the problems for the deaf and hard-of-hearing in the world of 1970. Scand. Audiology 2: 17–26, 1973.

Berger, K.: The Hearing Aid: Its Operation and Development. Detroit, National Hearing Aid Society, 1970.

Bergsma, D. (Ed.): Birth Defects: Atlas and Compendium. Baltimore, Williams & Wilkins, Published for the National Foundation—March of Dimes, 1973.

Bergstrom, L.: Personal communication, 1971.

Bergstrom, L., and Hemenway, W. G.: Otologic problems in submucous cleft palate. South. Med. J. 64: 1172–1177, 1971.

Bergstrom, L., Hemenway, W. G., and Downs, M. P.: A high risk registry to find congenital deafness. Otolaryngol. Clin. North Am. 4: 369–399, 1971.

Bergstrom, L., Hemenway, W. G., and Sando, I.: Pathological changes in congenital deafness. Laryngoscope 82: 1777–1792, 1972.

Bergstrom, L., and Stewart, J.: New concepts in congenital deafness. Otolaryngol. Clin. North. Am. (Symposium) 4: 431–443, 1971.

Berko, J., and Brown, R.: Psycholinguistic research methods. In Handbook of Research Methods in Child Development, edited by P. H. Mussen, p. 531. New York, John Wiley & Sons, 1960.

Berlin, C. I., and Catlin, F. I.: Manual of Standard Pure Tone Threshold Procedure, Programmed Instruction: Tactics for Obtaining Valid Pure Tone Clinical Thresholds. Johns Hopkins Med. Institutions, 1965.

Berlin, C. I., Hughes, L. F., Lowe-Bell, S. S., and Berlin, H. L.: Dichotic right ear advantage in children 5 to 13. In press, Cortex, 1974.

Berlin, C. I., and Lowe, S. S.: Temporal and dichotic factors in central auditory testing. In Handbook of Clinical Audiology, edited by J. Katz, p. 280. Baltimore, Williams & Wilkins, 1972.

Berlin, C. I., Lowe-Bell, S. S., Cullen, J. K., Jr., Thompson, C. L., and Loovis, C. F.: Dichotic speech perception: An interpretation of right ear advantage and temporal offset effects. J. Acoust. Soc. Am. 53:

699–709, 1973.

Berlin, C. I., Lowe-Bell, S. S., Cullen, J. K., Thompson, C. L., and Loovis, C. F.: Dichotic speech perception: An interpretation of right-ear advantage and temporal offset effects. J. Acoust. Soc. Am. 53: 699–709, 1973b.

Berlin, C. I., Lowe-Bell, S. S., Cullen, J. K., Thompson, C. L., and Stafford, M. R.: Is speech "special?" Perhaps the temporal lobectomy patient can tell us. J. Acoust. Soc. Am. 52: 702–705, 1972b.

Berlin, C. I., Lowe-Bell, S. S., Janetta, P. J., and Kline, D. G.: Central auditory deficits after temporal lobectomy. Arch. Otolaryngol. 96: 4–10, 1972c.

Berlin, C. I., Willett, M. E., Thompson, C. L., Cullen, J. K., Jr., and Lowe, S. S.: Voiceless versus voiced CV perception in dichotic and monotic listening. J. Acoust. Soc. Am. 47: 75–76, 1970.

Bess, J. C.: Ear canal collapse. Arch. Otolaryngol. 93: 408–412, 1971.

Bickford, R. G., Jacobsen, J. L., and Cody, T.: Nature of the averaged evoked potentials to sound and other stimuli in man. Ann. NY Acad. Sci. 112: 204–222, 1964.

Bjorkesten, G.: Unilateral acoustic tumors in children. Acta Psychiatr. Scand. 32: 1–5, 1957.

Black, F. O., Berstrom, L., Downs, M. P., and Hemenway, W. G.: Congenital Deafness: A New Approach to Early Detection Through a High Risk Register. Boulder, Colorado Associated University Press, 1971a.

Black, F. O., Sando, I., Wagner, J. A., and Hemenway, W. G.: Middle and inner ear abnormalities, 13–15 (D_1) trisomy. Arch. Otolaryngol. 93: 615–619, 1971b.

Black, J., and Hast, M.: Speech reception with a hearing signal. J Speech. Hear. Disord. 5: 70–75, 1962.

Bluestone, C. D., Beery, Q. C., and Paradise, J.: Audiometry and tympanometry in relation to middle ear effusions in children. Laryngoscope 83: 594–604, 1973.

Bocca, E., and Calearo, C.: Central hearing processes. In Modern Developments in Audiology, edited by J. Jerger, pp. 337–370. New York, Academic Press, 1963.

Bond, G. L.: Auditory and Speech Characteristics of Poor Readers. New York, Teachers College, Columbia University, Teachers' Contribution to Education #657, 1935.

Bordley, J. E., and Hardy, W. G.: A study in objective audiometry with the use of a psychogalvanic response. Ann. Otol. Rhinol. Laryngol. 58: 751–760, 1949.

Bordley, J. E., Ruben, R. J., and Lieberman, A. P.: Human cochlear potentials. Laryngoscope 74: 463–479, 1964.

Bornstein, H.: A description of some current sign systems designed to represent English. Am. Ann. Deaf 118: 454–463, 1973.

Bornstein, H., Kannapell, B. M., Saulnier, K. L., Hamilton, L. B., and Roy, H. L.: Signed English Basic Pre-School Dictionary; Little Red Riding Hood, Goldilocks and the Three Bears, etc. Washington, D.C., Gallaudet College Press, 1972.

Boyd, R. D.: CCD Development Progress Scale, Experimental Form, Manual and Directions, June, 1969.

Brackbill, Y.: Cumulative effects of continuous stimulation on arousal level in infants. Child Dev. 42: 17–26, 1971.

Brackbill, Y., Adams, G., Crowell, D. H., and Gray, M. L.: Arousal level in neonates and preschool children under continuous auditory stimulation. J. Exp. Child Psychol. 4: 178–188, 1966.

Brackbill, Y., and Downs, M. P.: Cited in Brackbill and Fitzgerald's "Development of the sensory analyzers during infancy." In Advances in Child Development and Behavior, edited by L. P. Lipsitt and H. Reese, pp. 4, 173–208. New York, Academic Press, 1969.

Brackbill, Y., and Fitzgerald, H. E.: Development of the sensory analyzers during infancy. In Advances in Child Development and Behavior, edited by L. P. Lipsitt and H. Reese, 4, 173–208. New York, Academic Press, 1969.

Bredberg, G., Engstrom, H., and Ades, H.: Cellular pattern and nerve supply of the human organ of Corti. Arch. Otolaryngol. 82: 462–469, 1965.

Bricker, D., and Bricker, W.: A programmed approach to operant audiometry for low-functioning children. J. Speech Hear. Disord. 34: 312–320, 1969.

Bridger, W. H.: Sensory discrimination and habituation in the human neonate. Am. J. Psychiatry 117: 991–996, 1961.

Briskey, R. J.: Binaural hearing aids and new innovations. In Handbook of Clinical Audiology, edited by J. Katz. Baltimore, Williams & Wilkins, 1972.

Briskey, R. J., and Sinclair, J.: The importance of low frequency amplification in deaf children. Audecibel (Winter), 7–20, 1966.

Brooks, D.: An objective method of detecting fluid in the middle ear. Int. Audiol. 7: 280–286, 1968.

Brooks, D.: The use of the electro-acoustic impedance bridge in the assessment of middle ear function. Int. Audiol. 8: 563–569, 1969.

Brooks, D.: Electroacoustic impedance bridge studies on normal ears of children. J. Speech Hear. Res. 14: 247–253, 1971.

Brooks, D. N.: Hearing screening: A comparative study of an impedance method and pure tone screening. Scand. Audiol. 2: 67–76, 1973.

Brooks, D. N.: Impedance measurement in screening for auditory disorders in children. Hearing Instruments (February) 20–21, 36, 1974.

Brown, J. B., Fryer, M. P., and Morgan, L. R.: Problems in reconstruction of the auricle. Plast. Reconstr. Surg. 43: 597–604, 1969.

Brown, K. S.: The genetics of childhood deafness. In Deafness in Childhood, edited by F. McConnell and P. H. Ward, pp. 177–202. Nashville, Vanderbilt University Press, 1967.

Brown, K. S., and Chung, C. S.: Genetic studies of deafness at the Clarke School for the Deaf, Northampton, Mass. In Report of the Proceedings of the International Congress on Education of the Deaf. Washington, D.C., U.S. Govt. Printing Office, 1964.

Bruner, J. S.: The cognitive consequences of early deprivation. In Sensory Deprivation, edited by P. Solomon, P. Kubansky, P. Leiderman, J. Mendelson, R. Trumbull, and D. Wexler, pp. 195–207. Cambridge, Harvard University Press, 1961.

Bruner, J. S.: Processes of Cognitive Growth: Infancy. Worcester, Clark University Press, 1968.

Bryden, M. P.: Attentional strategies and short-term memory in dichotic listening. Cognitive Psychol. 2: 99–116, 1971.

Butt, D. S., and Chreist, F. M.: A speechreading test for young children. Volta Review 70: 225–235, 1968.

Butterfield, E. C.: An extended version of modification of sucking with auditory feedback. Working Paper #43, Bureau of Child Research Laboratory, Children's Rehab. Unit, University of Kansas Medical Center, 1968.

Butterfield, G.: A note on the use of cardiac rate in the audiometric appraisal of retarded children. J. Speech Hear. Disord. 27: 378–379, 1962.

California Conference on Newborn Hearing Screening. Calif. Dept. of Public Health, Berkeley, and Public Health Service, HEW, Rockville, Md., 1971.

Carhart, R.: The usefulness of the binaural hearing aid. J. Speech Hear. Disord. 23: 41–51, 1958.

Carhart, R.: Monaural and binaural discrimination against competing sentences. Int. Audiology 4: 5–10, 1965.

Carhart, R.: Sensorineural hearing loss: An overview. Presented at the First International Conference on Electrical Stimulation of the Acoustic Nerve as a Treatment for Profound Sensorineural Deafness in Man, San Francisco, 1973.

Carhart, R., and Jerger, J.: Preferred method for clinical determination of pure tone thresholds. J. Speech Hear. Disord. 24: 330–345, 1959.

Carter, C. O.: An ABC of Medical Genetics. Boston, Little, Brown & Co., 1969.

Carver, W. F.: Hearing aids: A historical and technical review. In Handbook of Clinical Audiology, edited by J. Katz. Baltimore, Williams & Wilkins, 1972.

Chalfont, J. C., and Scheffelin, M. A.: Central Processing Dysfunction in Children. U.S. Dept. of HEW, Bethesda, Md., 1969.

Chomsky, N.: Aspects of the Theory of Syntax. Cambridge, Mass., M.I.T. Press, 1966.

Chung, C. S., Robinson, O. W., and Morton, N. E.: A note on deaf mutism. Ann. Hum. Genet. 23: 357–366, 1969.

Ciardi, J. T.: As I was saying. World Magazine, February 27, 1973.

Coats, A. C., and Dickey, J. R.: Non-surgical recording of human auditory-nerve action potentials and cochlear microphonics. Ann. Otol. Rhinol. Laryngol. 79: 844–852, 1970.

Cohen, A., Cohen, S. M., Levine, M., Maisel, R., Ruhm, H., and Wolfe, R. M.: Interdisciplinary pilot study of non-organic hearing loss. Ann. Otol. Rhinol. Laryngol. 72: 67–82, 1963.

Cohen, M. M., Rapin, I., Lyttle, M., and Schimmel, H.: Auditory evoked response (AER): Consistency of response in young sleeping children. Arch. Otolaryngol. 94: 214–217, 1971.

Cokely, D. R., and Gawlik, R.: A position paper on the relationship between manual English and Sign. The Deaf American, May, 7–9, 1973.

Condon, W. S., and Sander, L. W.: Neonate movement is synchronized with adult speech: Interactional participation and language structure. Science 183: 4120; 99–101, 1974.

Coombs, C. H.: Adaptation of galvanic response to auditory stimuli. J. Exp. Psychol. 22: 244–268, 1938.

Cooper, J. C.: More problems in instant medicine. Saturday Review, 56–61, 1967.

Corliss, E.: Facts about Hearing and Hearing Aids. A consumer's guide from the National Bureau of Standards, U.S. Dept. of Commerce. Washington, D.C., U.S. Govt. Printing Office, 1971.

Cornett, R. O.: Oralism vs manualism: Cued speech may be the answer. Hearing and Speech News 35: 6–9, 1967.

Crabtree, N., and Gerrard, J.: Perceptive deafness associated with severe neonatal jaundice. J. Laryngol. 64: 482–506, 1950.

Craig, W., Dodge, H. W., and Ross, P. J.: Acoustic neuromas in children: Report of two cases. J. Neurosurg. 11: 505–508, 1954.

Crispens, C. G., Jr.: Essentials of Medical Genetics. New York, Harper & Row, 1971.

Cullen, J. K., Ellis, M. S., Berlin, C. I., and Lousteau, R. J.: Human acoustic nerve action potential recordings from the tympanic membrane without anesthesia. Acta Otolaryngol. (Stockh.) 74: 15–22, 1972.

Cullen, J. K., and Thompson, C. L.: Release from masking in subjects with temporal lobe resections. Unpublished paper, Kresge Hearing Research Laboratory of the South, New Orleans, 1973.

Cunningham, G. C.: Biochemical screening programs and problems. In Earlier Recognition of Handicapping Conditions in Childhood: Proceedings of a Bi-Regional Institute, edited by E. M. Gold. University of California, Berkeley, School of Public Health, pp. 37–41, 1970.

Cunningham, G. C.: Conference on Newborn Hearing Screening. Calif. Dept. of Public Health, Berkeley, and Public Health Service, HEW, Rockville, Md., 1971.

Curren, J., and Ely, J.: Clearing the compression jungle. The Hearing Dealer 24: 16–34, 1973.

Davis, H.: Peripheral coding of auditory information. In Sensory Communication, edited by W. A. Rosenblith. Cambridge, MIT Press, 1961.

Danaher, E. M., and Pickett, J. M.: Relationship between the acoustic reflex and syllable discrimination. Presented at Convention of the American Speech and Hearing Association, San Francisco, 1972.

Darley, F. L.: Identification audiometry for school-age children: Basic procedures. J. Speech Hear. Disord. (Monograph Suppl.) #9, 26–34, 1961.

Davies, J.: Embryology of the Head and Neck in Relation to the Practice of Otolaryngology. Manual from Continuing Education Program. Rochester, American Academy of Ophthalmology and Otolaryngology, 1951.

d'Avignon, M., and Barr, B.: Ear abnormalities and cranial nerve palsy in thalidomide children. Arch. Otolaryngol. 80: 136–140, 1964.

Davis, H.: Biophysics and physiology of the inner ear. Physiol. Rev. 37: 1, 1957.

Davis, H.: The young deaf child: Identification and management. Acta Otolaryngol. [Suppl.] (Stockh.) 206: 94–99, 1965a.

Davis, H.: The young deaf child: Possibility of injury by amplified sound. Acta Otolaryngol. [Suppl.] (Stockh.) 206: 240–244, 1965b.

Davis, H.: Sedation of young children for electric response audiometry (ERA): Summary of a symposium. Audiology: J. Aud. Comm. 12: 55–57, 1973.

Davis, H., Hirsh, S. K., Shelnutt, J., and Bowers, C.: Further validation of evoked response audiometry (ERA). J. Speech Hear. Res. 10: 717–732, 1967.

Davis, H., Mast, T., Yoshie, N., and Zerlin, S.: The slow response of the human cortex to auditory stimuli: Recovery process. EEG Clin. Neurophysiol. 21: 105–113, 1966.

Davis, H., and Yoshie, N.: Human evoked cortical responses to auditory Stimuli. Physiologist 6: 164, 1963.

Davis, H., and Zerlin, S.: Acoustic relations of the human vertex potential. J. Acoust. Soc. Am. 39: 109–116, 1966.

Davis, P. A.: Effects of acoustic stimuli on the waking human brain. J. Neurophysiol. 2: 494–499, 1939.

Davis, R. C.: Factors affecting the galvanic response to auditory stimuli. Arch Psychol. (Frankf.) 18: 5–64, 1930.

Deatherage, B. H., and Hirsh, I. J.: Auditory localization of clicks. J. Acoust. Soc. Am. 31: 486–492, 1959.

DeHirsch, K., Jansky, J. J., and Langford, W. S.: Predicting Reading Failure. New York, Harper & Row, 1966.

Denenberg, V. H., and Morton, J. R. C.: Infantile stimulation, perpetual sexual-social interaction and emotionality. Anim. Behav. 12: 11–13, 1964.

Dennis, W.: Children of the Creche. Century Psychology Series. New York, Prentice-Hall, 1973.

Derbyshire, A. J., and Davis, H.: The action potential of the auditory nerve. Am. J. Physiol. 113: 476–504, 1935.

Derbyshire, A. J., and Farley, J. C.: Sampling auditory responses at the cortical level. Ann. Otol. Rhino. Laryngol. 68: 675–696, 1959.

Derbyshire, A. J., and McCandless, G. A.: Template for the EEG response to sound. J. Speech Hear. Res. 7: 95–102, 1964.

Detroit Tests of Learning Aptitude: Detroit, Bobbs-Merrill, 1935.

DiCarlo, L. M., and Gardner, E. F.: The efficiency of the Massachusetts pure-tone screening test as adapted for a university testing program. J. Speech Hear. Disord. 18: 175–182, 1953.

DiCarlo, L. M., Kindall, D. C., and Goldstein, R.: Diagnostic procedures for auditory disorders in children. Folia Phoniatr. (Basel) 14: 206–264, 1962.

Directory of programs and services for the deaf. Ann. Deaf 116: 214, 1971.

Dirks, D., and Carhart, R.: A survey of reactions from users of binaural and monaural hearing aids. J. Speech Hear. Disord. 27: 311–321, 1962.

Dodds, E., and Harford, E.: Modified earpieces and CROS for high frequency hearing loss. J. Speech Hear. Res. 11: 204–218, 1968.

Dodds, E., and Harford, E.: Follow-up report on modified earpieces and CROS for high frequency hearing losses. J. Speech Hear. Res. 13: 41–43, 1970.

Doerfler, L. G.: Neurophysiological clues to auditory acuity. J. Speech Hear. Disord. 13: 227–232, 1948.

Doerfler, L. G., and Kramer, J. C.: Unconditioned stimulus strength and the galvanic skin response. J. Speech Hear. Disord. 2: 184–192, 1959.

Doster, M.: Personal communication. Denver Public Schools Health Department, 1972.

Downs, M.: The familiar sounds test and other tests for hearing screening in children. J. Sch. Health 26: 77–87, 1956.

Downs, M.: Not Cleared for Hearing. Price Filmakers, Hollywood, (16 mm sound movie), 1965.

Downs, M. P.: Manual for organization and procedures of a newborn infant screening program. Hearing and Speech News 35: 26–36, 1967a.

Downs, M. P.: Testing hearing in infancy and early childhood. In Deafness in Childhood, edited by M. Freeman and P. H. Ward, Ch. 2, pp. 25–33. Nashville, Vanderbilt University Press, 1967b.

Downs, M. P.: The establishment of hearing aid use: A program for parents. Maico Audiological Library Series 4: 1967c

Downs, M. P.: The identification of congenital deafness. Trans. Am. Acad. Ophthalmol. Otolaryngol. 74: 1208–1214, 1970.

Downs, M. P.: Audiological evaluation of the congenitally deaf infant. Otolaryngol. Clin. North Am. 4: 347–358, 1971a.

Downs, M. P.: Auditory Screening of Infants (video tape): Nebraska Educational Television Council for Higher Education (NETCHE). Lincoln, University of Nebraska, 1971b.

Downs, M. P.: Maintaining children's hearing aids: The role of the parents. Maico Audiological Library Series 10: 1, 1971c.

Downs, M. P.: Overview of the management of the deaf child. Otolaryngol. Clin. North Am. 4: 223–226, 1971d.

Downs, M. P.: Relationship of pathology to function in congenital hearing loss. II. The auditory function in congenital hearing loss. Audiology: J. Aud. Comm. 11: 330–336, 1972b.

Downs, M. P.: Fitting the training program to the child. Fifth Danavox Symposium on Evaluation of Hearing Handicapped Children. Copenhagen, 1973.

Downs, M. P.: The Deafness Management Quotient. Hearing and Speech News 42: 8–28, 1974.

Downs, M. P., and Akin, J.: Unpublished research on a comparison between deaf and normal hearing infant vocalizations. Denver, 1973.

Downs, M. P., and Doster, M.: A hearing testing program for pre-school children. Rocky Mt. Med. J. 56: 37–40, 1959.

Downs, M. P., Doster, M. E., and Weaver, M.: Dilemmas in identification audiometry. J. Speech Hear. Disord. 30: 360–364, 1965.

Downs, M. P., and Hemenway, W. G.: Report on the hearing screening of 17,000 neonates. Int. Audiol. 8: 72–76, 1969.

Downs, M. P., and Silver, H. K.: The A.B.C.D.'s to H.E.A.R.: Early identification in nursery, office and clinic of the infant who is deaf. Clin. Pediatr. (Phila.) 11: 563–566, 1972.

Downs, M. P., and Sterritt, G. M.: Identification audiometry for neonates: A preliminary report. J. Aud. Res. 4: 69–80, 1964.

Downs, M. P., and Sterritt, G. M.: A guide to newborn and infant hearing screening programs. Arch. Otolaryngol. 85: 15–22, 1967.

Drake, C.: PERC Auditory Discrimination Test. Sherborn, Mass., Perc. Ed. and Research Center, 1965.

Dubnoff, B.: Early detection and remediation of learning disabilities. In Earlier Recognition of Handicapping Conditions in Childhood: Proceedings of a Bi-Regional Institute. University of California, Berkeley, School of Public Health, 131–140, 1970.

Dunlavy, A.: CROS: The new miracle worker. Audecibel (Fall issue), 1970.

Dupertius, S. M., and Musgrave, R. H.: Experiences with the reconstruction of the congenitally deformed ear. Plast. Reconstr. Surg. 23: 361–373, 1959.

Dykstra, R.: Auditory discrimination abilities and beginning reading achievement. Reading Research Quarterly, 1: 5–34, 1966.

Eagles, E. L., and Doerfler, L. G.: A study of hearing in children. II. Acoustic environment and audiometer performance. Trans. Am. Acad. Ophthalmol. Otolaryngol. 65: 238–296, 1961.

Eagles, E. L., Wishik, S. M., and Doerfler, L. G.: Hearing sensitivity and ear disease in children: A prospective study. Laryngoscope (Monograph) 1–274, 1967.

Edwards, E. P.: Kindergarten is too late. Saturday Review 60–79, 1968.

Efron, R.: Temporal perception, aphasia, and déjà vu. Brain 86: 403–424, 1963.

Eimas, P. D., Siqueland, E. R., Jusczyk, P., and Vigorit, J.: Speech perception in infants. Science 171: 303, 1972.

Eisenberg, R. B.: Auditory behavior in the human neonate. I. Methodologic problems and the logical design of research procedures. J. Aud. Res. 5: 159–177, 1965.

Eisenberg, R. B.: Auditory behavior in the human neonate: Functional properties of sound and their ontogenetic implications. Int. Aud. 8: 34–45, 1969.

Eisenberg, R. B.: The development of hearing in man: An assessment of current status. ASHA 12: 119–123, 1970.

Eisenberg, R. B., Coursin, D. B., and Rupp, N. R.: Habituation to an acoustic pattern as an index of differences among human neonates. J. Aud. Res. 6: 239–248, 1966.

Eisenberg, R. B., Griffin, E. J., Coursin, D. B., and Hunter, M. A.: Auditory behavior in the human neonate: A preliminary report. J. Speech Hear. Res. 7: 245–269, 1964.

Eliachar, I., and Northern, J.: Studies in tympanometry: Validation of the present technique for determining intra-tympanic pressures through the intact eardrum. Laryngoscope 84: 247–255, 1974.

Eliachar, I., Sando, I., and Northern, J.: Measurement of middle ear pressure in guinea pigs. Arch. Otolaryngol. 99: 172–176, 1974.

Elliot, G. B., and Elliot, K. A.: Some pathological, radiological and clinical implications of the precocious development of the human ear. Laryngoscope 74: 1160–1171, 1964.

Elliot, L. L., and Armbruster, V. B.: Some possible effects of the delay of early treatment of deafness. J. Speech Hear. Res. 10: 209–224, 1967.

English, G. M., Northern, J. L., and Fria, T. J.: Chronic otitis media as a cause of sensorineural hearing loss. Arch. Otolaryngol. 98: 17–22, 1973.

Erber, N.: Evaluation of special hearing aids for deaf children. J. Speech Hear. Disord. 36: 527–537, 1971.

Everberg, G.: Further studies on hereditary unilateral deafness. Acta Otolaryngol. (Stockh.) 51: 615–635, 1960.

Everett, N. B.: Functional Neuroanatomy. Philadelphia, Lea & Febiger, 1965.

Ewing, I. R., and Ewing, A. W. G.: The ascertainment of deafness in infancy and early childhood. J. Laryngol. Otol. 59: 309–338, 1944.

Fagan, J. F., III: Memory in the infant. J. Exp. Child Psycho. 9: 217–226, 1970.

Fagan, J. F., III: Infants' recognition memory for a series of visual stimuli. J. Exp. Child Psychol. 11: 244–250, 1971.

Falck, S. A.: Combined effects of noise and ototoxic drugs. Environ. Health Perspect. 5–22, 1972.

Fant, L. J., Jr.: An appraisal of the oral and combined methods of communication in the education of deaf children. Mimeographed manuscript prepared by Department of Education, Gallaudet College, Washington, D.C., 1963.

Fant, L. J., Jr.: Say It with Hands. Washington, D.C., Gallaudet College, 1964.

Fant, L. J., Jr.: Ameslan: An Introduction to the American Sign Language. Silver Spring, Md., National Association of the Deaf, 1972.

Fantz, R. L.: The origin of form perception. Sci. Am. 204: 66–72, 1961.

Fay, T. H.: Audiologic and otologic screening of disadvantaged children. In Otitis Media, edited by A. Glorig and K. Gerwin, pp. 163–170. Springfield, Ill., Charles C Thomas, 1972.

Federal Trade Commission, Complaint (D.8791, Hearing Aids), Charge #9, Released July 25, 1969.

Feinmesser, M., and Bauberger-Tell, L.: Evaluation of methods of detecting hearing impairment in infancy and early childhood. Presented at Conference on Newborn Hearing Screening, Bureau of Maternal and Child Health, San Francisco, 119–125, 1971. (Later personal correspondence, 1972.)

Feinmesser, M., and Zelig, S.: Congenital deafness associated with onychodystrophy. Arch. Otolaryngol. 74: 507–515, 1961.

Feldmann, H.: Experiments on binaural hearing in noise: The central nervous processing of acoustic information. Translations of the Beltone Institute for Hearing Research, 18 (July, 1965).

Feldman, R. M., and Goldstein, R.: Averaged evoked responses to synthetic syntax sentences (3S). J. Speech Hear. Res. 10: 689–696, 1967.

Fisher, B.: An investigation of binaural hearing aids. J. Laryngol. Otol. 73: 658–668, 1964.

Fisher, H. G., and Freedman, S. J.: The role of the pinna in auditory localization. J. Auditory Res. 8: 15–26, 1968.

Fleming, J. D.: The state of the apes. Psychology Today, 31–50, Jan. 1974.

Fletcher, H.: Speech and Hearing. New York, Van Nostrand, Inc., 1929.

Flower, R. M.: Auditory disorders and reading disorders. In Reading Disorders, edited by R. M. Flower, H. F. Gofman, and L. I. Lawson, pp. 81–102. Philadelphia, F. A. Davis Co., 1965.

Flower, R. M.: The evaluation of auditory abilities in the appraisal of children with reading problems. In Perception and Reading, edited by

H. K. Smith, pp. 21–24. Newark, Del. International Reading Association, 1968.

Ford, F. R.: Diseases of the Nervous System in Infancy, Childhood, and Adolescence, 5th Ed. Springfield, Ill., Charles C Thomas, Publisher, 1966.

Foust, K., and Gengel, R.: Speech discrimination by sensorineural hearing-impaired persons using a transposer hearing aid. Scand. Audiol. 2: 161–170, 1973.

Fowler, E. P., and Fletcher, H.: Three million deafened school children: Their detection and treatment. JAMA 87: 1877–1882, 1926.

Frankenburg, W.: Evaluation of screening procedures. In Earlier Recognition of Handicapping Conditions in Childhood: Proceedings of a Bi-regional Institute, edited by E. M. Gold. University of California, Berkeley, School of Public Health, pp. 42–51, 1970.

Frankenburg, W. K., and Dodds, J. B.: The Denver developmental screening test. J. Pediatr. 71: 181–191, 1967.

Fraser, G. R.: The genetics of congenital deafness. Otolaryngol. Clin. North Am. 4: 227–247, 1971.

Fraser, G. R., Froggatt, P., and James, T.: Congenital deafness associated with EKG abnormalities, fainting, attacks and sudden death: A recessive syndrome. Q. J. Med. 33: 361, 1964.

Freedman, A. M., and Kaplan, H. I.: Comprehensive Textbook of Psychiatry, pp. 1434–1438. Baltimore, Williams & Wilkins, 1967.

Freud, S.: Beyond the Pleasure Principle. London, Hogarth Press, 1948.

Friedlander, B. Z.: Receptive language development in infancy. Merrill-Palmer Quarterly of Behavior and Development 16: 7–51, 1970.

Friedlander, B., and DeLara, H. C.: Receptive language anomaly and language reading dysfunction in "normal" primary-grade school children. Psychol. in Schools 10: 12–18, 1973.

Froeschels, E., and Beebe, H.: Testing hearing of newborn infants. Arch. Otolaryngol. 44: 710–714, 1946.

Fromm, B., Nylen, C., and Zotterman, Y.: Studies in the mechanism of the Wever and Bray effect. Acta Otolaryngol. (Stockh.) 22: 477–486, 1935.

Fulton, R. T., and Lamb, L. E.: Acoustic impedance and tympanometry with the retarded: a normative study. Audiology 11: 199–208, 1972.

Fulton, R. T., and Lloyd, L. L. (Eds.): Audiometry for the Retarded with Implications for the Difficult-to-Test. Baltimore, Williams & Wilkins, 1969.

Furth, H. G.: Thinking without Language. New York, The Free Press, 1966.

Furusho, T.: A genetic study on the congenital deafness. Jap. J. Hum. Genet. 2: 35–58, 1957.

Gaeth, J. H., and Lounsbury, E.: Hearing aids and children in elementary schools. J. Speech Hear. Disord. 31: 283–289, 1966.

Gagne, R. M.: The Conditions of Learning. New York, Holt, Rinehart & Winston, 1965.

Galambos, R., and Davis, H.: The response of single auditory-nerve fibers to acoustic stimulation. J. Neurophysiol. 6: 39–57, 1943.

Galambos, R., and Davis, H.: Action potentials from single auditory-nerve fibers. Science 108: 513, 1948.

Galambos, R., Rosenberg, P. E., and Glorig, A.: The eyeblink response as a test for hearing. J. Speech Hear. Disord. 18: 373–378, 1953.

Galambos, R., Schwartzkopff, J., and Rupert, A.: Microelectrode study of superior olivary nuclei. Am. J. Physiol. 197: 527–536, 1959.

Gallagher, J. C.: Histology of the Temporal Bone. Washington, D.C., Armed Forces Institute of Pathology, 1967.

Gannon, R. P., and Tso, S. S.: The occult effect of kanamycin on the cochlea. Exerpta Medica 18: 98, 1969.

Gardner, H.: The forgotten lesson of Monsieur C. Psychology Today, Aug. 1973.

Gardner, M. B.: A pulse tone technique for clinical audiometric threshold measurements. J. Am. Speech Assoc. 19: 592–599, 1947.

Gardner, R. A., and Gardner, B. T.: Teaching sign language to a chimpanzee. Science 165: 664–672, 1969.

Garretson, M. D.: The need for multiple communication skills in the education process of the deaf. Rocky Mt. Leader 62: 1–8, 1963.

Geisler, C. D.: Electrical responses to acoustic clicks recorded from the human scalp. Quarterly Progress Report No. 57, Communications Biophysics Group. Cambridge, Mass., MIT 1960.

Gellis, S. S., and Feingold, M.: Atlas of Mental Retardation Syndromes. Washington, D.C., U.S. Dept. of HEW, 1968.

Gescheider, G. A.: Resolving of successive clicks by the ears and skin. J. Exp. Psychol. 71: 378–381, 1966.

Geschwind, N.: The anatomy of acquired disorders of reading. In Reading Disability: Progress and Research Needs in Dyslexia, edited by J. Money. Baltimore, Johns Hopkins, 1962.

Geschwind, N., and Levitsky, W.: Human brain: Left-right asymmetries in temporal speech region. Science 161: 186–187, 1968.

Gesell, A.: The psychological development of normal and deaf children in their preschool years. Volta Review 58: 117–120, 1956.

Giannini, M. J.: Rapid developmental screening check list. Committee on Children with Handicaps, Ch. III. New York, American Academy of Pediatrics, 1972.

Glorig, A.: Screening tests. In Audiometry, Principles and Practice, edited by A. Glorig, pp. 170–184. Baltimore, Williams & Wilkins, 1965.

Glorig, A., Moushegian, G., Bringewald, P., Rupert, A., and Gerkin, G. M.: Magnetically coupled stimulation of the ossicular chain: Measures in kangaroo rat and man. J. Acoust. Soc. 52: 694–696, 1972.

Goetzinger, C. P., Embrey, J. E., and Brooks, R.: Auditory assessment of cleft palate adults. Acta Otolaryngol. (Stockh.) 52: 551–557, 1960.

Gold, E. M.: Prevention of mental retardation. In Earlier Recognition of Handicapping Conditions in Childhood: Proceedings of a Bi-regional Institute, pp. 66–75. University of California, Berkeley, School of Public Health, 1970.

Goldman, R., Fristoe, M., and Woodcock, R. W.: Test of Auditory Discrimination. Minnesota, American Guidance Service, Inc., 1970.

Goldstein, R.: Detection and assessment of auditory disorder in children less than three years old: A critical review. Volta Review 57: 215–219, 1955.

Goldstein, R.: Electrophysiologic audiometry. In Modern Developments in Audiology, edited by J. Jerger, 1st Ed. New York, Academic Press, 1963.

Goldstein, R.: Pseudohypoacusis. J. Speech Hear. Disord. 31: 341–352, 1966.

Goldstein, R.: Auditory dysfunction associated with brain impairment. Postgrad. Med. 48: 83–85, 1970.

Goldstein, R.: Electroencephalic audiometry. In Modern Developments in Audiology, edited by J. Jerger, 2nd Ed., pp. 407–435. New York, Academic Press, 1973.

Goldstein, R., Landan, W. M., and Kleffner, F. R.: Neurological observations in a population of deaf and aphasic children. Ann. Otol. Rhinol. Laryngol. 69: 756–767, 1960.

Goldstein, R., McRandle, C. C., and Rodman, L. B.: Site of lesion in cases of hearing loss associated with Rh incompatibility: An argument for peripheral impairment. J. Speech Hear. Disord. 37: 447–450, 1972.

Goldstein, R., and Tait, C.: Critique of neonatal hearing evaluation. J. Speech Hear. Disord. 36: 3–18, 1971.

Goode, R. L.: An implantable hearing aid: State of the art. Trans. Am. Acad. Ophthalmol. Otolaryngol. 74: 128–139, 1970.

Goodhill, V.: Auditory pathway lesions resulting from Rh incompatibility. In Deafness in Childhood, Chap. 14, edited by F. McConnell and P. H. Ward. Nashville, Vanderbilt University Press, 1967.

Gorlin, R. J., and Pindborg, J. J.: Syndromes of Head and Neck. New York, McGraw-Hill, 1964.

Graham, F. K., Clifton, R. K., and Hatton, H. M.: Habituation of heart rate response to repeated auditory stimulation during the first five days of life. Child Dev. 39: 35–52, 1968.

Graham, M. D.: A longitudinal study of ear disease and hearing loss in patients with cleft lips and palates. Trans. Am. Acad. Ophthalmol. Otolaryngol. 67: 213–222, 1963.

Green, D. S.: Non-occluding earmolds with CROS and IROS hearing aids. Arch. Otolaryngol. 89: 96–522, 1969.

Greenberg, D. J., and Weizmann, F.: The measurement of visual attention in infants: A comparison of two methodologies. J. Exp. Child Psychol. 11: 234–243, 1971.

Greenway, E. B.: The communication needs of the deaf child. In Report of the Proceedings of the International Congress on the Education of the Deaf, pp. 433–439. Washington, D.C., Gallaudet College, 1964.

Griffing, T. S., Simonton, K. M., and Hedgecock, L. D.: Verbal auditory screening for pre-school children. Trans. Am. Acad. Ophthalmol. Otolaryngol. 71: 105–111, 1967.

Grings, W. W., Lowell, E. L., and Rushford, G. M.: Role of conditioning in GSR audiometry with children. J. Speech Hear. Disord. 24: 380–390, 1959.

Groen, J. J., and Hellema, A. C. M.: Binaural speech audiometry. Acta Otolaryngol. (Stockh.) 52: 397–414, 1960.

Groht, M. A.: Natural Language for Deaf Children. Washington, D.C., Gallaudet College Press, 1958.

Grossman, A. A., and Marcus, R. E.: Will County survey. Otolaryngological experiences in a hearing survey. J. Speech Hear. Disord. 14: 240–246, 1949.

Gustason, G., Pfetzing, D., and Zawolkow, E.: Signing Exact English. Rossmoor, Calif., Modern Signs Press, 1972.

Guyton, A. C.: Textbook of Medical Physiology, 4th Ed., pp. 264, 955. Philadelphia, W. B. Saunders, 1971.

Halfond, M. M., and Ballenger, J. J.: An audiologic and otorhinologic study of cleft lip and cleft palate cases. Arch. Otolaryngol. 64: 58–62, 1956.

Hall, J.: Cochlea and the cochlear nuclei in asphyxia. Acta Otolaryngol.

[suppl.] (Stockh.) 194: 1964.

Hall, J. G.: Diastrophic dwarfism with ossicle malformation. Paper presented at the Second Conference on the Clinical Delineation of Birth Defects, John Hopkins Medical Institutions, Baltimore, Md., May 30, 1969.

Hall, J. L., II: Binaural interaction in the accessory superior olivary nucleus of the cat. J. Acoust. Soc. 37: 814–823, 1965.

Hardy, J. B.: Viral infections in pregnancy: A review. Am. J. Obstet. Gynecol. 93: 1052–1065, 1965.

Hardy, J. B., Dougherty, A., and Hardy, W. F.: Hearing responses and audiometric screening in infants. J. Pediatr. 55: 382–390, 1959.

Hardy, W. G.: Problems of audition, perception, and understanding. Volta Bureau Reprint, 1956.

Hardy, W. G.: In Brain Mechanisms Underlying Speech and Language, edited by F. L. Darley. New York, Grune and Stratton, 1967.

Hardy, W. G., and Bordley, J. E.: Special techniques in testing the hearing of children. J. Speech Hear. Disord. 16: 122–131, 1951.

Hardy, W. G., and Pauls, M. D.: The test situation in PGSR audiometry. J. Speech Hear. Disord. 17: 13–24, 1952.

Hardy, W. G., and Pauls, M.: Significance of problems of conditioning in GSR audiometry. J. Speech Hear. Disord. 24: 123–126, 1959.

Harford, E., and Barry, J.: A rehabilitative approach to the problems of unilateral hearing impairment: The contralateral routing of signals (CROS). J. Speech Hear. Disord. 30: 121–128, 1965.

Harford, E., and Dodds, E.: The clinical application of CROS. Arch. Otolaryngol. 83: 455–464, 1966.

Harford, E. R., and Markle, D. M.: The atypical effect of a hearing aid on one patient with congenital deafness. Laryngoscope 65: 970–972, 1955.

Harris, J. D.: Monaural and binaural speech intelligibility and the stereophonic effect based on temporal cues. Laryngoscope 75: 428–446, 1965.

Harris, J. D.: The true goals and aspirations of audiology. Summary of the Symposium on Amplification for Sensorineural Hearing Loss, Twin Peaks, California, University of Redlands, 1971. In Harris on Audiology. Groton, Conn., J. Aud. Res., 1973.

Hart, B. O.: A child centered language program. Report of the Proceedings of the International Congress of the Education of the Deaf and of the 41st Meeting of the Convention of American Instructors of the Deaf. Gallaudet College, pp. 505–514. Washington, D.C., U.S. Govt. Printing Office, 1964.

Haskins, H.: A phonetically balanced test of speech discrimination for children. Unpublished Master's Thesis, 1949. (Cited by J. O'Neill and H. Oyer, in Applied Audiometry, New York, Dodd, Mead & Co., 1966.)

Haskins, H. L., and Hardy, W. G.: Clinical studies in stereophonic listening. Laryngoscope 70: 1427–1433, 1960.

Haug, O., Baccaro, P., and Guilford, F.: A pure-tone audiogram on the infant: The PIWI technique. Arch. Otolaryngol. 86: 101–106, 1967.

Hawkins, J. E., Jr.: Antibiotic insults to Corti's organ. In Sensorineural Hearing Processes and Disorders, edited by A. B. Graham. Boston, Little, Brown & Co., 1967a.

Hawkins, J. E., Jr.: Iatrogenic toxic deafness in children. In Deafness in Childhood, edited by F. McConnell, and P. H. Ward, pp. 156–168. Nashville, Vanderbilt University Press, 1967b.

Haynes, U.: A Developmental Approach to Casefinding with Special Reference to Cerebral Palsy, Mental Retardation and Related Disorders. Washington, D.C., Govt. Printing Office, 1967.

Health Information Series No. 140: Public Health Service Publication No. 1646, U.S. Dept. of HEW, 1971.

Hearing Aid Industry Conference (HAIC): Standard Method of Expressing Hearing Aid Performance, New York, 1961.

Heber, R., and Garber, H.: An experiment in the prevention of cultural-familial mental retardation. U.S. Dept. of HEW, Office of Education, Ed. Resources Inf. Center, Washington, D.C., ED 059762, PS 005367, 1970,.

Hemenway, W. G.: Relationship of pathology to function in congenital hearing loss. I: The pathology of congenital hearing loss. Audiology 11: 322–329, 1972.

Hemenway, W. G., and Bergstrom, L.: The pathology of acquired viral endolabyrinthitis. In Deafness in Childhood, edited by F. McConnell and P. H. Ward, pp. 91–122. Nashville, Vanderbilt University Press, 1967.

Hemenway, W. G., and Bergstrom, L. (Eds.): Symposium on Congenital Deafness. Otolaryngol. Clin. North Am. 4: 1971.

Hemenway, W. G., and Bergstrom, L.: Dysplasias of the inner ear. In Birth Defects, Atlas and Compendium, edited by D. Bergsma. Baltimore, Williams & Wilkins, published for the National Foundation—March of Dimes, 1972.

Hemenway, W. G., Sando, I., and McChesney, D.: Temporal bone pathology following maternal rubella. Arch. Klin. Exp. Ohren. Nasen.

Kehlkopfheilkd. 193: 287–300, 1969.

Hersch, B., and Amon, C.: An approach to reporting the diagnosis of hearing loss to parents of a hearing impaired child. Unpublished manuscript, University of Denver, 1973.

Hersch, L. B., and Solomon, M. A.: A comprehensive approach to understanding deafness. Am. Ann. Deaf 118: 34–36, 1973.

Hess, E. H.: Attitude and pupil size. Sci. Am. 212: 46–54, 1965.

HEW Monthly Vital Statistics Report: Advance Report: Final Natality Statistics, 1963. Washington, D.C., U.S. Dept. of HEW, Public Health Service, National Center for Health Statistics, 1964.

Hildyard, V. H., Stool, S. E., and Valentine, M. A.: Tuning fork tests as aid to screening audiometry. Arch. Otolaryngol., 78: 151–154, 1963.

Hildyard, V. H., and Valentine, M. A.: Collapse of the ear canal during audiometry. Arch. Otolaryngol. 75: 422–423, 1962.

Hilgard, E. R., and Marquis, D. G. (Revised by G. A. Kimble): Conditioning and Learning, 2nd Ed. New York, Appleton-Century-Crofts, 1961.

Hinchcliffe, R.: Epidemiological aspects of otitis media. In Otitis Media, edited by A. Glorig and K. Gerwin, pp. 36–43. Springfield, Ill., Charles C Thomas, Publisher, 1972.

Hirsh, I.: Comment reported in Proceedings of a Conference on Sensory Training Aids for the Hearing Impaired, edited by H. Levitt and P. Nye, National Academy of Engineering, Subcommittee on Sensory Aids, Washington, D.C., 1971.

Hirsh, J. E.: Effect of interaural time delay on amplitude of cortical responses evoked by tones. J. Neurophysiol. 31: 916–927, 1969.

Hodgson, W.: Audiological report of a patient with left hemispherectomy. J. Speech Hear. Disord. 32: 39–45, 1967.

Hodgson, W. R.: Testing infants and young children. In Handbook of Clinical Audiology, edited by J. Katz, pp. 498–519. Baltimore, Williams & Wilkins, 1972.

Hodgson, W., and Murdock, C.: Effects of the earmold on speech intelligibility in hearing aid use. J. Speech Hear. Res. 13: 290–297, 1970.

Hogan, D. D.: Autonomic responses as supplementary hearing measures. In Audiometry for the Retarded, edited by R. F. Fulton and L. L. Lloyd. Baltimore, Williams & Wilkins, 1969.

Holborow, C. A.: Deafness associated with cleft palate. Laryngoscope 76: 762–773, 1962.

Holm, V. A., and Kunze, L. H.: Effect of chronic otitis media on language and speech development. Pediatrics 43: 833–839, 1969.

Holmes, E. M.: The microtia ear. Arch. Otolaryngol. 49: 243–265, 1949.

Holmgren, L.: Can the hearing be damaged by a hearing aid? Acta Otolaryngol. (Stockh.) 28: 440, 1940.

Hopkinson, N. T.: Functional hearing loss. In Modern Developments in Audiology, edited by J. Jerger, 2nd Ed. New York, Academic Press, 1973.

Hord, D. J., Lubin, A., and Johnson, L. C.: The evoked heart rate response during sleep. Psychophysiology 3: 46–54, 1966.

House, W.: Multichannel electrical stimulation in man. Presented at the First International Conference on Electrical Stimulation of the Acoustic Nerve as a Treatment for Profound Sensorineural Deafness in Man, San Francisco, 1973.

Hsia, D. Y.: Biochemical aspects of handicapping conditions. In Earlier Recognition of Handicapping Conditions in Childhood: Proceedings of a Bi-Regional Institute, edited by E. M. Gold. University of California, Berkeley, School of Public Health, pp. 13–36, 1970.

Human Communication: The public health aspects of hearing, language, and speech disorders. U.S. Dept. of HEW, Public Health Service NINDB Monograph, 7, 1968.

Irwin, J. V., Hind, J. E. and Aronson, A.: Experience with GSR audiometry in a group of mentally deficient individuals. Train. Sch. Bull. (Vinel.) 54: 31, 1957.

Irwin, O. C.: Infant speech: Consonantal sounds according to manner of articulation. J. Speech Hear. Disord. 12: 402–404, 1947.

Irwin, O. C.: Infant speech, the effect of family occupational status and of age on use of sound frequency. J. Speech Hear. Disord. 13: 320–323, 1952.

Irwin, O. C.: Identification audiometry for school-age children: Basic procedures. J. Speech Hear. Disord. (Monograph) #9, 26–34, 1961.

Jaffe, B.: Hearing loss: Hope through research. PHS Publication #207, Health Information Series #,53, 1971a.

Jaffee, B. F.: Heredity and Congenital Factors Affecting Newborn Conductive Hearing. Berkeley, Calif., Conference Proceedings on Newborn Hearing Screening, State Dept. of Public Health, 1971b.

Jaffee, B., Hurtado, F., and Hurtado, E.: Tympanic membrane mobility in the newborn: With seven months' follow-up. Laryngoscope 80: 36–48, 1970.

Jepsen, O.: Middle ear muscle reflexes in man. In Modern Developments in Audiology, edited by J. Jerger. New York, Academic Press, 1963.

Jerger, J.: Auditory tests for disorders of the central auditory mechanisms. In Neurological Aspects of Auditory and Vestibular Disorders,

edited by W. S. Fields and B. R. Alford. Springfield, Ill., Charles C Thomas, Publisher, 1964.

Jerger, J.: Clinical experience with impedance audiometry. Arch. Otolaryngol. 92: 311–324, 1970.

Jerger, J.: Suggested nomenclature for impedance audiometry. Arch. Otolaryngol. 96: 1–3, 1972.

Jerger, J., Anthony, L., Jerger, S., and Mauldin, L.: Studies in impedance audiometry: III. Middle ear disorders. Arch. Otolaryngol. 99: 165–171, 1974b.

Jerger, J., Burney, P., Mauldin, L., and Crump, B.: Predicting hearing loss from the acoustic reflex. J. Speech Hear. Disord. 39: 11–22, 1974c.

Jerger, J., and Dirks, D.: Binaural hearing aids: An enigma. J. Acoust. Soc. 33: 537–538, 1961.

Jerger, J., Jerger, S., and Mauldin, L.: Studies in impedance audiometry: I. Normal and sensorineural ears. Arch. Otolaryngol. 96: 513–523, 1972.

Jerger, J., and Thelin, J.: Effects of electroacoustic characteristics of hearing aids on speech understanding. Bull. Prosthet. Res. 110: 159–197, 1968.

Jerger, J., Weikers, N. J., Sharbrough, F. W., and Jerger, S.: Bilateral lesions of the temporal lobe. Acta Otolaryngol. [Suppl.] (Stockh.) 258, 1969.

Jerger, S., Jerger, J., Mauldin, L., and Segal, P.: Studies in impedance audiometry: II. Children less than 6 years old. Arch. Otolaryngol. 99: 1–9, 1974a.

Johansson, B.: A new coding amplifier system for the severely hard of hearing. In Proceedings of the Third International Conference on Acoustics, Stuttgart, 1959, 2, 655–657, published 1961.

Johansson, B.: The use of the transposer for the management of the deaf child. Int. Audiology. 5: 362–372, 1966.

Johansson, B., Wedenberg, E., and Westin, B.: Measurement of tone response by the human fetus. Acta Otolaryngol., (Stockh.) 57: 188–192, 1964.

Johnsson, L., and Hawkins, J. E., Jr.: A direct approach to cochlear anatomy and pathology in man. Arch. Otolaryngol. 85: 43–57, 1967.

Johnston, P. W.: An efficient group screening test. J. Speech Hear. Disord. 17: 8–12, 1952.

Jones, H. E.: Conditioned psychogalvanic responses in infants. Psychol. Bull. 25: 183–184, 1928.

Jordan, O., Greisen, O., and Bentzen, O.: Treatment with binaural hearing aids. Arch. Otolaryngol. 85: 319–326, 1967.

Jordan, R. E., and Eagles, E. L.: The relation of air conduction audiometry to otologic abnormalities. Ann. Otol. Rhinol. Laryngol. 70: 819–827, 1961.

Jorgensen, M. B., and Kristensen, H. K.: Thalidomide induced aplasia of the inner ear. J. Laryngol. Otol. 78: 1095–1101, 1964.

Kagan, J.: Do infants think? Sci. Am. 226: 74–82, 1972.

Kagan, J., and Lewis, M.: Studies in attention in the human infant. Merrill-Palmer Quarterly of Behavior and Development 11: 101–119, 1965.

Kannapell, B. M., Hamilton, L. B., and Bornstein, H.: Signs for Instructional Purposes. Washington, D.C., Gallaudet College Press, 1969.

Kaplan, E. L.: The role of intonation in the acquisition of language. Doctoral dissertation, Cornell University, 1969.

Karmody, C. S., and Schuknecht, H. F.: Deafness in congenital syphilis. Arch. Otolaryngol. 83: 18–26, 1966.

Kasten, R. N.: Body and over the ear hearing aids. In Handbook of Clinical Audiology, edited by J. Katz. Baltimore, Williams & Wilkins, 1972.

Kasten, R., and Braunlin, R.: Traumatic hearing aid usage : A case study. Presented at the American Speech and Hearing Association Convention, 1970.

Katz, J. (Ed.): Handbook of Clinical Audiology. Baltimore, Williams & Wilkins, 1972.

Kearsley, R., Snider, M., Richie, R., and Talbot, N.: Study of relations between psychologic environment and child behavior. Am. J. Dis. Child. 104: 12–20, 1962.

Keen, R. C., Chase, W., and Graham, F. K.: Twenty-four hour retention by neonates of an habituated heart rate response. Psychon. Sci. 2: 265–266, 1965.

Keith, R.: Impedance audiometry with neonates. Arch. Otolaryngol. 97: 465–467, 1973.

Kenny, V.: A better way to teach deaf children. Harper's Magazine, pp. 61–65, March 1962.

Kidd, A. H., and Rivoire, J. L.: Perceptual Development in Children. New York, International Universities Press, 1966.

Kimmell, G. M., and Wahl, J.: The STAP (Screening Test for Auditory Perception). San Rafael, Calif., Academic Therapy Publications, 1969.

Kimura, D.: Cerebral dominance and the perception of verbal stimuli.

Can. J. Psychol. 15: 166–171, 1961.

Kinney, C. E.: Pathology of hereditary deafness. Ann. Otol., Rhinol. Laryngol. 59: 1117–1122, 1950.

Kinney, C. E.: The further destruction of partially deafened children's hearing by the use of powerful hearing aids. Ann. Otol. Rhinol. Laryngol. 70: 828–835, 1961.

Kinstler, D.: Care and maintenance of a child's hearing aid. The Voice of the California Speech and Hearing Association, February 1964.

Kirk, S. A., McCarthy, J. P., and Kirk, W. D.: The Illinois Test of Psycholinguistic Abilities, Urbana, University of Illinois Press, Rev. Ed. 1968.

Kittel, G., and Schmoll-Eskuche, G.: Statistische Erhebungen zur Atiologie Ererbter und fruh Erworbener Hochgradiger Perzeptionsstorungen. Arch. Ohren. Nasen. Kehlkopfheilkd. Z. Hals. Nasen. Ohrenheilkd. 181: 310–328, 1963.

Kleffner, F. R.: Hearing losses, hearing aids, and children with language disorders. J. Speech Hear. Disord. 38: 232–239, 1973.

Klockhoff, I.: Middle ear muscle reflexes in man: A clinical and experimental study with special reference to diagnostic problems in hearing impairment. Acta Otolaryngol. [Suppl.], (Stockh.) 164: 1–91, 1961.

Knight, C. H.: Auditory screening of the mentally retarded. Presented at the ASHA convention, 1973.

Knight, J. J.: Redetermination of optimum characteristics for a hearing aid with insert earphone. Int. Audiol. 6: 322–326, 1967.

Knox, A. W.: Electrodermal audiometry. In Handbook of Clinical Audiology, edited by J. Katz. Baltimore, Williams & Wilkins, 1972.

Kodman, F., Fein, A., and Mixon, A.: Psychogalvanic skin response audiometry with severe mentally retarded children. Am. J. Ment. Defic. 64: 131–136, 1959.

Kodman, P.: Successful binaural hearing aid users. Arch. Otolaryngol. 74: 302–314, 1961.

Koenig, W.: Subjective effects in binaural hearing. J. Acoust. Soc. 22: 61–62, 1950.

Kohl, H. R.: Language and Education of the Deaf. Publication of the Center for Urban Education, Policy Study #1, New York, 1966.

Konigsmark, B. W.: Hereditary deafness in man. New Engl. J. Med. 281: 713–720, 774–778, 827–832, 1969.

Konigsmark, B. W.: Hereditary deafness with external-ear abnormalities: A review. Johns Hopkins Med. J. 127: 228–244, 1970.

Konigsmark, B. W.: Hereditary and Congenital Factors Affecting Newborn Sensorineural Hearing. Berkeley, Calif., Conference Proceedings on Newborn Hearing. Screening, 1971a.

Konigsmark, B. W.: Syndromal approaches to the nosology of hereditary deafness. In Birth Defects, Original Article Series, edited by D. Bergsma, Vol. 7, 2–17, 1971b.

Konigsmark, B. W.: Genetic hearing loss with no associated abnormalities: A review. J. Speech Hear. Disord. 37: 89–99, 1972.

Krause, C. J., and McCabe, B. F.: Acoustic neuroma in a seven-year-old girl. Arch. Otolaryngol. 94: 359–363, 1971.

Kronvall, E. L., and Diehl, C. F.: The relationship of auditory discrimination to articulatory defects of children with no known organic impairment. J. Speech Hear. Disord. 19: 335–338, 1954.

Krug, R.: Teaching Syntax to Young Deaf Children. Boulder, Edumat Assoc., 1968.

Kryter, K. D., and Ades, H. W.: Studies on the function of the higher acoustic nervous centers in the cat. Am. J. Psychol. 56: 501–536, 1943.

Kubler-Ross, E.: On Death and Dying. New York, Macmillan, 1970.

Kushner, M., and Mencher, G.: Broad-band noise as a pre-test sensitizer in neonatal hearing screening. Presented at Convention of American Speech and Hearing Association, 1971.

Lamb, L. E., and Graham, J. T.: Influence of signal variables on the evoked response to sound. J. Speech Hear. Res. 10: 257–267, 1967.

Lamb, L. E., and Norris, T. W.: Acoustic impedance measurement. In Audiometry for the Retarded, edited by R. T. Fulton and L. L. Lloyd, Ch. 6, Baltimore, Williams & Wilkins, 1969.

Lamb, L., and Norris, T.: Relative acoustic impedance measurements with mentally retarded children. Am. J. Ment. Defic. 75: 51–56, 1970.

Langer, S. K.: Philosophy in a New Key. Cambridge, Harvard University Press, 1957.

Lawrence, M. M., and Feind, C. R.: Vestibular responses to rotation in the newborn infant. Pediatrics, 12: 300–306, 1953.

Lempert, J., Meltzer, P. E., Wever, E. G., and Lawrence, M.: The cochleogram and its clinical application: Concluding observations. Arch. Otolaryngol. 51: 307–311, 1950.

Lempert, J., Wever, E. G., and Lawrence, M.: The cochleogram and its clinical application. Arch. Otolaryngol. 45: 61–67, 1947.

Lenneberg, E. H.: Biological Foundations of Language. New York, John Wiley & Sons, 1967.

Lerner, J. W.: Children with Learning Disabilities: Theories, Diagnosis and Teaching Strategies. Boston, Houghton Mifflin Co., 1971.

Leshin, G. J.: Childhood non-organic hearing loss. J. Speech Hear. Disord. 25: 290–292, 1960.

Levitt, H., and Nye, P. W.: Sensory Training Aids for the Hearing Impaired. Proceedings of a Conference, Easton, Md., 1970. Published by the National Academy of Engineering, Subcommittee on Sensory Aids, Washington, D.C., 1971.

Lewis, J. L.: Semantic processing of unattended messages using dichotic listening. J. Exp. Psychol. 85: 225–228, 1970.

Lewis, M., and Goldberg, S.: Perceptual-cognitive development in infancy: A generalized expectancy model as a function of the mother-infant interaction. Merrill-Palmer Quarterly of Behavior and Development 15: 81–100, 1969.

Libby, R. E.: Symposium on the achievement of optimal amplification for the hearing impaired child. The Hearing Dealer 13–25, June 1973.

Liden, G., and Kankkonen, A.: Visual reinforcement audiometry. Acta Otolaryngol (Stockh.) 67: 281–292, 1961.

Liden, G., Peterson, J. L., and Bjorkman, G.: Tympanometry: A method for analysis of middle-ear function. Acta Otolaryngol. (Stockh.) 263: 218–224, 1970.

Lieberman, P.: Primate vocalizations and human linguistic ability. Unpublished paper, University of Connecticut, Dept. of Linguistics, 1968.

Lieberman, P., Harris, K. S., Wolff, P., and Russell, L. H.: Newborn infant cry and non-human primate vocalization. J. Speech Hear. Res., 1974, in press.

Liebman, J., and Graham, J. T.: Changes in the parameters of the averaged auditory evoked potentials related to the number of data samples analyzed. J. Speech Hear. Res. 10: 782–785, 1967a.

Liebman, J., and Graham, J. T.: Frequency and intensity effects of bone conduction signals on averaged evoked auditory potentials. J. Aud. Res. 7: 157–162, 1967b.

Lilly, D. J.: Acoustic impedance at the tympanic membrane. In Handbook of Clinical Audiology, edited by J. Katz. Baltimore, Williams & Wilkins, 1972.

Lilly, D. J.: Measurement of acoustic impedance at the tympanic membrane. In Modern Developments in Audiology, edited by J. Jerger, 2nd Ed. New York, Academic Press, 1973.

Lindsay, J. R.: Labyrinthitis of viral origin. In Sensorineural Hearing Process and Disorders, edited by A. B. Graham. Boston, Little, Brown & Co., 1967a.

Lindsay, J. R.: Congenital deafness of inflammatory origin. In Deafness in Childhood, edited by McConnell and Ward, pp. 142–155. Nashville, Vanderbilt University Press, 1967b.

Lindsay, J. R.: Inner ear histopathology in genetically determined congenital deafness. In Birth Defects, Part IX, Ear. Baltimore, Williams & Wilkins, published for National Foundation—March of Dimes, 1971a.

Lindsay, J. R.: Inner ear pathology in congenital deafness. Otolaryngol. Clin. North Am. (Symposium) 4: 2 1971b.

Lindsay, J. R.: Profound childhood deafness, inner ear pathology. Ann. Otol. Rhinol. Laryngol. (Suppl. 5) 82, 1973.

Lindsay, J. R., and Hemenway, . W. G.: Inner ear pathology due to measles. Ann. Otol. Rhinol. Laryngol. 63: 754–771, 1954.

Lindsley, D. B.: Emotion. In Handbook of Experimental Psychology, edited by S. S. Stevens. New York, John Wiley & Sons, 1951.

Ling, D.: The education and general background of children with defective hearing. Unpublished research associateship thesis, Cambridge University, Institute of Education, 1959.

Ling, D.: Three experiments on frequency transposition. Am. Ann. Deaf 113: 283–294, 1968.

Ling, D.: Comment on "a portable diagnostic speech audiometry unit." J. Speech Hear. Disord. 35: 310, 1970.

Ling, D.: Rehabilitation of cases with deafness secondary to otitis media. In Otitis Media, edited by A. Glorig and K. S. Gerwin, Ch. 23. Springfield Ill., Charles C Thomas, Publisher, 1972.

Ling, D., and Druz, W. S.: Transposition of high frequency speech sounds by partial vocoding of the speech spectrum: Its use by deaf children. J. Aud. Res. 7: 133–144, 1967.

Ling, D., Ling, A. H., and Doehring, D. G.: Stimulus response and observer variables in the auditory screening of newborn infants. J. Speech Hear. Res. 13: 9–18, 1970.

Ling, D., and Maretic, H.: Frequency transposition in the teaching of speech to deaf children. J. Speech Hear. Res. 14: 37–46, 1971.

Linthicum, F. H.: Surgery of congenital deafness. Otolaryngol. Clin. North Am. (Symposium) 4: 2, 1971.

Lipsitt, L. P., and Levy, N.: Electrotactual threshold in the neonate. Child Dev. 30: 547–554, 1959.

Lloyd, L. L.: Behavioral audiometry viewed as an operant procedure. J. Speech Hear. Disord. 31: 128–135, 1966.

Lloyd, L. L., and Norris. T. W.: Relative acoustic impedance measurements with mentally retarded children. Am. J. Ment. Defic. 75: 51–56, 1970.

Lloyd, L. L.: Operant conditioning audiometry with retarded children. In Differential Diagnosis of Speech and Hearing Problems of Mental Retardates, pp. 103–121. Washington, D.C., Catholic University of America Press, 1968.

Lloyd, L. L.: Audiological aspects of mental retardation. In International Review of Research in Mental Retardation, edited by N. R. Ellis, pp. 311–374. New York, Academic Press, 1970.

Lloyd, L. L., and Reid, M. J.: The incidence of hearing impairment in an institutionalized mentally retarded population. Am. J. Ment. Defic. 71: 746–763, 1967.

Lloyd, L. L., Spradlin, J. E., and Reid, M. J.: An operant audiometric procedure for difficult-to-test patients. J. Speech Hear. Disord. 33: 236–245, 1968.

Lounsbury, E. W., Osborn, C. D., Schuneman, J. W., and Viscomi, G. J.: Air-Bone Gap Measurements in Identification Audiometry. Lansing, Michigan Dept. of Public Health, 1965.

Lowe, S. S., Cullen, J. K., Thompson, C. L., Berlin, C. I., Kirkpatrick, L. L., and Ryan, J. T.: Dichotic and monotic simultaneous and time-staggered speech. J. Acoust. Soc. Am. 47: 76, 1970.

Luke, J.: A comparative investigation of language abilities among children with limited auditory impairment. Master's thesis, Colorado State University, Ft. Collins, 1965.

Luria, A. R.: The Mentally Retarded Child. Oxford, Pergamon Press, 1963.

Luria, A. R.: Higher Cortical Functions in Man. New York, Basic Books, 1966a.

Luria, A. R. (University of Moscow—translated by B. Haigh): Human Brain and Psychological Processes. New York, Harper & Row, 1966b.

Lybarger, S.: Some comments on CROS. Natl. Hear. Aid J. 21: 8–33, 1968.

Lybarger, S.: Earmolds. In Handbook of Clinical Audiology, edited by J. Katz. Baltimore, Williams & Wilkins, 1972.

Lybarger, S. F.: Advantages and limitations of the "Y" cord. Hear. Aid J., pp. 6 and 34, April 1973.

MacCollum, D. W.: The lop ear. JAMA 110: 1427–1430, 1938.

Mackintosh, H. K. (Ed.): Children and Oral Language. Joint publication of the Association for Childhood Education International, Association for Supervision and Curriculum Development, International Reading Association, and the National Council of Teachers of English, 1964.

Macrae, J. H.: TTS and recovery from TTS after use of powerful hearing aids. J. Acoust. Soc. Am. 43: 1445–1446, 1968a.

Macrae, J. H.: Recovery from TTS in children with sensorineural deafness. J. Acoust. Soc. Am. 44: 1451, 1968b.

Macrae, J. H., and Farrant, R. H.: The effect of hearing aid use on the residual hearing of children with sensorineural deafness. Ann. Otol. Rhinol. Laryngol. 74: 409–419, 1965.

Magown, H. W.: Commentary. In Brain Mechanisms Underlying Speech and Language, edited by F. Darley and C. Millikan, pp. 199–201. New York, Grune & Stratton, 1967.

Marcus, R. E.: Vestibular function and additional findings in Waardenburg's syndrome. Acta Otolaryngol. [Suppl.] (Stockh.) 229, 1968.

Martensson, B.: Dominant hereditary nerve deafness. Arch. Otolaryngol. 52: 270–274, 1960.

Martin, E. M., Osberger, M. J., and Pickett, J. M.: Discrimination of formant frequency transitions in synthetic vowels. J. Speech Hear. Res. 16: 439–451, 1973.

Martin, E., and Pickett, J. M.: Sensorineural hearing loss and upward spread of masking. J. Speech Hear. Res. 13: 426–437, 1970.

Masterton, R. B., and Diamond, I. T.: Effects of auditory cortex ablation on discrimination of small binaural time differences. J. Neurophysiol. 27: 15–36, 1964.

Matkin, N. D.: Some essential features of a pediatric audiological evaluation. Talk presented to the Eighth Danavox Symposium, Copenhagen, June 1973.

Matkin, N. D., and Carhart, R.: Auditory profiles associated with Rh incompatibility. Arch. Otolaryngol. 84: 502–513, 1966.

Matkin, N. D., and Carhart, R.: Hearing acuity and Rh incompatability: Electrodermal thresholds. Arch. Otolaryngol. 87: 383–388, 1968.

Matkin, N., and Thomas, J.: The utilization of CROS hearing aids by children. Maico Audiological Library Series 10: 8, 1972.

Matz, G. J., and Naunton, R. F.: Ototoxicity of chloroquine. Arch. Otolaryngol. 88: 370–372, 1968.

Matzker, J.: Two new methods for the assessment of central auditory functions in cases of brain disease. Ann. Otol. Rhinol. Laryngol. 68: 1185–1197, 1959.

McCaffrey, A.: Speech perception in infancy. Personal communication cited in Friedlander, 1970.

McCandless, G. A.: Clinical application of evoked response audiometry. J. Speech Hear. Res. 10: 468–478, 1967.

McCandless, G. A.: Electroencephalic audiometry. In Audiological Assessment, edited by D. E. Rose, pp. 405–422. Englewood Cliffs, N.J., Prentice-Hall, 1971.

McCandless, G. A., and Best, L.: Summed evoked responses using pure tone stimuli. J. Speech Hear. Res. 9: 266–272, 1966.

McCandless, G. A., and Rose, D. E.: Evoked cortical responses to stimulus change. J. Speech Hear. Res. 13: 624–634, 1970.

McClellan, M. S., Strong, J. P., Vautier, T., and Blatt, I.: Otitis media in the newborn. Arch. Otolaryngol. 85: 380–382, 1967.

McClure, W. J.: The ostrich syndrome and educators of the deaf. The Kentucky Standard 100: 5 (Kentucky School for the Deaf, Danville), 1973.

McDonough, E. R.: Fanconi anemia syndrome. Arch. Otolaryngol. 92: 284–285, 1970.

McFarlan, D.: The voice test of hearing. Arch. Otolaryngol. 5: 1–5, 1927.

McLay, K., and Maran, A. G. D.: Deafness and the Klippel-Feil syndrome. J. Laryngol. Otol. 83: 175–184, 1969.

Meadow, K. P.: Parental response to the medical ambiguities of congenital deafness. J. Health Soc. Behav. 9: 299–309, 1968.

Meadow, K. P.: The effect of early manual communication and family climate. Doctoral dissertation. Berkeley. University of California, 1968.

Meier, J.: Screening and Assessment of Young Children at Developmental Risk. Dept. HEW Publication #(OS) 73–90. Washington, D.C., U.S. Govt. Printing Office, March 1973.

Melloni, B. J.: Some Pathological Conditions of Eye, Ear, Throat: An Atlas. Chicago: Abbott Laboratories, 1957.

Melnick, W., Eagles, E. L., and Levine, H. S.: Evaluation of a recommended program of identification audiometry with school-age children. J. Hear. Disord. 29: 3–13, 1964.

Mencher, G. T.: Screening infants for auditory deficits: University of Nebraska Neonatal Hearing Project. Audiology: J. Aud. Comm. (Suppl.) 11: 69, 1972.

Mencher, G. T.: Infant hearing screening: The state of the art. Maico Audiological Library Series, Vol. 12, No. 7., 1974.

Mencher, G., and Derbyshire, A.: Unpublished research. Lincoln, Neb., 1972.

Mencher, G. T., and McCulloch, B. F.: Auditory screening of kindergarten children using the VASC. J. Speech Hear. Disord. 35: 241–247, 1970.

Mengel, M. C., Konigsmark, B. W., and McKusick, V. A.: Two types of congenital recessive deafness. Eye Ear Nose Throat Mon. 48: 301–305, 1969.

Menyuk, P.: The Development of Speech. Indianapolis and New York, Bobbs-Merrill Co., 1972.

Messing, E. S.: Auditory perception: What is it? In Successful Programming: Many Points of View, edited by J. J. Arena, pp. 439–452. San Rafael, Calif., 5th Annual Con. Pro., Association of Children with Learning Disabilities, Academic Therapy Press, 1969.

Metz, O.: The acoustic impedance measured on normal and pathological ears. Acta Otolaryngol. [Suppl.] (Stockh.) 63, 1946.

Metz, O.: Threshold of reflex contractions of muscles of middle ear and recruitment of loudness. Arch. Otolaryngol. 55: 536–543, 1952.

Meyerson, L.: Hearing for speech in children: A verbal audiometric test. Acta Otolaryngol. [Suppl.] (Stockh.) 128: 1–165, 1956.

Michels, M. W., and Randt, C. T.: Galvanic skin response in the differential diagnosis of deafness. Arch. Otolaryngol. 65: 302–311, 1947.

Michelson, R. P.: The results of electrical stimulation of the cochlea in human sensory deafness. Ann. Otol. Rhinol. Laryngol. 80: 914–919, 1971a.

Michelson, R. P.: Electrical stimulation of the human cochlea: A preliminary report. Arch. Otolaryngol. 93: 317–323, 1971b.

Miles, A. C.: Cued speech. American Education, November 1967.

Miller, G. A., and Nicely, P. E.:1955 analysis of perceptual confusions among some English consonants. J. Am. Speech Assoc. 27: 338–352, 1955.

Miller, M. H., and Polisar, I. A.: Audiological Evaluation of the Pediatric Patient (2nd Printing). Springfield, Ill., Charles C Thomas, Publisher, 1971.

Milner, B.: Laterality effects in audition. In Interhemispheric Relations and Cerebral Dominance, edited by V. B. Mountcastle. Baltimore, Johns Hopkins Press, 1962.

Milner, B., Taylor, L., and Sperry, R. W.: Lateralized suppression of dichotically presented digits after commissural section in man. Science 161: 184–186, 1968.

Mindel, E. D., and Vernon, M.: They Grow in Silence: The Deaf Child and His Family, p. 23. Silver Spring, Md., National Association of the Deaf, 1971.

Moffat, S.: Helping the Child Who Cannot Hear. The Public Affairs

Committee, Public Affairs Pamphlet #479, 381 Park Ave., South, New York, 1972.

Moffitt, A. B.: Speech perception in infants. Doctoral dissertation, University of Minnesota, 1968.

Moffitt, A. B.: Speech perception by 20 to 24 week old infants. Paper presented at March Meeting of Society for Research in Child Development, Santa Monica, Calif., 1969.

Monroe, H. J.: A comparative Rorschach investigation of functional and non-functional hearing impairment. Unpublished doctoral dissertation, University of Denver, 1957.

Moody, P. A.: Introduction to Evolution. New York, Harper & Brothers, 1953.

Morgan, C. T.: Physiological Psychology, 3rd Ed. New York, McGraw-Hill, 1965.

Moss, J. W., Moss, M., and Tizard, J.: Electrodermal response audiometry with mentally defective children. J. Speech Hear. Res. 4: 41–47, 1961.

Moya, F., and Thorndyke, V.: Passage of drugs across the placenta. Am. J. Obstet. Gynecol. 84: 1778–1798, 1963.

Murai, J. I.: Speech developments of infants. Psychologica 3: 27–35, 1960.

Murai, J. I.: The sounds of infants. Studia Phonologica 3: 21–24, 1964.

Murphy, K. P.: Ascertainment of deafness in children. Panorama 3, 1962a.

Murphy, K. P.: Development of hearing in babies. Child Family 1, 1962b.

Murphy, K. P., and Smyth, C. N.: Response of fetus to auditory stimulation. Lancet 1: 972–973, 1962.

Myatt, B., and Landes, B.: Assessing discrimination loss in children. Arch. Otolaryngol. 77: 359–362, 1963.

Myklebust, H.: Auditory Disorders in Children. New York, Grune and Stratton, Inc., 1954.

Nagafuchi, M.: Development of dichotic and monaural hearing abilities in young children. Acta Otolaryngol. (Stockh.) 69: 409–414, 1970.

Nager, G. T.: Congenital aural atresia: Anatomy and surgical management. Birth Defects, Part IX, Ear. Baltimore, Williams & Wilkins, published for National Foundation—March of Dimes, 1971.

Nakazima, S.: A comparative study of the speech development of Japanese and American English in childhood. Studia Phonologica 3: 27–39, 1962.

Nassif, R., and Harboyan, G.: Madelung's deformity with conductive hearing loss. Arch. Otolaryngol. 91: 175–178, 1970.

Naunton, R. F.: The effect of hearing aid use upon the user's residual hearing. Laryngoscope 67: 569–576, 1957.

Neff, W. D.: The effects of partial section of the auditory nerve. J. Comp. Physiol. Psychol. 40: 203–216. 1947.

Neff, W. D.: Neural mechanisms of auditory discrimination. In Sensory Communications, edited by W. A. Rosenblith, pp. 259–278. Cambridge, MIT Press, 1961.

Neisser, A.: Cognitive Psychology. Appleton-Century-Crofts, Meredith Publishing Co., 1967.

Nelson, J. M.: Agnosia, Aproxia, Aphasia: Their Value in Cerebral Localization, 2nd Ed. New York, Hafner Publishing Co., 1948.

Newby, H.: Audiology, 2nd Ed. New York, Appleton-Century-Crofts, 1964.

Newhart, H. A.: A new pure tone audiometer for school use. Arch. Otolaryngol. 28: 777–779, 1938.

Newhart, H. A., and Reger, S. N.: Manual for a School Hearing Conservation Program, 2nd rev. Rochester, AAOO, 1956.

Niemeyer, W., and Sesterhenn, G.: Calculating the hearing threshold from the stapedial reflex threshold for different sound stimuli. Presented at the International Society of Audiology, Budapest, 1972.

Northern, J. L.: Clinical application of acoustic impedance measurements. Otolaryngol. Clin. North Am. (Symposium on Congenital Deafness) 4: 359–368, 1971a.

Northern, J. L. (Ed.): Audiometric Assistant Training Guide. U.S. Dept. HEW, Office of Education, Manpower Development and Training Program. Washington, D.C., National Association of Hearing and Speech Agencies, 1971b.

Northern, J. L.: The current status of implantable hearing aids. Hear. Aid J. 26: 15–32, 1973a.

Northern, J. L.: Clinical measurement procedures. In Handbook of Impedance Audiometry, edited by J. Jerger. New York, American-Electromedics Corp., 1974, in press.

Northern, J., and Bergstrom, L.: Impedance audiometry. Eye Ear Nose Throat Mon. 52: 404–406, 1973.

Northern, J. L., Downs, M. P., Lybarger, S. F., and Traynor, R.: Y-cord vs binaural hearing. Presented at the Third International Hearing Aid Seminar, San Diego, 1973.

Northern, J. L., and Hattler, K. W.: Earmold influence on aided speech identification tasks. J. Speech Hear. Res. 13: 162–172, 1970.

Northern, J. L., McChord, W., Jr., Fischer, E., and Evans, P.: Hearing services in residential schools for the deaf. Maico Audiological Library Series, XI, 4, 1972.

Northern, J. L., Teter, D. L., and Krug, R. F.: Characteristics of manually communicating deaf adults. J. Speech Hear. Disord. 36: 71–76, 1971.

Office of Demographic Studies, Summary of Selected Characteristics of Hearing Impaired Students, United States: 1969–70, Annual Survey of Hearing Impaired Children and Youth, Series D, No. 5, 1971.

Omerod, F. C.: The pathology of congenital deafness. J. Laryngol. Otol. 74: 919, 1960.

O'Neill, J. J., and Oyer, H. J.: Psychogalvanic skin resistance audiometry. In Applied Audiometry, edited by O'Neill and Oyer. New York, Dodd, Mead, and Co., 1966.

Ornitz, E. M., Ritvo, E. R., Carr, E. M., La Franchi, S., and Walter, R. D.: The effect of sleep onset on the auditory averaged evoked response. EEG Clin. Neurophysiol. 23: 335–341, 1967.

Ornstein, R. E.: Right and left thinking. Psychol. Today, May 1973.

Pannbacker, M.: Hearing loss and cleft palate. Cleft Palate J. 6: 50–56, 1969.

Paparella, M. M., and Brady, D. R.: Sensorineural hearing loss in chronic otitis media and mastoiditis. Arch. Otolaryngol. 74: 108–115, 1970.

Paparella, M. M., and Suguira, S.: The pathology of suppurative labyrinthitis. Ann. Otol. Rhinol. Laryngol. 75: 554–586, 1967.

Paradise, J. L., and Bluestone, C. D.: Diagnosis and management of ear disease in cleft palate infants. Trans. Am. Acad. Ophthalmol. Otolaryngol. 73: 709–714, 1969.

Patten, B. M.: Human Embryology, 3rd Ed. New York, McGraw-Hill, 1968.

Pearson, A. A., Jacobson, A. D., VanCalcar, R., and Sauter, R. W.: The Development of the Ear. Rochester, Section on Instruction, Home Study Courses, American Academy of Otolaryngology and Ophthalmology, 1970.

Penfield, W., and Rasmussen, T.: The Cerebral Cortex of Man. New York, Hafner Publishing Co., 1968.

Penfield, W., and Roberts, L.: Speech and Brain Mechanisms. Princeton, Princeton University Press, 1959.

Perlman, H. B., and Case, T. J.: Electrical phenomena of the cochlea in man. Arch. Otolaryngol. 34: 710–718, 1941.

Peterson, D. M., and Schimke, R. N.: Hereditary cup-shaped ears and the Pierre Robin syndrome. J. Med. Genet. 5: 52–55, 1968.

Peterson, G. E., and Lehiste, I.: Revised CNC lists for auditory testing. J. Speech Hear. Disord. 27: 62, 1962.

Pollack, D.: Educational Audiology for the Limited Hearing Infant. Springfield, Ill., Charles C Thomas, Publisher, 1970.

Pollack, D.: The development of an auditory function. Otolaryngol. Clin. North Am. Symposium on Congenital Deafness 4: 319–335, 1971.

Portmann, M., and Aran, J. M.: Electro-cochleographic sur le nourrissons et le jeune enfant. Acta Otolaryngol. (Stockh.) 71: 253–261, 1971.

Portmann, M., Aran, J. M., and Lagourge, P.: Testing for recruitment by electrocochleography. Ann. Otol. Rhinol. Laryngol. 82: 36–43, 1973.

Powell, R. N.: Poverty, the greatest handcapping condition in childhood. In Earlier Recognition of Handicapped Conditions in Childhood, edited by A. Oglesby and H. Sterling, pp. 141–148. University of California, Berkeley, School of Public Health, 1970.

Premack, A. J., and Premack, D.: Teaching language to an ape. Sci. Am. 227: 92–99, 1972.

Price, L., and Goldstein, R.: Averaged evoked responses for measuring auditory sensitivity in children. J. Speech Hear. Disord. 31: 248–256, 1966.

Price, L., Rosenblut, B., Goldstein, R., and Shepherd, D.C.: The averaged evoked response to auditory stimulation. J. Speech Hear. Res. 9: 361–370,1966.

Proctor, C. A., and Lawrence, M.: The development of sensory cell innervation in the inner ear. University of Michigan Medical Bulletin 25: 37–48, 1959.

Proctor, C. A., and Proctor, B.: Understanding hereditary nerve deafness. Arch. Otolaryngol. 85: 23–40, 1967.

Quigley, S. P., and Frisina, D.: Institutionalized and Psychoeducational Development in Deaf Children. Council For Exceptional Children Research Monograph, Series A, 3, 1961.

Ramaiya, J. J.: A study of binaural hearing aid performance. Unpublished Master's thesis directed by F. McConnell, Vanderbilt University, Nashville, 1971.

Rapin, I.: Evoked responses to clicks in a group of children with communication disorders. Ann. N.Y. Acad. Sci. 112: 182–203, 1964.

Rapin, I.: Description submitted in response to request from the author. Albert Einstein College of Medicine, 1972.

Rapin, I., and Bergman, M.: Auditory evoked responses in uncertain diagnoses. Arch. Otolaryngol. 90: 307–314, 1969.

Reddell, R. C., and Calvert, D. R.: Selecting a hearing aid by interpreting audiologic data. J. Auditory Res. 6: 445–452, 1966.

Reger, S. N., and Newby, H. A.: A group pure tone hearing test. J. Speech Hear. Disord. 12: 61–66, 1947.

Reichstein, J., and Rosenstein, J.: Differential diagnosis of auditory defects: A review of the literature. Except. Child. 31: 73–82, 1964.

Reis, P.: Academic Achievement Test Results of a National Testing Program for Hearing Impaired Students. Office of Demographic Studies, Gallaudet College, Washington, D.C., 1973a.

Reis, P.: Personal communication, 1936b.

Reisen, A. H.: The development of visual perception in man and chimpanzee. Science 106: 107–108, 1947.

Reisen, A. H.: Effects of stimulus deprivation on the development and atrophy of the visual sensory system. Am. J. Orthopsychiatry 30: 23–36, 1960.

Reisen, A. H.: Excessive arousal effects of stimulation after early sensory deprivation. In Sensory Deprivation, edited by P. Solomon, P. Kiebansky, P. Leiderman, J. Mendelson, R. Trumbull, and D. Wexler, pp. 34–41. Cambridge, Harvard University Press, 1967.

Reneau, J. P., and Mast, B. S.: Telemetric EEG audiometry instrumentation for use with the profoundly retarded. Am. J. Ment. Defic. 72: 506–511, 1968.

Renvall, U., Liden, G., Jungert, S., and Nilsson, E.: Impedance audiometry as screening method in school children. Scand. Audiol. 2: 133–140, 1973.

Richards, G. B., and Kartye, J. P.: Comparison of three types of ear tips used for impedance audiometry. Arch. Otolaryngol. 97: 437–440, 1973.

Richards, I. D. G., and Roberts, C. J.: The AT RISK infant. Lancet 2: 711–714, 1967.

Richmond, J. B.: Children's Hospital, Boston. Talk before the Conference on Screening and Assessment of Young Children at Developmental Risk, The President's Committee on Mental Retardation, October 1972.

Ridgeway, J.: Dumb children. The Saturday Review, August, 19–21, 1969.

Rintelmann, W., Harford, E., and Burchfield, S.: A special case of auditory localization: CROS for blind persons with unilateral hearing loss. Arch. Otolaryngol. 91: 284–288, 1970.

Rittmanic, P. A.: The mentally retarded and mentally ill. In Audiological Assessment, edited by D. E. Rose, pp. 369–401. Englewood Cliffs, N.J., Prentice Hall, 1971.

Roberts, C.: Can hearing aids damage hearing? Acta Otolaryngol. (Stockh.) 69: 123–125, 1970.

Robertson, E. O., Peterson, J. L., and Lamb, L. E.: Relative impedance measurements in young children. Arch. Otolaryngol. 88: 162–168, 1968.

Robinson, A.: Genetic and chromosomal disorders. In Current Pediatric Diagnosis and Treatment, edited by C. H. Kempe, H. K. Silver, and D. O'Brien. Los Altos, Calif., Lange Medical Publications, 1972.

Robinson, G. D., and Cambon, K. G.: Hearing loss in infants of tuberculous mothers treated with streptomycin during pregnancy. N. Engl. J. Med. 271: 949–951, 1964.

Rogers, B. O.: Microtic, lop, cup, and protruding ears. Plast. Reconstr. Surg. 41: 208–231, 1968.

Rojskjaer, C.: Presented at the Fifth International Congress of Audiology, Bonn, 1960.

Romer, A. S.: The Vertebrate Body. Philadelphia, W. B. Saunders, 1962.

Ronis, B. J.: Cochlear potentials in otosclerosis. Laryngoscope 78: 212, 1966.

Rose, D. E., Galambos, R., and Hughes, J. R.: Microelectrode studies of the cochlear nuclei of the cat. Johns Hopkins Med. J. 104: 211–251, 1959.

Rose, D. E., Keating, L. W., Hedgecock, L. D., Schreurs, K. K., and Miller, K. E.: Aspects of acoustically evoked responses. Arch. Otolaryngol. 94: 347–350, 1971.

Rose, D. E., Keating, L. D., Hedgecock, K. E., Miller, K., and Schreurs, K. K.: A comparison of evoked response audiometry and routine clinical audiometry. Audiology 11: 238–243, 1972.

Rose, D. E., and Ruhm, H. B.: Some characteristics of the peak latency and amplitude of the acoustically evoked response. J. Speech Hear. Res. 9: 412–422, 1966.

Rosen, J.: The place of GSR audiometry in work with young children. Volta Rev. 58: 387–391, 1956.

Rosenzweig, M. R., and Rosenblith, W. A.: Responses to auditory stimuli at the cochlea and at the auditory cortex. Psychol. Monographs 67: 1–26, 1953.

Ross, M.: Changing concepts in hearing aid candidacy. Eye Ear Nose Throat Mon. 48: 27–34, 1969.

Ross, M.: Classroom acoustics and speech intelligibility. In Handbook of Clinical Audiology, edited by J. Katz. Baltimore, Williams & Wilkins, 1972.

Ross, M., and Lerman, J.: Hearing aid usage and its effect upon residual hearing: A review of the literature and an investigation. Arch. Otolaryngol. 86: 57–62, 1967.

Ross, M., and Lerman, J.: A picture identification test for hearing-impaired children. J. Speech Hear. Res. 13: 44–53, 1970.

Ross, M., and Truex, E. H., Jr.: Protecting residual hearing in hearing aid user. Arch. Otolaryngol. 82: 616–617, 1957.

Roswell, F., and Chall, J.: Auditory Blending Test. New York, Essay Press, 1963.

Rozanov, T. V.: Specific features of the development of thinking in deaf children. Fifth Danavox Symposium. Copenhagen, 1973.

Rozin, P., Poritsky, S., and Sotsky, R.: American children with reading problems can easily learn to read English represented by Chinese characters. Science 171: 1264–1267, 1971.

Ruben, R. J.: Anatomical diagnosis of non-conductive deafness by physiological tests. Arch. Otolaryngol. 78: 47–51, 1963.

Ruben, R. J.: Cochlear potentials as a diagnostic test in deafness. In Sensorineural Hearing Processes and Disorders, edited by A. B. Graham, pp. 313–337. Boston, Little, Brown & Co., 1967.

Ruben, R. J., Bordley, J. E., and Lieberman, A. T.: Cochlear potentials in man. Laryngoscope 71: 1141–1164, 1961.

Ruben, R. J., Bordley, J. E., Nager, G. T., Sekula, J., Knickerbocker, G. G., and Fisch, U.: Human cochlear responses to sound stimuli. Ann. Otol. Rhinol. Laryngol. 169: 459, 1960.

Ruben, R. J., Knickerbocker, G. G., Sekula, J., Nager, G. T., and Bordley, J. E.: Cochlear microphonics in man. Laryngoscope 69: 665, 1959.

Ruben, R. J., Lieberman, A. T., and Bordley, J. E.: Some observations on cochlear potentials and nerve action potentials in children. Laryngoscope 5: 545, 1962.

Ruben, R. J., and Walker, A. E.: The VIIIth nerve action potentials in Meniere's disease. Laryngoscope 11: 1456–1464, 1963.

Ruhm, H. B., and Carhart, R.: Objective speech audiometry: A new method based on electrodermal response. J. Speech Hear. Res. 1: 169–178, 1958.

Rupp, R. R.: An approach to the communicative needs of the very young hearing impaired child. J. Acad. Rehab. Audiology 4: 11–22, 1971.

Ruppert, E. S., Buerk, E., and Pfordresher, M. F.: Hereditary hearing loss with saddle nose and myopia. Arch. Otolaryngol. 92: 95–98, 1970.

Sanchez-Longo, L. P., and Forster, F. M.: Clinical significance of impairment of sound localization. Neurology (Minneap.) 8: 119–125, 1958.

Sando, I., Baker, B., Black, F. O., and Hemenway, W. G.: Persistence of stapedial artery in trisomy 13–15 syndrome. Arch. Otolaryngol. 96: 441–447, 1972.

Sando, I., Bergstrom, L., Wood, R. P., II, and Hemenway, W. G.: Temporal bone findings in trisomy 18 syndrome. Arch. Otolaryngol. 91: 552–559, 1970.

Sando, I., Hemenway, W. G., and Morgan, R. W.: Histopathology of the temporal bones in mandibulofacial dysostosis Trans. Am. Acad. Ophthalmol. Otolaryngol. 72: 913–924, 1968.

Sando, I., and Wood, R. P.: Congenital middle ear anomalies. Otolaryngol. Clin. North Am. (Symposium) 4: 291–318. 1971.

Sank, D., and Kallman, F. J.: The role of heredity in total early deafness. Volta Rev. 65: 461–470, 1963.

Sataloff, J.: Pitfalls in routine hearing testing. Arch. Otolaryngol. 73:717–726, 1961.

Schein, J. D.: The Deaf Community Study of Washington, D.C. Washington, D.C., Gallaudet College Press, 1965.

Schein, J. D.: Another accolade for Ameslan. The Deaf American, 14, May 1973.

Schlesinger, H. S., and Meadow, K. P.: Emotional support to parents. Monograph on Parent Programs in Child Development Centers, edited by D. L. Lillie, pp. 13–25. Chapel Hill, University of North Carolina, 1972a.

Schlesinger, H. S., and Meadow, K. P.: Sound and Sign; Childhood Deafness and Mental Health. Berkeley, University of California Press, 1972b.

Schuknecht, H. F.: Pathology of sensorineural deafness of genetic origin. In Deafness in Childhood, edited by F. McConnell and P. H. Ward, pp. 69–90. Nashville, Vanderbilt University Press, 1967.

Schuchman, G.: An ear level hearing aid for bilateral atresia. Arch. Otolaryngol. 94: 87–88, 1971.

Schulman, C. A.: Effects of auditory stimulation on heart rate in premature infants as a function of level of arousal, probability of CNS damage, and conceptional age. Dev. Psychobiology 2: 172–183, 1970a.

Schulman, C. A.: Heart rate response habituation in high-risk premature infants. Psychophysiology 6: 690–694, 1970b.

Schulman, C. A., Smith, C. R., Weisinger, M., and Fay, T. H.: The use of heart rate in the audiological evaluation of non-verbal children: I. Evaluation of children at risk for hearing impairment. Neuropaediatrie 2: 187–196, 1970.

Schulman, C. A., and Wade, G.: The use of heart rate in the audiological evaluation of non-verbal children: II. Clinical trials on an infant population. Neuropaediatrie 2: 197–205, 1970.

Scottish Council for Research in Education. Hearing defects in school children. London, University of London Press, 1956.

Scouten, E. L.: The place of the Rochester method in American education of the deaf. Report of the Proceedings of the International Congress on the Education of the Deaf, 429–433, 1964.

Screening Test for Auditory Perception (STAP): Academic Therapy Publications, 1969.

Semeritskaya, F. M.: Rhythm and its disturbance in various motor lesions. Candidate dissertation. Institute of Psychology, Moscow, 1945.

Shambaugh, G. E.: Surgery of the Ear, 2nd Ed. Philadelphia, W. B. Saunders, 1967.

Sheridan, M. D.: Manual for the Stycar Hearing Test. Mere, Upton, Park, Slough, Bucks: National Foundation for Ed. Research in England and Wales, 1957.

Shimizu, H., Hardy, W., and Hardy, M. P.: Some basic consideration of EDR audiometry. In Sensorineural Hearing Processes and Disorders, edited by A. B. Graham, pp. 295–304. Boston, Little, Brown & Co., 1967.

Siegenthaler, B., and Haspiel, G.: Development of two standardized measures of hearing for speech by children. Cooperative Research Program, Project #2372, United States Office of Education, 1966.

Silver, H. K., and Ott, J. E.: The child health associate. A new health professional to provide comprehensive health care to children. Pediatrics 51: 1–7, 1973.

Silverman, S. R., and Lane, H. S.: Deaf children. In Hearing and Deafness, 3rd Ed., edited by H. Davis and S. R. Silverman. New York, Holt, Rhinehart, and Winston, 1970.

Simmons, F. B.: Electrical stimulation of the auditory nerve in man. Arch. Otolaryngol. 84: 2–54, 1966.

Simmons, F. B.: Solicited statement from Doctor Simmons to author (CRIB-O-GRAM). January 1973.

Skinner, P. H.: Electroencephalic response audiometry. In Handbook of Clinical Audiology, edited by J. Katz. Baltimore, Williams & Wilkins, 1972.

Sloane, H. N., and MacAulay, B. D.: Operant Procedures in Remedial Speech and Language Training. New York, Houghton, Mifflin, 1968.

Smith, C. R.: Habilitation procedures for the hard-of-hearing. Nat. Hear. Aid J.: October 1967.

Smith, D. W.: Recognizable Patterns of Human Malformation. Philadelphia, W. B. Saunders, 1970.

Smith, K.: An experimental study of the effects of systematic reinforcement on the discrimination responses of normal and hearing impaired children. Unpublished doctoral dissertation, University of Kansas, Lawrence, 1969.

Sohmer, H., and Feinmesser, M.: Cochlear action potentials recorded from the external ear in man. Ann. Otolaryngol. 76: 427–435, 1967.

Sohmer, H., and Feinmesser, M.: Routine use of electrocochleography (cochlear audiometry) on human subjects. Audiology 12: 167–173, 1973.

Sparks, R., Goodglass, H., and Nickel, B.: Ipsilateral versus contralateral extinction in dichotic listening resulting from hemispheric lesions. Cortex 6: 249–260 1970.

Spencer, E.: An investigation of the maturation of various factors of auditory perception in pre-school children. Unpublished doctoral disseration, Northwestern University, Evanston, Ill., 1958.

Spitz, R. A.: A Genetic Field Theory of Ego Formation: Its Implications for Pathology. New York, International Universities Press, 1959.

Spitz, R. A. (In collaboration with W. G. Cobliner): The first year of life: A psychoanalytic study of normal and deviant development of object relations. New York, International Universities Press, 1965.

Spoendlin, H.: The innervation of the organ of Corti. J. Laryngol. Otol. 81: 717–738, 1967.

Spoendlin, H.: Innervation patterns in the organ of Corti of the cat. Acta Otolaryngol. (Stockh.) 67: 239–254, 1969.

Spradlin, J. E., Locke, W. J., and Fulton, R. T.: Conditioning and Audiological assessment. In Audiometry for the Retarded: With Implications for the Difficult-to-Test, edited by R. T. Fulton and L. L. Lloyd. Baltimore, Williams & Wilkins, 1969.

Spreng, M., and Keidel, W. D.: Separierung von Cerebroaudiogramm (CAG), Neuroaudiogramm (NAG), und Otoaudiogramm (OAG) in der Objecktiven Audiometrie. Arch. Klin. Exp. Ohren. Nasen. Kehlkopfheilk. 189: 225, 1967.

Statten, P., and Wishart, D. E. S.: Pure-tone audiometry in young children: Psychogalvanic-skin-resistance and peep-show. Ann. Otol. Rhinol. Laryngol. 65: 511–534, 1956.

Stechler, G.: Newborn attention as affected by medication during labor.

Science 144: 315–317, 1964.

Stevens, S. S., and Warshofsky, F.: Sound and Hearing. Life Science Library. New York, Time-Life Books, 1965.

Stevenson, A. C., and Cheeseman, E. A.: Hereditary deaf mutism, with special reference to Northern Ireland. Ann. Hum. Genet. 20: 177–207, 1956.

Stewart, J. L., Pollack, D., and Downs, M. P.: A unisensory program for the limited hearing child. ASHA 6: 151–154, 1964.

Stewart, J. M.: The pediatric management of the congenitally deaf child. Otolaryngol. Clin. North Am. (Symposium on Congenital Deafness) 4: 337–345, 1971.

Stewart, J. M.: Genetic counseling. In Maternity Nursing Today, edited by J. Clausen, M. Flook, B. Ford, M. Green, and E. Popiel. New York, McGraw-Hill, 1973.

Stewart, J. M.: Unpublished report of a study under a grant from the National Foundation of Birth Defects. Denver, 1974.

Stewart, J. M., and Bergstrom, L.: Familial hand abnormality and sensori-neural deafness, a new syndrome. J. Pediatr. 78: 102–110, 1971.

Stewart, K.: A new instrument for detecting the galvanic skin response. J. Speech Hear. Disord. 19: 169–173, 1954a.

Stewart, K.: Some basic considerations in applying the GSR technique to the measurement of auditory sensitivity. J. Speech Hear. Disord. 19: 174–183, 1954b.

Stewart, V. J. H.: A comparison of COR audiometry, play audiometry and evoked response audiometry with young children. Unpublished master's thesis, University of Colorado, Boulder, 1970.

Stokoe, W. C.: Sign Language Structure: An Outline of the Visual Communication System of the American Deaf. Buffalo, N.Y., University of Buffalo Press, 1960.

Stokoe, W. C., Casterline, D. C., and Croneberg, C. G.: A Dictionary of American Sign Language on Linguistic Principles. Washington, D.C., Gallaudet College Press, 1965.

Stool, S., and Randall, P.: Unexpected ear disease in infants with cleft palate. Cleft Palate J. 4: 99–103, 1967.

Storer, T. I., and Usinger, R. L.: General Zoology, New York, McGraw-Hill, 1957.

Strauss, R. B.: Premedication in clinical audiometry. Arch. Otolaryngol. 68: 354–363, 1958.

Stuckless, E. R., and Birch, J. W.: The influence of early manual communication on the linguistic development of deaf children. Am. Ann. Deaf 3: 452–460, 499–504, 1966.

Studdert-Kennedy, M., and Shankweiler, D.: Hemispheric specialization for speech perception. J. Acoust. Soc. 48: 579–594, 1970.

Survey of Hearing Impaired Children and Youth. Gallaudet College Office of Demographic Studies. Washington, D.C., series D, 9: 1971.

Sussman, H. M.: The laterality effect in lingual-auditory tracking. J. Opt. Soc. Am. 49: 1874–1880, 1971.

Suzuki, T.: Problems in electric response audiometry (ERA) during sedation. Audiology 12: 129–136, 1973.

Suzuki, T., and Ogiba, Y.: Conditioned orientation audiometry. Arch. Otolaryngol. 74: 192–198, 1961.

Suzuki, T., and Origuchi, K.: Averaged evoked response audiometry (ERA) in young children during sleep. Acta Otolaryngol. [Suppl.] (Stockh.) 252: 19–28, 1969.

Suzuki, T., and Taguchi, K.: Cerebral evoked response to auditory stimuli in waking man. Ann. Otol. Rhinol. Laryngol. 74: 128–139, 1965.

Suzuki, T., and Taguchi, K.: Cerebral evoked response to auditory stimuli in young children during sleep. Ann. Otol. Rhinol. Laryngol. 77: 102–110, 1968.

Tasaki, I.: Nerve impulses in individual auditory nerve fibers of the guinea pig. J. Neurophysiol. 17: 97–122, 1954.

Templin, M. C.: Certain Language Skills in Children: Their Development and Inter-Relationships. University of Minnesota Press, 1957.

Templin, M.: Vocabulary problems of the deaf child. Int. Audiology 5: 349, 1966.

Tervoort, B.: Development of languages and the critical period. The young deaf child: Identification and management. Acta Otolaryngol. [Suppl.] (Stockh.) 206: 247–251, 1964.

Teter, D. L., Aspinall, K. B., and Stewart, V.: The fitting of high frequency emphasis hearing aids: Some comments and two case reports, J. Colo. Speech Hear. Assoc., Nov. 1969.

Teter, D. L., and Newell, R. C.: The acoustically Evoked responses: Instrumentation and Methodology. Biomedical Sciences Instrumentation, Eighth International Symposium, Denver, Colorado, May 1970.

Thompson, C. L., and Hughes, L. F.: Effects of stimulus intensity in competing message tasks: I. Equal intensity dichotic stimuli. Report of a research project supported in part by USPHS grant NS-07005 (Unpublished), 1973.

Thompson, C. L., Stafford, M. R., Cullen, J. K., Hughes, L. F., Lowe-Bell,

S. S., and Berlin, C.: Interaural intensity differences in dichotic speech perception. Paper presented at the 83rd meeting of the Acoustical Society of America, Buffalo, 1972.

Thorner, M., and Remein, O. R.: Principles and procedures in the evaluation of screening for disease. Public Health Monograph #67, May 1967.

Tibbling, L.: The rotatory nystagmus response in children. Acta Otolaryngol., (Stockh.) 68: 459–467, 1969.

Transactions of National Conference on Newborn Hearing Screening. California State Dept. of Public Health, 1971.

Travis, L. E., and Silverman, R. S.: Education of deaf children. Handbook on Speech Pathology and Audiology. New York, Appleton-Century-Crofts, 1971.

Turnure, C.: Response to voice of mother and stranger by babies in the first year. Presented at meeting of the Society for Research in Child Development, Santa Monica, March 1969.

Uhr, L., and Miller, J. G.: Drugs and Behavior. New York, John Wiley & Sons, 1960.

Van Bergeijk, W. A.: Variation on a theme of Bekesy: A model of binaural interaction. J. Acoust. Soc. Am. 34: 1431–1437, 1962.

Van Bergeijk, W. A., Pierce, J. R., and David, E. E.: Waves and the Ear. Garden City, N.Y., Doubleday and Co., 1960.

Ventry, I.: A case for psychogenic hearing loss. J. Speech Hear. Disord. 33: 89–92, 1968.

Ventry, I. M., Chaiklin, J. B., and Boyle, W. F.: Collapse of the ear canal during audiometry. Arch. Otolaryngol. 73: 727–731, 1961.

Ventry, I., Chaiklin, J., and Dixon, R. (Eds.): Hearing: A Book of Readings, pp. 410–413. New York, Appleton-Century-Crofts, 1971.

Vernon, J.: Round window stimulation in man. Presented at the First International Conference on Electrical Stimulation of the Acoustic Nerve as a Treatment for Profound Sensorineural Deafness in Man, San Francisco, 1973.

Vernon, J., Mahoney, T., Sliming, A., Kaufmann, M., and Jacobson, M.: A pizoelectric implantable hearing aid. (cited in J. L. Northern: Current status of implantable hearing aids. Hear. Aid J. 26: 6, 1973.

Vernon, M.: Tuberculous meningitis and deafness. J. Speech Hear. Disord. 32: 177–181, 1967a.

Vernon, M.: Meningitis and Deafness: The problem, its physical, audiological, and educational manifestations in deaf children. Laryngoscope 77: 1856–1874, 1967b.

Vernon, M., and Koh, S. D.: Effects of early manual communication on achievement of deaf children. Am. Ann. Deaf 115: 527–536, 1970.

Victoreen, J. A.: Hearing Enhancement. Springfield, Ill., Charles C Thomas, Publisher, 1960.

Victoreen, J. A.: A Guide to Applied Otometric Procedures. Colorado Springs, Vicon Instrument Co., 1973a.

Victoreen, J. A.: Basic Principles of Otometry. Springfield, Ill., Charles C Thomas, Publisher, 1973b.

Waldon, E. F.: Audio-reflexometry in testing hearing of very young children. Audiology 12: 14–20, 1973.

Wampler, D. W.: Linguistics of Visual English. Santa Rosa, Calif., 2322 Maher Drive, #35, 1971.

Ward, P. H., Lindsay, J. R., and Warner, N. E.: Cytomegalic inclusion disease affecting the temporal bone. Laryngoscope 75: 628–636, 1965.

Warkany, J.: Congenital Malformations. Chicago, Year Book Medical Publishers, 1971.

Watson, D. O.: Talk with Your Hands. Winneconne, Wis., 1964.

Watson, L., and Tolan, T.: Hearing Tests and Hearing Instruments. Baltimore, Williams & Wilkins, 1949.

Weaver, M.: Personal communication, 1972.

Weaver, M., and Downs, M. P.: Ear, nose, and throat. In Current Pediatric Diagnosis and Treatment, 2nd Ed., edited by C. H. Kempe, H. K. Silver, and D. O'Brien. Los Altos, Calif. Lange Medical Publications, 1972.

Weber, H. J., McGovern, F. J., and Zink, D.: An evaluation of 1000 children with hearing loss. J. Speech Hear. Disord. 32: 343–354, 1967.

Wedenberg, E.: Auditory tests on newborn infants. Acta Otolaryngol. (Stockh.) 45: 5, 1956.

Wedenberg, E.: Auditory tests on newborn infants. In Conference on Newborn Hearing Screening, edited by G. C. Cunningham, pp. 126–130. California State Dept. of Public Health, 1971.

Weinstein, R. L., Kliman, B., and Scully, R. E. Familial syndrome of primary testicular insufficiency with normal virilization, blindness, deafness, and metabolic abnormalities. New Engl. J. Med. 281: 969–977, 1969.

Weir, R. H.: Some questions on the child's learning of phonology. In The Genesis of Language, edited by F. Smith and G. Miller, pp. 153–169. Cambridge, MIT Press, 1966.

Wepman Test of Auditory Discrimination, 1958. Language Research Associates.

West, R.: A critique for the rationales of tests for hearing. J. Speech Hear. Disord. 5: 19–24, 1940.

Wever, E. G., and Bray, C. W.: Auditory nerve impulses. Science 71: 215, 1930.

Wever, E. G., and Lawrence, M.: Physiological Acoustics. Princeton, N.J., Princeton University Press, 1954.

Wever, E. G., and Neff, W. D.: A further study of the effects of partial section of the auditory nerve. J. Comp. Physiol. Psychol. 40: 217–226, 1947.

Whetnall, E.: Binaural hearing. J. Laryngol. Otol. 78: 1079, 1964.

Wilber, L. A., Goodhill, V., and Hogue, A. C.: Comparative acoustic impedance measures. Presented to the American Speech and Hearing Association, 1970.

Wiley, T.: Filtered speech audiometry for children. Masters thesis, Colorado State University, Fort Collins, 1968.

Williams, H. L., Teas, D. I., and Morlock, H. C.: Evoked responses to clicks and electroencephalographic stages of sleep in man. Science 138: 685–686, 1962.

Wolff, P. H.: The causes, controls, and organization of behavior in the neonate. Psychol. Issues 5: 1–99, 1966.

Wood, R. P.: Otitis media. Personal communication, Division of Otolaryngology, University of Colorado School of Medicine, Denver, 1972.

World Health Organization: The early detection and treatment of handicapping defects in young children. Report on a Working Group Convened by the Regional Office for Europe of the World Health Organization, 1967.

Yoshie, N.: Auditory nerve action potential responses to clicks in man. Laryngoscope 78: 198–215, 1968.

Yoshie, N., and Ohashi, T.: Clinical use of cochlear nerve action potential responses in man for differential diagnosis of hearing losses. Acta Otolaryngol. [Suppl.] (Stockh.) 252: 71–87, 1969.

Yoshie, N., Ohashi, T., and Suzuki, T.: Nonsurgical recording of auditory nerve action potentials in man. Laryngoscope 77: 76–85, 1967.

Yoshie, N., and Yamaura, K.: Cochlear microphonic responses to pure tones in man recorded by a non-surgical method. Acta Otolaryngol. [Suppl.] (Stockh.) 252: 37–69, 1969.

Young, W. E.: The retention of reading comprehension and relation to hearing comprehension and retention. J. Exp. Education 5: 30–39, 1936.

Yules, R. B.: Hearing in cleft palate patients. Arch. Otolaryngol. 91: 319–323, 1970.

Zeaman, D., Deane, G., and Wegner, N.: Amplitude and latency characteristics of the conditioned heart response. J. Physiol. 38: 235–250, 1954.

Zeaman, D., and Wegner, N.: The role of drive reduction in the classical conditioning of an autonomically mediated response. J. Exp. Psychol. 48: 349–354, 1954.

Zeaman, D., and Wegner, H.: Cardiac reflex to tones of threshold intensity. J. Speech Hear. Disord. 21: 71–75, 1956.

Zelazo, P. R.: Smiling to social stimuli: Eliciting and conditioning effects. Dev. Psychol. 4: 32–42, 1971.

Zemlin, W. R.: Speech and Hearing Science. Englewood Cliffs, N.J., Prentice-Hall, 1968.

Zenith Hearing Aid Sales Corporation: Hearing Aids and Their Components, Chicago, 1965.

Zigmund, N.: Intrasensory and intersensory processes in normal and dyslexic children. Unpublished doctoral dissertation, Northwestern University, Evanston, Ill., 1966.

Zigmund, N.: Maturation of auditory processes in children with learning disabilities. In Introduction to Learning Disabilities, edited by L. Tarnpol. Springfield, Ill., Charles C Thomas, Publisher, 1973.

Zink, G. D.: Hearing aids children wear: A longitudinal study of performance. Volta Rev. 74: 41–51, 1972.

Zink, G. D., and Alpiner, J. G.: Hearing aids: One aspect of a state public school hearing conservation program. J. Speech Hear. Disord. 33: 329–344, 1968.

Zurif, E. B., and Sait, P. E.: The laterality effect in lingual-auditory tracking. J. Acoust. Soc. 49: 1874–1880, 1970.

Zwislocki, J.: An acoustic method for clinical examination of the ear. J. Speech Hear. Res. 6: 303–314, 1963.

AUTHOR INDEX

SUBJECT INDEX